Concise System of Orthopaedics and Fractures

To our students, past and present
  who have immeasurably enriched our lives

To Violet Apley and Joan Solomon
  who have shared the trials and joys of teaching and writing

Concise System of Orthopaedics and Fractures

Second edition

A. Graham Apley

MB BS, FRCS, FRCSEd(Hon)
Consulting Orthopaedic Surgeon, St Thomas' Hospital, London;
Emeritus Consultant Orthopaedic Surgeon, St Peter's Hospital, Chertsey, Surrey;
Former Editor, *Journal of Bone and Joint Surgery* (British Issue)

Louis Solomon

MB ChB, MD, FRCS, FRCSEd
Emeritus Professor of Orthopaedic Surgery, University of Bristol;
Emeritus Professor of Orthopaedic Surgery, University of the Witwatersrand,
Johannesburg

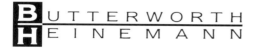
BUTTERWORTH
HEINEMANN

Butterworth-Heinemann
Linacre House, Jordan Hill, Oxford OX2 8DP
225 Wildwood Avenue, Woburn, MA 01801-2041
A division of Reed Educational and Professional Publishing Ltd

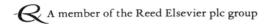 A member of the Reed Elsevier plc group

OXFORD AUCKLAND BOSTON
JOHANNESBURG MELBOURNE NEW DELHI

First published 1988
Revised reprint 1989
Reprinted 1991, 1992, 1993
Second edition 1994
Reprinted 1997 (twice), 1998, 1999

British Library Cataloguing in Publication Data
Apley, A. Graham
    Concise System of Orthopaedics and
    Fractures. - 2Rev.ed
    I. Title II. Soloman, Louis
    617.3

ISBN 0 7506 1767 5

Library of Congress Cataloguing in Publication Data
Apley A. Graham (Alan Graham)
    Concise system of orthopaedics and fractures/A. Graham Aply,
    Louis Solomon, - 2nd ed.
    p. cm.
    A bridgement of: Apley's system of orthopaedics and fractures/A.
    Graham Apley, Louis Solomon. 7th ed.
    1. Orthopaedics 2. Fracture fixation. I. Solomon, Louis.
    II. Apley A Graham (Alan Graham). Apley's system of orthopaedics
    and fractures. III. Title
    617.dc20

Composition by Scribe Design, Gillingham, Kent
Printed and bound in the United Kingdom at the University Press, Cambridge

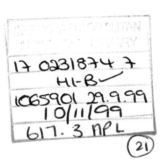
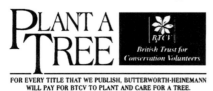

Contents

Preface

Ever since the first edition of the *Concise System* was published in 1988 we have been collecting comments from reviewers, from students and from teachers. Some have asked for more detail, others for less; all have urged us to preserve the format and the style. We hope we have satisfied the conservationists; as for the rest, we have simplified some sections and amplified others, aiming to reflect the changing face of orthopaedics.

We have included a brief description of the common non-operative procedures used in orthopaedics, which is needed by many doctors and many allied professionals. Another change from the earlier edition is the provision of more detail regarding the management of acute injuries – a subject so important and so rapidly growing that enlargement was a must. In addition, we have taken account of the increasing use of sophisticated diagnostic techniques and of key-hole surgery. Despite these additions we have tried to remain concise, to combine brevity with accuracy, to preserve the systematic approach and to describe even complex topics in simple words. Those wanting more information on any particular subject can refer to the corresponding section in the larger companion volume, *Apley's System of Orthopaedics and Fractures* (Seventh edition).

We hope that our readers – undergraduate students, young doctors, those in the allied health disciplines, practitioners who need to be masters of all trades, and specialists (even orthopaedic specialists) who want to refresh their memories – will find this relatively short version of a large subject enlivening and enlightening.

AGA
LS

Part 1   General Orthopaedics

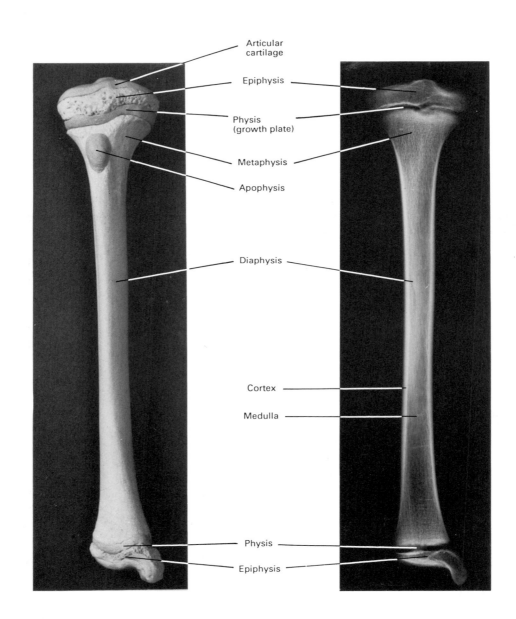

Articular
cartilage

Epiphysis

Physis
(growth plate)

Metaphysis

Apophysis

Diaphysis

Cortex

Medulla

Physis

Epiphysis

Diagnosis in orthopaedics 1

'Information consists of differences that make a difference'
Gregory Bateson

Orthopaedics is concerned with bones, joints, muscles, tendons and nerves – the skeletal system and all that makes it move. Conditions that affect these structures fall into seven easily remembered pairs:

1. *Congenital and developmental abnormalities.*
2. *Infection and inflammation.*
3. *Arthritis and rheumatic disorders.*
4. *Metabolic dysfunction and degeneration.*
5. *Tumours and lesions that mimic them.*
6. *Sensory disturbance and muscle weakness.*
7. *Injury and mechanical derangement.*

Diagnosis is the identification of disease. It begins with the systematic gathering of information – from the patient's history, the physical examination, x-ray appearances and special investigations. It should, however, never be forgotten that every orthopaedic disorder is part of a larger whole – a patient who has a mind and a personality, a job and hobbies, a family and a home; all have a bearing upon the disorder and its treatment.

Symptoms

Carefully and patiently compiled, the history can be every bit as informative as examination or laboratory tests. In orthopaedics the important symptoms are *pain, stiffness, swelling, deformity, altered sensibility* and *loss of function*. We need to know whether they appeared suddenly or gradually, how long they have been present, whether they are constant or intermittent, severe or mild – and whether anything makes them better or worse.

SYMPTOMS

Pain
Stiffness
Swelling
Deformity
Change in sensibility
Loss of function

Pain

Pain is the most common symptom. Its precise location is important, so ask the patient to point to where it hurts. But don't assume that the site of pain is always the site of pathology; often pain is 'referred'.

Referred pain Pain arising in or near the skin is usually localized accurately. Pain arising in deep structures is more diffuse and is sometimes of unexpected distribution; thus, hip disease may manifest with pain in the knee (so might an obturator hernia!). This is not because sensory nerves connect the two sites; it is due to inability of the cerebral cortex to distinguish between sensory messages from embryologically related sites.

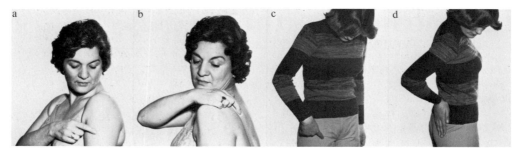

1.1 'Point to where it hurts'   In (a) and (b) the complaint would be of 'shoulder' pain, in (c) and (d) of 'hip' pain. The likely diagnoses are (a) supraspinatus tendinitis, (b) cervical spondylosis, (c) a disorder of the hip joint itself, (d) a prolapsed lumbar disc.

Stiffness

Stiffness may be generalized (typically in rheumatoid arthritis and ankylosing spondylitis) or localized to a particular joint. Patients often have difficulty distinguishing stiffness from painful movement; limited movement should never be assumed until verified by examination.

Locking is the sudden inability to complete a certain movement; it suggests a mechanical block, e.g. due to a loose body or a torn meniscus. Unfortunately, patients use the term for any painful limitation of movement; much more reliable is a history of *'unlocking'* when the offending body suddenly moves out of the way.

Swelling

Swelling may be in the soft tissues, the joint or the bone; to the patient they are all the same. It is important to establish whether the swelling followed an injury, whether it appeared rapidly (probably a haematoma or a haemarthrosis) or slowly (soft tissue inflammation or a joint effusion), whether it is painful (acute inflammation, infection – or a tumour!) and whether it is constant or comes and goes.

Deformity

The common deformities are well described in terms such as round shoulders, spinal curvature, knock knees, bow legs, pigeon toes and flat feet. Some 'deformities' are merely variations of the normal (e.g. short stature or wide hips); others disappear spontaneously with growth (e.g. flat feet or bandy legs in an infant). However, if the deformity is *progressive* it may be serious.

Weakness

Muscle weakness may be associated with any joint dysfunction. It may also suggest a more specific neurological disorder.

Instability

The patient complains that the joint 'gives way' or 'jumps out'. If this happens repeatedly it suggests ligamentous deficiency, recurrent subluxation or some internal derangement like a loose body.

Change in sensibility

Tingling or numbness signifies interference with nerve function – pressure from a neighbouring structure (e.g. a prolapsed intervertebral disc), local ischaemia (e.g. nerve entrapment in a fibro-osseous tunnel) or a peripheral neuropathy. It is important to establish its exact distribution; from this we can tell whether the fault lies in a peripheral nerve or in a nerve root.

Loss of function

Functional disability is more than the sum of individual symptoms and its expression depends upon the needs of the patient. The patient may say 'I can't sit for long' rather than 'I have backache', or 'I can't put my socks on' rather than 'my hip is stiff'. Moreover, what to one patient is merely inconvenient may, to another, be incapacitating. Thus a lawyer or a teacher may readily tolerate a stiff knee provided it is painless and does not impair walking; but to a plumber or a parson the same disorder might spell economic or spiritual disaster.

Past history

Patients should always be asked about previous accidents, illnesses, operations and drug therapy. They may give vital clues to the present disorder.

Examination

Examination begins from the moment we set eyes on the patient; we should be observing his appearance, his posture and his gait. A limp may be due to a short leg, instability of a joint, or pain.

When we proceed to the structured examination, the patient must be suitably undressed; no mere rolling up of a trouser leg is sufficient. If one limb is affected, both must be exposed so that they can be compared.

We examine first the good limb, then the bad. The student is often inclined to rush in with both hands – a temptation which must be resisted. Only by proceeding in a purposeful, orderly way can we avoid missing important signs. The system we use is simple but comprehensive:

LOOK   FEEL   MOVE.

- ● LOOK
  - first at the *skin*: for scars, colour changes and abnormal creases.
  - then at the *shape*: is there swelling, wasting or a lump? Is a normally straight bone bent?
  - and then the *position*: many joint disorders and nerve lesions have characteristic deformities. Limbs are three-dimensional, so look for deformities in 3 planes.

EXAMINATION

LOOK:	Skin
	Shape
	Position
FEEL:	Skin
	Soft tissues
	Bones and joints
MOVE:	Active
	Passive
	Abnormal

- ● FEEL
  - *the skin*: is it warm or cold; moist or dry; and is sensation normal?
  - *the soft tissues*: is there a lump, and where does it arise? Are the pulses normal?
  - *the bones and joints*: Are the outlines normal? Is the synovium thickened? Is there excessive joint fluid?

Tenderness is always important, and if localized is often diagnostic. If you know precisely *where* it is, you're halfway to knowing *what* it is.

- ● MOVE
  - *active*: ask the patient to move the joint, and test for power.

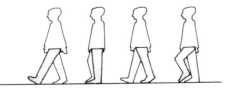

1.2 The gait cycle Follow the left leg through the four stages of the gait cycle: heel strike; stance phase; toe-off; and swing phase.

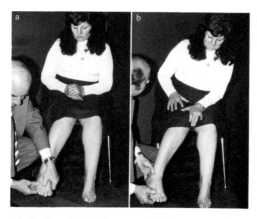

1.3 Feeling for tenderness   (a) How not to do it. It is better to watch the patient's face (b), and to stop the moment she feels pain.

Pronation and supination: these, too, are rotatory movements, but the terms are applied only to movements of the forearm and the foot.

Circumduction: a composite movement made up of a rhythmic sequence of all the other movements. This is possible only for ball-and-socket joints (hip, shoulder).

Certain specialized movements, such as opposition of the thumb, lateral flexion and rotation of the spine, and inversion and eversion of the foot, will be described under the relevant regions.

While testing movement, feel for crepitus: *joint crepitus* is usually coarse and fairly diffuse; *tendon crepitus* is fine and precisely localized to the affected tendon sheath.

Neurological examination

If the symptoms include either weakness or a change in sensibility, a complete neurological examination of the part is mandatory.

Deformities

The word 'deformity' may be applied to a person, a bone or a joint. Shortness of stature is a kind of deformity; it may be due to shortness of the limbs or of the trunk, or both. An individual bone may also be abnormally short; this is rarely important in the upper limbs, but it is in the lower.

– *passive*: record the range of movement in each physiological plane.
– *abnormal*: is the joint unstable? Is there movement at an old fracture site?

Flexion/extension: movements in the sagittal plane, e.g. at the knee, elbow, ankle and the joints of the fingers and toes.

Adduction/abduction: movements in the coronal plane, towards or away from the midline.

External (lateral) rotation and internal (medial) rotation: rotational movements around a longitudinal axis.

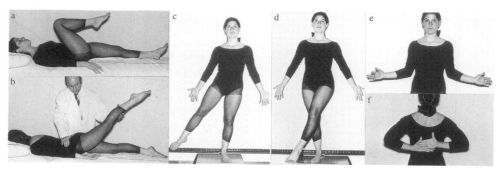

1.4 Active movements   (a) Flexion, (b) extension, (c) abduction and (d) adduction at the hip, (e) external (lateral) and (f) internal (medial) rotation at the shoulder.

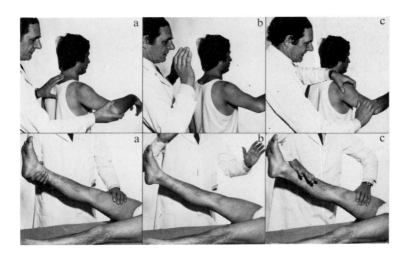

If a limb appears to be crooked it is important to establish whether the deformity is in the bone or in the joint.

SIX CAUSES OF BONE DEFORMITY
1. Congenital disorders (e.g. pseudarthrosis)
2. Bone softening (e.g. rickets, osteomalacia)
3. Dysplasia (e.g. multiple exostosis)
4. Growth plate injury (e.g. epiphyseal separation)
5. Fracture malunion
6. Paget's disease

SIX CAUSES OF JOINT DEFORMITY
1. Skin contracture (e.g. burn)
2. Fascial contracture (e.g. Dupuytren's)
3. Muscle contracture (e.g. Volkmann's)
4. Muscle imbalance (e.g. asymmetrical paralysis)
5. Joint instability (e.g. torn ligament, or dislocation)
6. Joint destruction (e.g. arthritis)

A joint may be held in an unnatural position either because of faulty alignment

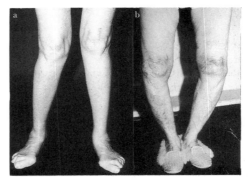

1.6 Valgus and varus (a) Valgus deformity in rheumatoid arthritis; (b) varus with osteoarthritis.

or because it lacks full movement. The more common deformities have special names.

Varus and valgus It may seem pedantic to replace 'bow legs' and 'knock knees' with 'genu varum' and 'genu valgum'. But comparable colloquialisms are not available for deformities of the elbow, hip or big toe; and, besides, the formality is justified by the need for clarity and consistency. *Varus* means that the part distal to the joint is displaced towards the midline, *valgus* away from it.

Kyphosis and lordosis Seen from the side, the spine has a series of curves – convex posteriorly in the dorsal region (kyphosis), and convex anteriorly in the cervical and lumbar regions (lordosis). Excessive curvature constitutes a kyphotic or lordotic deformity.

Scoliosis Seen from behind, the spine is straight. Any curvature in this (coronal) plane is called scoliosis.

'Fixed' deformity This does *not* mean that the joint is unable to move; it means that a particular movement cannot be completed. Thus, the knee may flex fully but not extend fully – at the limit of its extension it is still 'fixed' in a certain amount of flexion. In the spine a fixed deformity is called a *structural deformity*; it differs from a *postural deformity*, which the patient himself can, if properly instructed, correct by his own muscular effort.

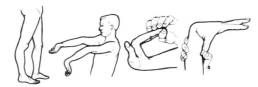

1.7 Generalized joint hypermobility Being double-jointed is not an unmixed blessing. Recurrent dislocation and painful joints are possible sequels. (Redrawn from *Journal of Bone and Joint Surgery* vol. 25B, page 704, by courtesy of Miss R. Wynne-Davies, and the Editor.)

acrobats – but they do have a tendency to recurrent dislocation (e.g. of the shoulder or patella).

Severe joint laxity is a feature of certain rare disorders such as Marfan's syndrome and osteogenesis imperfecta.

Stiff joints

It is convenient to distinguish three grades of joint stiffness.

All movements absent Surgical fusion of a joint is called *arthrodesis*; pathological fusion is called *ankylosis*. Acute suppurative arthritis typically ends in bony ankylosis; tuberculous arthritis often heals by fibrosis and causes fibrous ankylosis.

All movements limited Restriction of movement in all directions is characteristic of non-infective arthritis and is usually due to synovial swelling or capsular fibrosis.

One or two movements limited Limitation of movement in some directions with full movement in others suggests a mechanical block or joint contracture.

Lax joints

Generalized joint hypermobility occurs in about 5 per cent of people and is familial. Hypermobile joints are not necessarily unstable – as witness the controlled performances of

Bony lumps

A bony lump may be due to faulty development, injury, inflammation or a tumour. Although x-ray examination is essential, the clinical features can be highly informative.

Size A large lump attached to bone, or a lump which is getting bigger, is nearly always a tumour.

Site A lump near a joint is most likely to be a tumour (benign or malignant); a lump in the shaft may be fracture callus, inflammatory new bone or a tumour.

Shape A benign tumour has a well-defined margin; malignant tumours, inflammatory lumps and callus have a vague edge.

Consistency A benign tumour feels bony hard; malignant tumours often give the impression that they can be indented.

Tenderness Lumps due to active inflammation, recent callus or a rapidly growing sarcoma are tender.

Multiplicity Multiple bony lumps are uncommon: they occur in hereditary multiple exostosis and in Ollier's disease.

X-ray examination

The process of reading x-ray films should be as methodical as clinical examination. It is seductively easy to be led astray by some flagrant anomaly; systematic study is the only safeguard against missing other important signs.

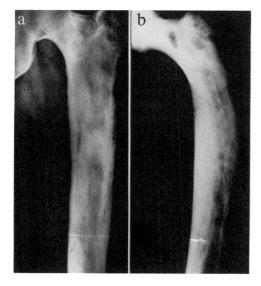

1.8 Shape and density Both these bones are wider than normal and have abnormal architecture. In (a) chronic osteomyelitis the bone is straight; in (b) Paget's disease the bone is bent.

Start with a general orientation: identify the part, the particular view and, if possible, the type of patient; try to visualize the living person, the age, build and sex. Then examine, in sequence, the *soft tissues*, the *bones*, the *joints*, the *surrounding tissues*.

Soft tissues Unless examined early, these are liable to be forgotten. Look for variations in shape (swelling or wasting) and variations of density (e.g. calcification).

Bones Look for deformity or local irregularities; examine the cortices for areas of destruction or new bone formation; then look for areas of reduced density (osteoporosis or destruction), or increased density (sclerosis). Remember that 'vacant' areas are not necessarily cysts; any tissue that is radiolucent may look 'cystic'.

Joints The radiographic 'joint' consists of the articulating bones and the 'space' between them. The 'joint space' is, of course, illusory; it is occupied by radiolucent articular cartilage. Look for narrowing of this space, which signifies loss of cartilage thickness, and examine the bone ends for flattening, erosion, cavitation or sclerosis – all features of arthritis. The joint margins may show osteophytes (typical of osteoarthritis) or erosions (typical of rheumatoid arthritis).

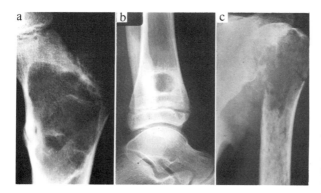

1.9 'Vacant' areas in bone may be (a) well-defined like scooped out cavities (probably a solitary cyst), (b) surrounded by dense new bone (a chronic abscess with bone reaction) or (c) ragged or 'moth-eaten' (malignant disease).

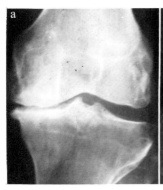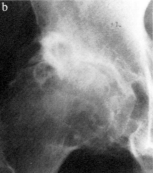

1.10 Joint x-rays (a) The lateral compartment of this knee is normal; in the medial compartment some articular cartilage has worn away and the joint 'space' is therefore reduced. (b) In this osteoarthritic hip the superior joint space is virtually obliterated and there are juxta-articular cysts with reactive sclerosis.

Special imaging techniques

CONTRAST RADIOGRAPHY Radio-opaque liquids may be used to outline cavities during x-ray examination (air or gas can be used in the same way). Common examples are sinography (outlining a sinus), arthrography (outlining a joint) and myelography (outlining the spinal theca).

TOMOGRAPHY Tomography provides an image 'focused' on a selected plane and may show changes that are obscured by the overlapping images in conventional x-ray films. It is particularly useful for detecting changes in the spine.

COMPUTED TOMOGRAPHY (CT) This method is capable of recording bone and soft tissue outlines in cross-section. It is particularly useful for displaying the shape of the spinal canal and for mapping the spread of tumours into the soft tissues. The computed data can be reconstructed as a three-dimensional image.

RADIONUCLIDE SCANNING* A bone-seeking radioisotope compound (^{99m}technetium methylene diphosphonate) is injected intravenously and its presence in the tissues is recorded with a gamma camera or rectilinear scanner. Increased uptake during the blood phase (immediately after injection) signifies a hyperaemia; activity during the bone phase (about 3 hours later) suggests

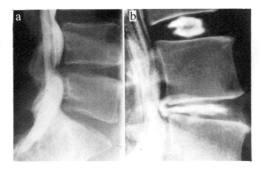

1.11 Contrast radiography (a) Myelography outlines the spinal theca; the contrast medium has been indented by a bulging disc. (b) Contrast material can be injected into the disc itself; in this discogram the upper disc is normal, but the lower is degenerate, allowing injected material to escape.

new bone formation. This information is valuable in the diagnosis of stress fractures (which often do not show on x-ray), bone infection and bone tumours.

DIAGNOSTIC ULTRASOUND Ultrasound scanning produces images of tissues that show up poorly on x-ray, e.g. soft tissue haematomas, joint effusions or cartilage outlines.

MAGNETIC RESONANCE IMAGING (MRI) This depends upon the response of atoms and molecules to a magnetic field and does not involve ionizing radiation. MR images are similar to those of CT scans, but with

* X-rays are history, scanning is news.

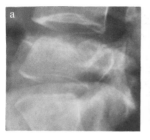
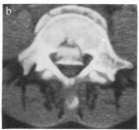
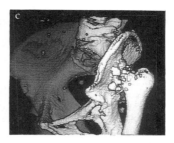

1.12 Computed tomography　The plain x-ray (a) shows a fracture of the vertebral body, but one cannot tell precisely how the bone fragments are displaced. The computed tomograph (b) shows clearly that they are dangerously close to the cauda equina. (c) Three-dimensional CT reconstruction of a congenital hip dislocation.

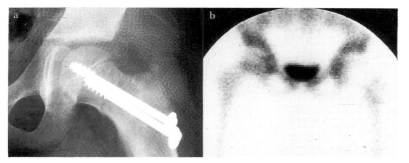

1.13 Radionuclide scanning　(a) This fractured femoral neck in a child has resulted in loss of the blood supply, as shown by (b) the void in the left hip on the technetium scan.

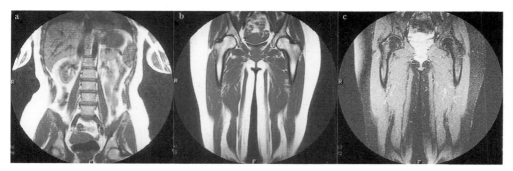

1.14 Magnetic resonance imaging　(a, b) T_1-weighted and (c) STIR (short tau inversion recovery) sequences of the torso and thigh areas, showing the contrasting definition and brightness of the various structures and tissues.

clearer differentiation of tissues. Moreover, sectional 'cuts' can be obtained in almost any plane. This is particularly useful in the diagnosis of brain and spinal cord lesions.

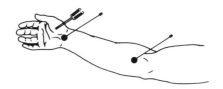

Electrodiagnosis

1.15 Electrodiagnosis Electrodes at different levels are used to stimulate the median nerve and one in the thenar muscle records contraction. If the distance between the electrodes is measured and the time interval (from stimulation to muscle contraction) is recorded, conduction velocity can be calculated.

Nerve and muscle function can be studied by electrical methods. Two types of investigation are employed: nerve conduction and electromyography.

Nerve conduction

The time interval between stimulation of a motor nerve and muscle contraction can be measured accurately. If the test is repeated at two points a fixed distance apart along the nerve, the conduction velocity between these points can be determined. Normal values are about 40–60 m per second. Sensory nerve conduction can be measured in a similar way.

Conduction velocity is slowed in peripheral nerve damage or compression, and the site of the lesion can be established by taking measurements in different segments of the nerve.

If the nerve is divided, there is no response to stimulation of the nerve and an abnormal response to galvanic stimulation of the muscle (the 'reaction of degeneration'). By plotting the voltage against the duration of stimulus necessary to produce contraction, a *strength/duration curve*, can be obtained, which reflects the degree of muscle innervation after nerve injury. Serial examinations will show whether recovery is taking place.

Electromyography

Electromyography does not involve electrical stimulation. Instead, an electrode in the muscle is used to record motor unit activity at rest and when attempts are made to contract the muscle. Normally there is no electrical activity at rest, but on voluntary contraction characteristic oscilloscopic patterns appear. Changes in these patterns can identify certain neuropathic and myopathic disorders.

Infection

Infection may reach the bones and joints via the *blood stream* from a distant site, or by *direct invasion* from a skin puncture, operation or an open fracture. Depending on the type of organism, the site of infection and the host response, the result may be a pyogenic osteomyelitis or arthritis, a chronic granulomatous reaction (classically seen in tuberculosis), or an indolent response to an unusual organism (e.g. a fungal infection).

Acute haematogenous osteomyelitis

Acute osteomyelitis almost invariably occurs in children, when adults are affected it may be because of compromised host resistance due to debilitation, disease or drugs (e.g. immuno-suppressive therapy). The causal organism is usually *Staphylococcus aureus*, although in young children *Haemophilus influenzae* is not uncommon. Patients with sickle-cell anaemia are prone to develop salmonella bone infections. Unusual organisms are also found in heroin addicts.

The blood stream is invaded, perhaps from a minor skin abrasion or a boil. In adults the source of infection may be an arterial line or a dirty needle and syringe. The organisms usually settle in the metaphysis at the growing end of a long bone, possibly because the hairpin arrangement of capillaries slows down the rate of blood

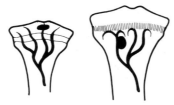

2.1 Acute osteomyelitis In infants infection may settle near the very end of the bone; joint infection and growth disturbance easily follow. In children, metaphyseal infection is usual; the growth disc acts as a barrier to spread.

flow. In young infants the epiphysis may be involved, while in adults infection may appear almost anywhere.

Pathology

INFLAMMATION The earliest change is an acute inflammatory reaction. The intraosseous pressure rises, causing intense pain and obstruction of blood flow.

SUPPURATION By the second day pus appears in the medulla and forces its way along the Volkmann canals to the surface, where it forms a subperiosteal abscess. It then spreads along the shaft, to re-enter the bone at another level, or bursts out into the soft tissues. In infants, infection often extends into the epiphysis and thence into the joint. In older children the physis is a

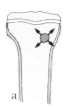
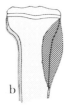
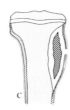

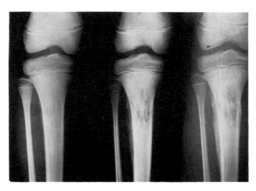

2.2 Acute osteomyelitis (a) Infection in the metaphysis may spread towards the surface, to form a subperiosteal abscess (b). Some of the bone may die, and is encased in periosteal new bone as a sequestrum (c). The encasing involucrum is sometimes perforated leading to sinuses.

2.3 Acute osteomyelitis The first x-ray, 2 days after symptoms began, is normal – it always is; metaphyseal mottling and periosteal changes were not obvious until the second film, taken 14 days later; eventually much of the shaft was involved.

barrier to direct spread but where the metaphysis is partly intracapsular (e.g. at the hip, shoulder or elbow) pus may discharge through the periosteum into the joint.

NECROSIS The rising intraosseous pressure, vascular stasis, infective thrombosis and periosteal stripping increasingly compromise the blood supply; by the end of a week there is usually evidence of necrosis. Pieces of bone may separate as sequestra which act as foreign-body irritants, causing persistent discharge through a sinus until they escape or are removed. However, the larger sequestra remain entombed in cavities of bone.

NEW BONE FORMATION New bone forms from the deep layer of the periosteum. With time the new bone thickens to form an involucrum enclosing the infected tissue and sequestra. If the infection persists, pus may discharge through perforations (cloacae) in the involucrum and track by sinuses to the skin surface; the condition is now established as a chronic osteomyelitis.

RESOLUTION If infection is controlled and intraosseous pressure released, the bone will heal though it may remain thickened.

Clinical features

The patient, usually a child, presents with pain, malaise and a fever; in neglected cases toxaemia may be marked. Sometimes a history of a preceding skin lesion, an injury or a sore throat may be obtained.

ACUTE OSTEOMYELITIS

Pain
Fever   } Unless modified
Inflammation   by antibiotics
Acute tenderness
X-RAYS NORMAL DURING FIRST 10 DAYS

The limb is held still and there is acute 'fingertip' tenderness near one of the larger joints. Even the gentlest manipulation is painful and joint movement is restricted. Local redness, swelling, warmth and oedema are later signs and signify the presence of pus.

In infants, and especially in the newborn, the constitutional disturbance can be misleadingly mild; the baby simply fails to thrive and is drowsy but irritable. Suspicion should be aroused by a history of birth difficulties or umbilical artery catheterisation.

X-RAY *For the first 10 days x-rays show no abnormality.* Later there is rarefaction of the metaphysis and periosteal new bone formation. With healing there is sclerosis. Sometimes sequestra are seen, separated from the surrounding bone.

INVESTIGATIONS   There is usually a leucocytosis and the blood culture may be positive. In doubtful cases radioisotope bone scanning is helpful and may show increased activity long before x-ray changes appear.

Complications

Spread   Infection may spread to the joint (septic arthritis) or to other bones (metastatic osteomyelitis).

Growth disturbance   If the physis is damaged there may later be shortening or deformity.

Persistent infection   Treatment must be prompt and effective. 'Too little too late' may result in chronic osteomyelitis.

Treatment

ANTIBIOTICS   Blood and, if possible, aspiration material are sent immediately for culture, but the prompt administration of antibiotics is so vital that the result is not awaited. Initially the choice of antibiotics is based on the findings from direct examination of the aspirate and a 'best guess' at the most likely pathogen; a more appropriate drug can be substituted once the organism is identified and its antibiotic sensitivity is known.

Older children and previously fit adults,   who probably have a staphylococcal infection, are started on flucloxacillin and fusidic acid, intravenously for the first 3 or 4 days and then – once their condition begins to improve – orally for another 3–6 weeks.

In children under 4 years   (who have a high incidence of haemophilus infection) and in any case in which *Gram-negative organisms* are seen in the smear, it is advisable to start with one of the cephalosporins.

ANALGESICS   Osteomyelitis is extremely painful; adequate and repeated analgesics must be given.

SPLINTAGE   Complete bed rest is essential. A splint is desirable but should not conceal the affected area. With acute osteomyelitis of the upper femur, traction is needed to prevent hip dislocation.

DRAINAGE   If antibiotics are given early, drainage may not be necessary. If a subperiosteal abscess can be detected (overlying oedema is a useful sign), or if pyrexia and local tenderness persist for more than 24 hours after adequate antibiotics, the pus should be let out; this will also allow the organism to be identified.

Subacute haematogenous osteomyelitis

Osteomyelitis may present in a relatively mild form, presumably because the organism is less virulent or the patient more resistant. The distal femur and the proximal and distal tibia are the favourite sites. The patient is usually a child or adolescent who has had pain near one of the large joints for several weeks. The typical x-ray picture is of a small, oval cavity surrounded by sclerotic bone – the classic **Brodie's abscess** – but sometimes the lesion is more diffuse. A small abscess is easily mistaken for an osteoid osteoma and the diagnosis may be made only when the lesion is explored.

If the condition is troublesome, the abscess is opened under antibiotic cover.

Post-traumatic and postoperative osteomyelitis

An open fracture may become infected; this is the usual cause of osteomyelitis in adults. Many different organisms are involved but *Staphylococcus aureus* is the most common offender.

The patient is feverish and develops pain and swelling over the fracture site; the wound is inflamed and there may be a seropurulent discharge. Blood tests show a leucocytosis and an increased sedimentation rate. A wound swab should be examined and cultured for organisms.

The essence of treatment is prophylaxis: thorough debridement of open fractures, the provision of drainage by leaving the wound open, and antibiotics. For established infection, regular wound dressing is required. Loose or ineffectual implants should be removed; stable implants are left undisturbed until the fracture has united. If the fracture is unfixed and unstable, an external fixator can be applied.

Postoperative infection is not uncommon; the incidence in general hospitals is 3–5%. Predisposing factors are debility, chronic disease (e.g. rheumatoid arthritis), previous infection, corticosteroid therapy, difficult or long operations, haematoma formation, wound tension and tight dressings or plasters. There is also an increased risk with the use of foreign material (metal, plastic or cement) for joint replacement or for the internal fixation of fractures. Prophylaxis is the key; the cleanest possible surgical environment, a meticulous technique, careful haemostasis and suction drainage. In all high-risk situations prophylactic antibiotics are essential.

Treatment is the same as for post-traumatic infection.

Chronic osteomyelitis

This used to be a common sequel to acute haematogenous osteomyelitis; nowadays it more frequently follows an open fracture or operation.

An area of bone has been destroyed by the acute infection leaving sequestra surrounded by dense sclerosed bone. The imprisoned sequestra provoke a chronic seropurulent discharge which escapes through a sinus. Bacteria may remain dormant for years giving rise to recurrent flares of acute infection.

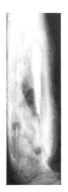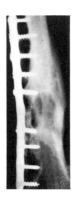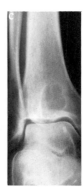

2.4 Chronic osteomyelitis Chronic bone infection, with a persistent sequestrum, may be a sequel to acute osteomyelitis (a). More often it follows an open fracture or operation (b). Occasionally it presents as a Brodie's abscess (c).

Clinical features

The patient presents because pain, pyrexia, redness and tenderness have recurred (a 'flare'), or with a discharging sinus. X-rays show areas of bone rarefaction surrounded by sclerosis, and sometimes sequestra. A sinogram may help to localize the site. Bone scans are useful in revealing hidden foci of infection.

Treatment

Treatment is usually conservative. A sinus may be painless and need a dressing simply to protect the clothing; a flare often settles with a few days' rest, although if an abscess presents it should be incised. Most antibiotics fail to penetrate the barrier of fibrous tissue plus bone sclerosis. Fucidic acid and the cephalosporins are exceptions and may be useful. Sequestrectomy should be performed only if a sequestrum is radiologically visible and surgically accessible. After sequestrectomy the 'dead space' should be irrigated with antibiotic solution and allowed to fill with granulation tissue. More dramatic procedures involving bone grafts and muscle flaps are sometimes used.

Acute suppurative arthritis

Cause and pathology

The causal organism is usually *Staphylococcus aureus*; in children under 3 years *Haemophilus influenzae* is fairly common. The joint is invaded through a penetrating wound, by eruption of a bone abscess or by blood spread from a distant site. As infection spreads through the joint, articular cartilage is destroyed. Pus may burst out of the joint to form abscesses and sinuses. Later, with healing, the raw articular surfaces may adhere, producing fibrous or bony ankylosis.

Clinical features

The usual features are acute pain and swelling in a single large joint – commonly the hip in children and the knee in adults. However, any joint can be affected. The patient becomes ill, with a rapid pulse and swinging fever. The white cell count is raised and blood culture may be positive.

Many of the local signs can be elicited only in superficial joints. The skin looks red, the joint is held flexed and it is swollen. There is superficial warmth, diffuse tenderness and fluctuation. All movements are grossly restricted and often completely abolished by pain and spasm (pseudoparesis).

The diagnosis can be confirmed by aspiration and examination of the pus for organisms.

X-RAY may show widening of the joint space and soft tissue swelling; ultrasonography will reveal a joint effusion. In late cases there are signs of subarticular bone destruction.

Complications

Dislocation A tense effusion may cause dislocation.

Epiphyseal destruction In neglected infants the largely cartilaginous epiphysis may be destroyed, leaving an unstable pseudarthrosis.

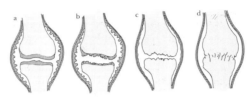

2.5 Acute suppurative arthritis In the early stage (a) there is an acute synovitis with a purulent joint effusion. (b) Soon the articular cartilage is attacked by bacterial and cellular enzymes. If the infection is not arrested, the cartilage may be completely destroyed (c); healing then leads to bony ankylosis (d).

Growth disturbance Physeal damage may result in shortening or deformity.

Ankylosis If articular cartilage is eroded, healing may lead to ankylosis.

Treatment

The first priority is to aspirate the joint and examine the fluid. Treatment is then started without further delay and follows the same lines as for acute osteomyelitis.

ANTIBIOTICS Systemic antibiotics should be started as soon as joint fluid and blood samples have been taken for culture; once the bacterial sensitivity is known the appropriate drug is substituted. Injections are continued for several weeks and are followed by oral antibiotics for a further 3–4 weeks.

SPLINTAGE The joint must be rested either on a splint or in a widely split plaster. At the hip, the joint should be held abducted and 30° flexed.

DRAINAGE Under anaesthesia, pus is drained and the joint washed out. This is best done by open operation, but in a superficial joint it can be achieved by repeated aspiration and irrigation.

Once the patient's general condition is good and the joint is no longer inflamed, gentle and gradually increasing movements are encouraged. But if articular cartilage has been destroyed, the aim is to keep the joint immobile in the optimum position while ankylosis is awaited.

Tuberculosis

Tuberculosis is again on the increase; bones or joints are affected in about 5% of patients. *Mycobacterium tuberculosis* has a predilection for the vertebral bodies and the large synovial joints.

Pathology

Infection reaches the skeleton by haematogenous seeding from the lung or intestine. There is a chronic inflammatory reaction, characteristically leading to caseation. Spread into soft tissues leads to a subacute abscess (the so-called 'cold abscess'). Infected material may discharge to the surface leaving a chronic sinus. Secondary pyogenic infection may follow.

If the articular surfaces have been destroyed there will be fibrous ankylosis and permanent loss of function.

Clinical features

The patient, usually a child or young adult, complains of pain and (in a superficial joint)

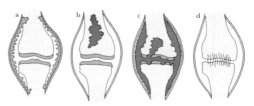

2.6 Tuberculous arthritis   The disease may begin as synovitis (a) or osteomyelitis (b), both of which can resolve. From either it may extend to become a true arthritis (c); not all the cartilage is destroyed, and healing is usually by fibrous ankylosis (d).

swelling. Muscle wasting is characteristic and synovial thickening is often striking. Movements are limited in all directions. As articular erosion progresses the joint becomes stiff and severely deformed; in late cases there may be a sinus.

In tuberculosis of the spine, pain may be deceptively slight. Consequently the patient may not present until there is a visible abscess or until collapse causes a localized kyphosis (gibbus). Occasionally the presenting feature is weakness or loss of sensibility in the lower limbs.

X-RAYS show soft tissue swelling and rarefaction of the bone. In the early stages the joint space is retained but later there is narrowing and irregularity with bone erosion on both sides of the joint. Cystic lesions may appear in the bone.

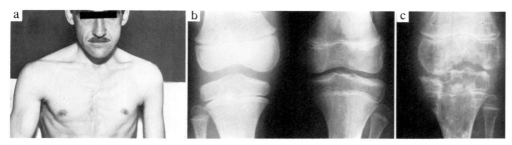

2.7 Tuberculosis   A characteristic feature of tuberculosis is wasting of muscle (a). The knees in (b) show osteoporosis on the left, due to synovitis. This often resolves with treatment, but if cartilage and bone are destroyed (c), healing is by fibrosis.

Diagnosis

Except in areas where tuberculosis is common, diagnosis may often be delayed simply because the disease is not suspected. In many respects it resembles rheumatoid arthritis. Features suggesting tuberculosis should trigger more active investigation; these are:

- involvement of only one joint
- the long history
- marked synovial thickening
- marked muscle wasting
- periarticular osteoporosis

The ESR is usually raised and the Mantoux test is positive.

Synovial biopsy for histological examination and culture is often necessary.

Treatment

The mainstay of treatment is antituberculous *chemotherapy*, using a combination of drugs (e.g. rifampicin and isoniazid) for 6 months or more. If chemotherapy is started early, the joint may heal and function be completely restored.

Local measures include rest, traction and – occasionally – operation. Splintage should be continued for several months, by which time it is usually clear whether the joint has been saved. If the articular surfaces are destroyed, the joint is immobilized until all signs of disease activity have disappeared. If the disease remains quiescent, arthrodesis – or even joint replacement – may be considered.

Rheumatic disorders 3

These are a group of conditions which cause chronic pain, swelling and tenderness of joints and tendon sheaths. Although characterized by a persistent arthritis, they are essentially systemic diseases affecting connective tissues throughout the body.

Rheumatoid arthritis

Rheumatoid arthritis (RA) affects about 3 per cent of the population, women three times more often than men. It usually starts in the fourth or fifth decade.

Cause

The cause is unknown, but it is believed that some antigen – possibly a virus – sets off a chain of events culminating in a chronic inflammatory disorder in which abnormal

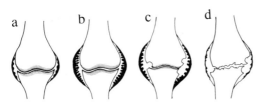

3.1 Pathology of rheumatoid arthritis (a) The normal joint. (b) Stage 1 – synovitis and joint swelling. (c) Stage 2 – early joint destruction with periarticular erosions. (d) Stage 3 – advanced joint destruction and deformity.

immunological reactions are prominent. These include the production of antibodies (both IgG and IgM) to the body's own IgG. Such 'autoantibodies' appear as serum rheumatoid factors (RF) in 80% of patients with RA, and they can also be demonstrated in the synovium.

The abnormal immune response may be genetically predetermined, for patients with RA show increased frequencies of HLA-DR4.

Pathology

Although tissues throughout the body are affected, the brunt of the attack falls on synovium. The pathological changes, if unchecked, proceed in three stages.

Stage 1: synovitis Synovial membrane becomes inflamed and thickened, giving rise to a cell-rich effusion. Although painful and swollen, the joints and tendons are still intact and the disorder is potentially reversible.

Stage 2: destruction Persistent inflammation causes tissue destruction. Articular cartilage is eroded and tendon fibres may rupture.

Stage 3: deformity The combination of articular destruction, capsular stretching and tendon rupture leads to progressive instability and deformity.

The most characteristic extra-articular lesion is the *rheumatoid nodule*, a small granuloma occurring under the skin (especially over bony prominences), on tendons, in the sclera and in viscera.

Other systemic features are *lymphadenopathy, vasculitis, muscle weakness* and *visceral disease* affecting the lungs, heart, kidneys, brain and gastrointestinal tract.

Clinical features

The usual pattern is the insidious emergence of a symmetrical polyarthritis affecting mainly the hands and feet, together with early morning stiffness and a general lack of well-being.

During stage 1 (synovitis) there is typically swelling, increased warmth and tenderness of the proximal finger joints and the wrists, as well as of the tendon sheaths around these joints. Later the disease may 'spread' to the elbows, shoulders, knees, ankles and feet. Occasionally the condition begins in one of the larger joints.

In stage 2 (destruction) joint movements are limited and isolated tendon ruptures appear. Subcutaneous nodules may be felt over the olecranon process; although they occur in only 25 per cent of patients, they are pathognomonic of RA.

In stage 3 (deformity) the diagnosis is obvious at a glance. Fingers are deviated ulnarwards, often with subluxation or dislocation of the metacarpophalangeal joints; elbows cannot be straightened and the shoulders have lost abduction; knees may be swollen and held in flexion and valgus; the toes are clawed and there are painful callosities under the metatarsal heads. Muscle wasting is often severe. About a third of all patients develop pain and stiffness in the cervical spine.

In long-standing cases there may be vasculitis and peripheral neuropathy. Marked visceral disease is rare.

X-RAYS   *In stage 1* x-rays show only soft tissue swelling and periarticular osteoporosis. *In stage 2* there is narrowing of the 'joint space' and marginal bony erosions, especially around the wrists and the proximal joints of the hands and feet. *In stage 3* articular destruction and joint deformity are obvious.

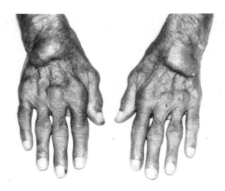

3.2 Rheumatoid arthritis – early features   This patient, with a 3-month history of joint pains, has swelling of the proximal interphalangeal joints ('spindling'), of some metacarpophalangeal joints and extensor tendon sheaths, and of both wrists. The changes are remarkably symmetrical.

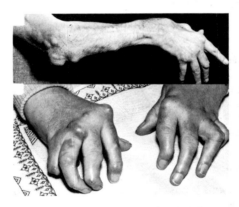

3.3 Rheumatoid arthritis – late features   There are subcutaneous nodules on the extensor surfaces and characteristic deformities of the hands.

INVESTIGATIONS   In active phases the ESR is raised and C-reactive protein is present. Serological tests for rheumatoid factor are positive in 80 per cent of patients; sometimes antinuclear factors also are present.

Diagnosis

The minimal criteria for diagnosing RA are: (1) bilateral, symmetrical polyarthritis involving (2) the proximal joints of the hands

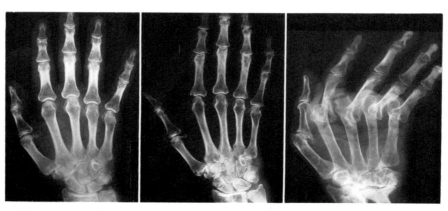

3.4 Rheumatoid arthritis – sequence of changes The progress of disease is well shown in this patient's x-rays. First there was only soft-tissue swelling and periarticular osteoporosis; later juxta-articular erosions appeared; ultimately the joints became unstable and deformed.

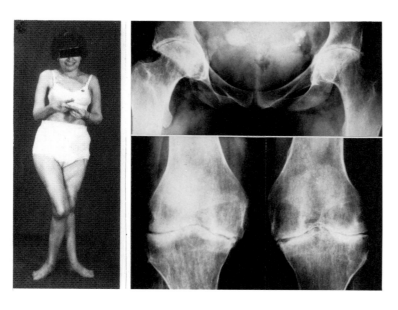

3.5 Rheumatoid arthritis The acute phase is over, but the patient is left with secondary osteoarthritis of the hips and knees.

or feet, present for (3) at least 6 weeks. If, in addition, there are subcutaneous nodules or periarticular erosions on x-ray, the diagnosis is certain. *A positive test for rheumatoid factor in the absence of the above features is not sufficient to diagnose RA, nor does a negative test exclude the diagnosis if all the other features are present.* The chief value of the rheumatoid factor tests is in assessing prognosis; high titres herald more serious disease.

In the differential diagnosis of polyarthritis several disorders must be considered.

Heberden's arthropathy affects the *distal* interphalangeal joints and causes nodular swellings with radiologically obvious osteophytes.

Reiter's disease affects the large joints and the lumbosacral spine. There is a history of urethritis or colitis and often also conjunctivitis.

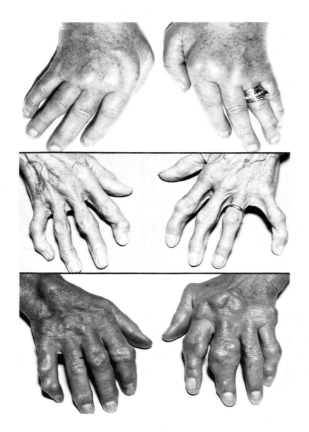

3.6 Rheumatoid arthritis – differential diagnosis These three patients all presented with painful swollen finger joints. In the upper figure it is the proximal joints which are enlarged and deformed (rheumatoid arthritis); in the middle figure the distal joints are the worst (Heberden's osteoarthritis); in the lower the asymmetrical nodules are actually large tophi (gout).

Ankylosing spondylitis may involve the peripheral joints, but it is primarily a disease of the sacroiliac and intervertebral joints, causing back pain and progressive stiffness.

Polyarticular gout affects large and small joints, and tophi on fingers and toes may be mistaken for rheumatoid nodules.

Seronegative polyarthritis is a feature of a number of conditions vaguely related to rheumatoid arthritis: psoriatic arthritis, juvenile chronic arthritis (Still's disease), systemic lupus erythematosus and other connective-tissue diseases.

Polymyalgia rheumatica occurs mostly in middle-aged or elderly women, causing marked postinactivity stiffness and weakness. Pain is most severe around the pectoral and pelvic girdles; tenderness is in muscles rather than joints. The ESR is almost always high. This is a form of giant-cell arteritis and carries the risk of temporal arteritis resulting in blindness. Corticosteroids provide rapid and dramatic relief of all symptoms.

Course*

In 80 per cent of patients RA follows a periodic course, with intermittent 'flares' during which symptoms and signs of inflammation are more severe. With time these attacks occur less frequently and the disease may become almost quiescent; by then, however, the joints are often permanently damaged.

In 5 per cent there is relentless progression of the disease with increasing inflammatory

*RA does not burn itself out – it burns itself in.

activity, joint destruction, muscle wasting and visceral involvement.

In 10 per cent – usually men over 55 – symptoms start explosively but, rather paradoxically, the condition tends to subside and follows a relatively mild course.

In the fortunate few the condition settles after the first or second attack and does not recur.

Complications

JOINT RUPTURE   Occasionally the joint lining ruptures and synovial contents spill into the soft tissues. Treatment is directed at the underlying synovitis – i.e. splintage and injection of the joint, with synovectomy as a second resort.

INFECTION   Patients with rheumatoid arthritis – and even more so those on corticosteroid therapy – are susceptible to infection. Sudden clinical deterioration, or increased pain in a single joint, should alert one to the possibility of septic arthritis and the need for joint aspiration.

Treatment

The management of rheumatoid arthritis is guided by four simple injunctions: (1) *stop the synovitis*; (2) *prevent deformity*; (3) *reconstruct*; (4) *rehabilitate*. A multidisciplinary approach is needed from the beginning; the physician, surgeon, physiotherapist, occupational therapist, orthotist and social worker must co-operate as a team.

TREATMENT OF RA

1 Stop the synovitis
2 Prevent deformity
3 Reconstruct
4 Rehabilitate

● 1. STOP THE SYNOVITIS

Anti-inflammatory drugs   Mild to moderate synovitis can be controlled with non-steroidal anti-inflammatory drugs; these are not curative, do not influence the progress of erosions and do not lower the ESR, but they do control pain and stiffness and therefore improve function. Side effects (rashes, gastrointestinal symptoms, peptic ulceration) are common but reversible.

Disease-modifying drugs   Gold, penicillamine and immunosuppressive drugs have a direct action on the immunopathological process and can control disease progress. However, they all have unpredictable – and potentially lethal – side effects on the kidney, liver and haemopoietic system. They are, therefore, usually introduced only when other measures have failed; but in severe cases with florid synovitis, high ESR and strongly positive rheumatoid factor tests (when simpler measures are likely to fail) they may be used much earlier. Their effects must always be monitored by regular blood tests and by liver and renal function tests. Dosage should be adjusted with great caution; the rule is: 'Start low, go slow'.

Corticosteroids   So effectively do these relieve joint pain and stiffness that their use is a constant temptation; a temptation to be resisted, however, because of their adverse effects on metabolism, adrenal function, bone structure and soft-tissue integrity. With experience and discipline they can be used during severe, incapacitating exacerbations or to help weather the storm while waiting for gold or penicillamine to take effect.

Rest and splintage   No drug will reduce joint inflammation more effectively than rest and immobilization. This is ideally indicated for acute exacerbations but night splints can be used intermittently at any stage of the disease.

Intra-articular injections   Corticosteroids, cytotoxic drugs and radiocolloids are effective when injected into inflamed joints or tendon sheaths. However, they should be used sparingly, for repeated injections can cause tissue damage.

Synovectomy   Even at an early stage of the disease, if all other measures fail, operative

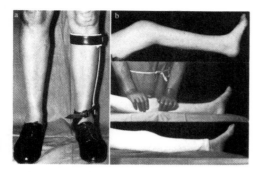

3.7 Treatment of rheumatoid arthritis   (a) Splintage to rest inflamed joints may, if started early, halt the progress of deformity. (b) An early fixed deformity of the knee can be corrected by gentle manipulation and temporary plaster splintage.

synovectomy is justified. With the appearance of increasingly potent drugs, this is seldom called for.

● 2. PREVENT DEFORMITY

Physiotherapy Inflamed joints must be rested, but should also be put through a passive range of movement each day. As disease activity subsides, active exercises are encouraged.

Operation Tendon rupture and joint instability are preludes to progressive deformity.

They should be treated whenever they occur – either by permanent splintage or by operation (tendon suture or replacement).

● 3. RECONSTRUCT

Advanced joint destruction, instability and deformity are clear indications for reconstructive surgery, often combined with synovectomy of the joint or tendons. Arthrodesis, osteotomy and replacement all have their place and are considered in the appropriate chapters. NB. If an operation is needed, always check the cervical spine for instability.

● 4. REHABILITATE

Rehabilitation should not be seen as a rearguard action; it accompanies all stages of treatment from the start, and includes functional assessment, special training, social integration and psychological adjustment.

A full understanding of the patient's specific needs must influence treatment. Some patients are well motivated and crave to return to work and domestic independence; others are passive and dependent. For the one group mechanical aids, special utensils, adjustment of home and work space are essential adjuncts to medical and surgical treatment; for the other, the support of family and friends may be all that they want.

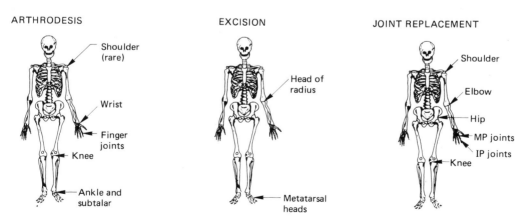

3.8 Operations for rheumatoid arthritis   Sites where each may be useful

Ankylosing spondylitis

Like rheumatoid arthritis, this is a generalized chronic inflammatory disease – but its effects are seen mainly in the spine and sacroiliac joints. It is characterized by pain and stiffness of the back, with variable involvement of the hips and shoulders and (more rarely) the peripheral joints. Its prevalence is about 0.2% in western Europe, but is much lower in Japanese and Negroid peoples. Males are affected more frequently than females (estimates vary from 2 : 1 to 10 : 1) and the usual age at onset is between 15 and 25 years.

Cause

The disease tends to run in families; close relatives may have either classic ankylosing spondylitis or one of the other 'spondarthritides' such as Reiter's disease, psoriatic arthritis or enteropathic arthritis. The fact that all these conditions are associated with a particular tissue type, the HLA-B27, suggests a common genetic predisposition; the specific clinical syndrome is probably triggered by some recent event – often genitourinary or bowel infection.

Pathology

The disease starts as an inflammation of the sacroiliac and vertebral joints and ligaments. Sometimes the hips and shoulders also are affected, and very occasionally the peripheral joints.

Pathological changes follow a fairly constant sequence: inflammation – granulation tissue formation – erosion of articular cartilage or bone – replacement by fibrous tissue – ossification of the fibrous tissue – ankylosis.

If many vertebrae are involved, the spine may become absolutely rigid. If the costovertebral joints are involved, respiratory excursion is diminished.

Clinical features

Most patients are young men who complain of persistent backache and stiffness, often worse in the early morning or after inactivity. About 10 per cent have pain in peripheral joints.

The most typical sign is stiffness of the spine. All movements are diminished, but loss of extension is both the earliest and the most severe. The 'wall test' is useful: if a healthy person stands with his back to a wall, his heels, buttocks, scapulae and occiput can all touch the wall simultaneously; if extension is seriously diminished, this is impossible. In advanced cases the entire spine may be rigid ('poker back') and chest expansion is decreased to well below the normal 7 cm.

If the hips are involved, they also may go on to complete ankylosis.

Occasionally, peripheral joints are swollen and tender. Some patients complain of painful heels and have tenderness at the insertion of the tendo Achillis.

Extraskeletal manifestations include ocular inflammation, aortic valve disease, carditis and pulmonary fibrosis.

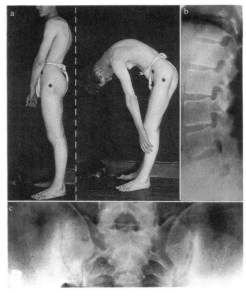

3.9 Ankylosing spondylitis – early The early features are (a) a stiff spine, (b) 'squaring' of the lumbar vertebrae, and (c) bilateral sacroiliac erosion.

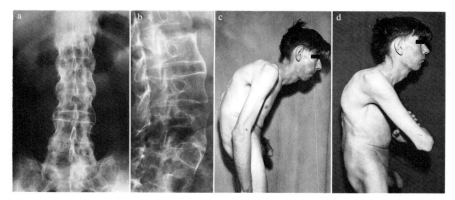

3.10 Ankylosing spondylitis – late   (a–c) Bony bridges (syndesmophytes) between the vertebral bodies convert the spine into a rigid column ('bamboo spine'). (d) After spinal osteotomy this man's back is still rigid, but his posture, function and outlook are vastly improved.

X-RAYS   The cardinal sign is fuzziness or frank erosion of the sacroiliac joints. Later these joints become sclerosed and, eventually, completely ankylosed.

Ossification across the intervertebral discs produces bony bridges (syndesmophytes) spanning the gaps between adjacent vertebral bodies. Bridging at several levels gives the appearance of a 'bamboo spine'.

Peripheral joints may show erosive arthritis resembling that of RA.

INVESTIGATIONS   The ESR is usually elevated during active phases of the disease. HLA-B27 is present in 90 per cent of cases.

Treatment

There is no specific treatment. Pain may be controlled by analgesics and non-steroidal anti-inflammatory drugs; above all the patient must be encouraged to exercise and keep moving. Postural training can prevent serious deformity; if ankylosis is inevitable, let it at least be in good position.

Stiffness of the hips can be treated by joint replacement, although this seldom provides more than moderate mobility. Severe flexion deformity of the spine may be reduced by vertebral osteotomy.

Seronegative spondarthritis

A number of conditions usually associated with seronegative polyarthritis (i.e. without serum rheumatoid factors) may show changes in the spine and sacroiliac joints indistinguishable from those of ankylosing spondylitis. The best defined of these conditions are *psoriatic arthritis*, *Reiter's disease* and the arthritis that sometimes accompanies *ulcerative colitis* or *Crohn's disease*; together with classic *ankylosing spondylitis* they are often grouped as the 'seronegative spondarthritides'.

The exact relationship between these disorders is unknown, but they share certain important features: (1) the characteristic spondylitis and sacroiliitis occur in all of them; (2) they are all associated with HLA-B27; (3) they show familial aggregation; and (4) there is considerable overlap within families, some members having one disorder and close relatives another.

Psoriatic arthritis

About 4 per cent of patients with chronic polyarthritis have psoriasis; not all, however, have psoriatic arthritis, which is a distinct entity and not simply 'RA plus psoriasis'. Unlike RA, psoriatic arthritis affects men and women equally and tends to run in families. The arthritis is not as clearly symmetrical as in RA and – in marked contrast to the latter – it occurs mainly in the *interphalangeal* joints of the fingers and toes. Bone destruction may be so severe that the digits are completely flail or badly deformed ('arthritis mutilans'). About a quarter of the patients develop sacroiliac and vertebral changes like those of ankylosing spondylitis. HLA-B27 occurs in about 60 per cent of those with overt sacroiliitis.

General treatment aims at controlling the skin disorder with topical preparations, and

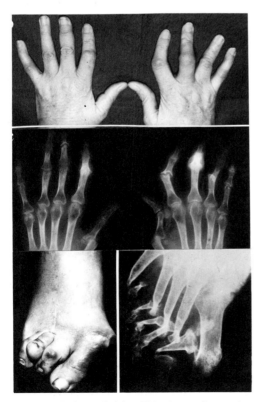

3.11 Psoriatic arthritis This is a destructive arthritis affecting the interphalangeal joints of the fingers and toes.

alleviating joint symptoms with non-steroidal anti-inflammatory drugs. In resistant forms of arthritis, immunosuppressive agents have proved effective.

Local treatment consists of judicious splintage to prevent undue deformity, and surgery for unstable joints.

Reiter's disease and reactive arthritis

'Classic' Reiter's disease is a clinical triad: polyarthritis, conjunctivitis and non-specific urethritis. However, the term is now used more loosely for a *reactive arthritis* associated with non-specific urogenital or bowel infection. It is probably the most common type of large-joint polyarthritis in young men. Familial aggregation, overlap with other forms of seronegative spondarthritis in first-degree relatives, and an increased frequency of HLA-B27 in all these disorders point to a genetic predisposition. *Lymphogranuloma venereum* and *Chlamydia trachomatis* have been implicated as urogenital infective agents, but arthritis also occurs with bowel infection due to *Shigella, Salmonella* or *Yersinia enterocolitica.*

The joints themselves are not infected; the synovitis is the end stage of an abnormal immune response to infection elsewhere or to its products.

Clinical features

Reiter's disease affects mainly large joints, especially the knee and ankle. Often it starts as an acute arthritis with marked effusion suggesting gout or a mechanical derangement. Tenosynovitis and plantar fasciitis are common. Backache and stiffness, due to sacroiliitis and spondylitis, occur in the majority of patients at some stage. Although the disease is said to be self-limiting, 80 per cent of patients continue to have symptoms for many years.

Typically there is a history of *urethritis, prostatitis, cervicitis* or diarrhoea. *Ocular lesions* include conjunctivitis, episcleritis and uveitis.

X-rays are at first normal, but after many months may show an erosive arthritis. Sacroiliac and vertebral changes are similar to those of ankylosing spondylitis.

Special investigations   Tests for HLA-B27 are positive in 75 per cent of patients with sacroiliitis. The ESR may be high in the active phase. The causative organism can sometimes be isolated from urethral fluids or faeces, and tests for antibodies may be positive.

Diagnosis

If the condition affects only one or two joints it is usually mistaken for gout or infective arthritis. Examination of the synovial fluid for organisms and crystals will help to exclude these disorders.

Treatment

General treatment is indicated for active urogenital or bowel infection; a short course of antibiotics is usually sufficient, but for *Chlamydia* tetracycline daily for 6 months is recommended.

Local treatment is non-specific and palliative: rest and splintage if arthritis is severe, and then prolonged administration of anti-inflammatory agents while waiting for spontaneous remission.

Juvenile chronic arthritis ('Still's disease')

Juvenile chronic arthritis (JCA) is the preferred term for non-infective inflammatory joint disease of more than 3 months' duration in children under 16 years. It embraces a group of disorders in all of which pain, swelling and stiffness of the joints are common features.

The prevalence is about 1 per 1000 children, and boys and girls are affected with equal frequency.

The cause is probably similar to that of rheumatoid disease: an abnormal immune response to some antigen in children with a particular genetic predisposition. However, rheumatoid factor is usually absent.

Clinical features

JCA occurs in several characteristic forms.

Systemic JCA   This, the classic Still's disease, is usually seen below the age of 3 years. It starts with intermittent fever, rashes and malaise; there may also be lymphadenopathy, splenomegaly and hepatomegaly. Joint swelling occurs some weeks or months after the onset; fortunately, it usually resolves when the systemic illness subsides but it may go on to progressive arthritis. Rheumatoid factor tests are negative.

Pauciarticular JCA   This is by far the commonest form of JCA. It usually occurs below the age of 6 years and is more common in girls. Only a few joints are involved and there is no systemic illness. The child presents with pain and swelling of medium sized joints (knees, ankles, elbows and wrists); rheumatoid factor tests are negative. A serious complication is chronic iridocyclitis, which occurs in about 50 per cent.

Polyarticular seropositive JCA   This is usually seen in older children – mainly girls – and it resembles classic RA, with multiple small-joint involvement, progressive articular destruction and positive tests for rheumatoid factor. The term 'juvenile rheumatoid arthritis' can be used for this group.

Seronegative spondarthritis   In older children – usually boys – the condition may take the form of sacroiliitis and spondylitis; hips and knees are sometimes involved as well. Tests for HLA-B27 are often positive and this should probably be regarded as 'juvenile ankylosing spondylitis'.

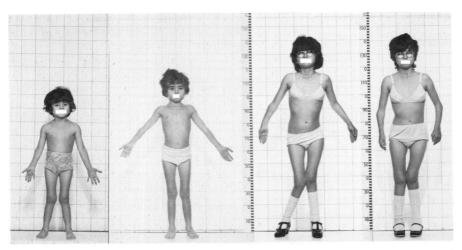

3.12 Juvenile chronic arthritis This young girl developed JCA when she was 5 years old. Here we see her at 6, 9 and 14 years of age. The arthritis became inactive, leaving her with a knee deformity, which has been treated by osteotomy. Her eyes, too, were affected by iridocyclitis. (Courtesy of Mr Malcolm Swann and Dr Barbara Ansell.)

Complications

Stiffness Whilst most patients recover good function, some permanent loss of movement is common.

Growth defects There is general retardation of growth, sometimes aggravated by prolonged corticosteroid therapy.

Iridocyclitis This is most common in pauciarticular disease; untreated it may lead to blindness.

Amyloidosis In children with long-standing active disease there is a serious risk of amyloidosis, which may be fatal.

Treatment

General treatment is similar to that of rheumatoid arthritis. Corticosteroids should be used only for severe systemic disease and chronic iridocyclitis unresponsive to topical therapy.

Local treatment aims to prevent stiffness and deformity. Night splints are useful for the wrists, hands, knees and ankles; prone lying for some period each day may prevent flexion contracture of the hips. Between periods of splinting, active exercises are encouraged.

Fixed deformities may need correction by serial plasters; when progress is no longer being made, joint capsulotomy may help.

For painful, eroded joints operation is indicated. Useful procedures include custom-designed arthroplasties of the hip and knee (even in children), and arthrodesis of the wrist or ankle.

CHRONIC ARTHRITIS

Rheumatoid arthritis
Many joints, often symmetrical
Proximal finger joints
Subcutaneous nodules
Erosive arthritis

Reactive arthritis (Reiter's disease)
Several large joints
Spondylitis
Urethritis, colitis, conjunctivitis

Osteoarthritis
Few joints, asymmetrical
Distal finger joints
Hypertrophic arthritis

The systemic connective tissue diseases

'Systemic connective tissue disease' is a collective term for a group of closely related conditions that have features which overlap with those of rheumatoid disease. Like RA, these are 'autoimmune disorders', probably triggered by viral infection in genetically predisposed individuals.

Systemic lupus erythematosus is the best known. It occurs mainly in young females and may be difficult to differentiate from RA. Although joint pain is usual, it is often overshadowed by systemic symptoms such as malaise, anorexia, weight loss and fever. Characteristic clinical features are skin rashes (especially the 'butterfly rash' of the face), Raynaud's phenomenon, peripheral vasculitis, splenomegaly, and disorders of the kidney, heart, lung, eyes and central nervous system. Anaemia, leucopenia and elevation of the ESR are common. Tests for antinuclear factor are always positive.

Corticosteroids are indicated for severe systemic disease and may have to be continued for life. Progressive joint deformity is unusual and the arthritis can almost always be controlled by anti-inflammatory drugs, physiotherapy and intermittent splintage.

A curious complication of systemic lupus is avascular necrosis (usually of the femoral head). This may be due in part to the corticosteroid treatment, but the disease itself seems to predispose to bone ischaemia.

Crystal deposition disorders 4

The crystal deposition disorders are a group of conditions characterized by the presence of crystals in and around the joints, bursae and tendons. Three clinical conditions in particular are associated with this phenomenon: gout, calcium pyrophosphate dihydrate (CPPD) deposition disease and hydroxyapatite deposition. In each of these conditions, crystal deposition has three distinct consequences: (1) it may be inert and asymptomatic; (2) it may induce an acute inflammatory reaction; or (3) it may result in slow destruction of the affected tissues.

Gout

This is a disorder of purine metabolism characterized by hyperuricaemia and recurrent attacks of acute synovitis due to urate crystal deposition. Late changes include cartilage degeneration. It is much more common in men (20:1) and is rarely seen before the menopause in women. Two forms are recognized: (1) *primary* (95 per cent), an inherited disorder with overproduction or underexcretion of uric acid; and (2) *secondary* (5 per cent), resulting from acquired conditions that cause uric acid overproduction (e.g. myeloproliferative disorders) or underexcretion (e.g. renal failure).

Pathology

Crystals of monosodium urate are deposited in and around the joint and appear in synovial fluid. They excite attacks of acute inflammation. In chronic gout urate deposits produce tophi in bursae, tendons, cartilage and periarticular bone. Joint surfaces may be damaged, leading to degenerative arthritis. Urate calculi appear in the urine, and crystal deposition in the kidney parenchyma may cause renal failure.

Clinical features

Patients are usually men over the age of 30 years. Often there is a family history of gout.

The acute attack The sudden onset of severe joint pain which lasts for a week or two is typical of acute gout. This is usually spontaneous but may be precipitated by minor trauma, operation, unaccustomed exercise or alcohol. The commonest sites are the metatarsophalangeal joint of the big toe, the ankle and finger joints, and the olecranon bursa. The skin looks red and shiny and there is considerable swelling. The joint feels hot and extremely tender, suggesting a cellulitis or septic arthritis. Sometimes the only feature is acute pain and tenderness in the heel or the sole of the foot.

Hyperuricaemia is present at some stage, although not necessarily during an acute attack. The diagnosis can be established beyond doubt by finding the characteristic birefringent crystals in the synovial fluid.

Chronic gout Recurrent acute attacks may eventually merge into polyarticular gout. Tophi may appear around joints, over the

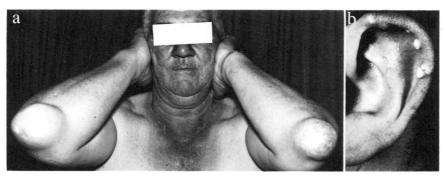

4.1 Gout This man with chronic gout declares his diagnosis at a glance, (a) with his rubicund face, bulging olecranon bursae, and (b) tophi.

olecranon and in the pinna of the ear. A large tophus can ulcerate and discharge its chalky material. Joint erosion causes chronic pain, stiffness and deformity. Renal lesions include calculi and parenchymal disease.

X-rays

During the acute attack x-rays show only soft-tissue swelling. Chronic gout may show asymmetrical, punched-out 'cysts' in the periarticular bone, joint space narrowing and secondary osteoarthritis.

Differential diagnosis

Infection Cellulitis, septic bursitis, an infected bunion or septic arthritis must all be excluded, if necessary by immediate joint aspiration.

Rheumatoid arthritis Polyarticular gout affecting the fingers may be mistaken for rheumatoid arthritis, and elbow tophi for rheumatoid nodules. In difficult cases biopsy will establish the diagnosis.

Treatment

The acute attack should be treated by resting the joint and giving indomethacin, diclofenac or naproxen in large doses.

Between attacks, attention should be given to simple measures such as losing weight,

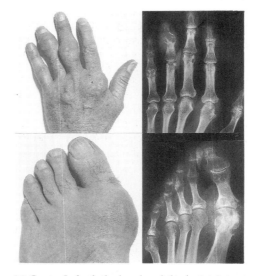

4.2 Gout In both the hand and the foot, joints are asymmetrically swollen; x-rays show large periarticular excavations, which are filled with uric acid deposits.

cutting out alcohol and eliminating diuretics. Interval therapy is indicated if attacks recur at frequent intervals, if there are tophi or if renal function is impaired. Asymptomatic hyperuricaemia does not call for treatment. Uricosuric drugs (probenecid or sulphinpyrazone) can be used if renal function is normal. Allopurinol, a xanthine oxidase inhibitor, is usually preferred. *These drugs*

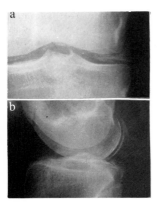
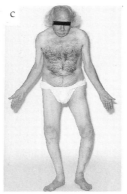
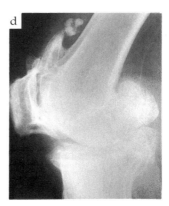

4.3 Pyrophosphate arthropathy   (a, b) Chondrocalcinosis, with calcification of menisci and deposition of crystals in the articular cartilage. (c) This middle-aged man presented with osteoarthritis in several large joints, including the elbow and ankle where osteoarthritis is uncommon; note also (d) the large trailing osteophytes in the patellofemoral joint.

should never be started during an acute attack, and they should always be covered by an anti-inflammatory preparation or colchicine, otherwise they may actually precipitate an acute attack.

GOUT AND PSEUDOGOUT

Gout
Smaller joints
Intense pain
Inflammation
Hyperuricaemia
Uric acid crystals

Pseudogout
Large joints
Moderate pain
Swelling
Chondrocalcinosis
Calcium pyrophosphate crystals

Calcium pyrophosphate arthropathy (pseudogout; chondrocalcinosis)

Chondrocalcinosis   The deposition of calcium pyrophosphate dihydrate (CPPD) crystals in

cartilage – is common, especially in the elderly. It is usually regarded as evidence of cartilage ageing or degeneration; occasionally, however, it is associated with a metabolic disorder (e.g. hyperparathyroidism or haemochromatosis).

Pseudogout   Although chondrocalcinosis is usually asymptomatic, the patient may present with an acute non-septic synovitis resembling gout. The knee is the usual site but other large joints can be involved. X-ray may show calcification of articular cartilage or menisci. Diagnosis is confirmed by finding the characteristic positively birefringent crystals in the synovial fluid.

Chronic pyrophosphate arthropathy   Older patients sometimes present with polyarticular osteoarthritis. In these cases it is difficult to tell whether the CPPD deposition has caused the arthritis or merely aggravated an underlying degenerative condition.

Treatment

The treatment of pseudogout is similar to that of classic gout: rest, non-steroidal anti-inflammatory drugs, joint aspiration and intra-articular injection of corticosteroid. Chronic pyrophosphate arthropathy is treated like osteoarthritis.

Calcium hydroxyapatite (HA) deposition disorders

Minute deposits of hydroxyapatite crystals in periarticular soft tissues may give rise to an acute, painful reaction; this is seen most commonly in the shoulder. Treatment is by non-steroidal anti-inflammatory drugs or by local injection of corticosteroids.

Osteoarthritis and related disorders

5

Osteoarthritis

Osteoarthritis is a degenerative joint disorder in which there is progressive loss of articular cartilage accompanied by new bone formation and capsular fibrosis. It is defined as *primary* when no cause is obvious, and *secondary* when it follows a demonstrable abnormality.

Cause

The most obvious thing about osteoarthritis is that it increases in frequency with age. This does not mean that it is an expression of senescence; it simply shows that osteoarthritis takes

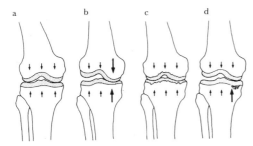

5.1 Osteoarthritis – causal factors In the normal joint (a) the forces are evenly distributed. The remaining diagrams show the three ways in which cartilage may be damaged; (b) deformity increases the stress in a localized area by concentrating the load at this point; (c) cartilage which has been weakened by some preceding disorder is unable to bear even normal loads; (d) if the subarticular bone is abnormal it may be unable to support the cartilage adequately.

many years to develop. To be sure, cartilage ageing does occur, resulting in splitting and flaking of the surface, but these changes are not progressive and they do not cause symptomatic arthritis.

Osteoarthritis results from a disparity between the stress applied to articular cartilage and the ability of the cartilage to withstand that stress. This may be due to an abnormal increase in load over a small area of cartilage (e.g. pressure from a torn piece of meniscus), undue weakening of the cartilage (an ill-understood phenomenon), abnormal support by subchondral bone, or a combination of these. The subsequent sequence of changes is still disputed, but at an early stage there appears to be damage to the collagen meshwork and loss of proteoglycans from the cartilage matrix. Structural damage follows.

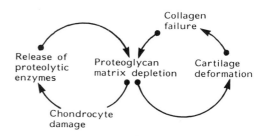

Pathology

The cardinal features are: (1) progressive cartilage destruction; (2) subarticular cyst formation; (3) remodelling of the bone ends

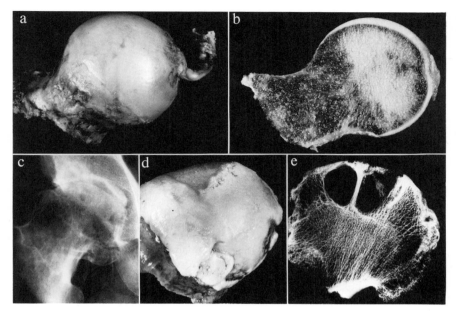

5.2 Osteoarthritis – pathology (a) Normal ageing causes slight degeneration of the articular surface, but the coronal section (b) shows that the cartilage thickness is well preserved even in old age. By contrast, in progressive osteoarthritis (lower row) the weight-bearing area is severely damaged: the x-ray (c) shows cartilage loss at the superior pole and cysts in the underlying bone; the specimen (d) shows that the top of the head was completely denuded of cartilage; and a fine-detail x-ray of the specimen (e) shows that the subchondral bone plate has been perforated.

with osteophyte formation; and (4) capsular fibrosis.

The earliest morphological change is softening of the articular cartilage. The normally smooth and glistening surface becomes frayed, or *fibrillated*, and eventually it is worn away to expose the underlying bone.

The subarticular bone reacts to these changes in two ways. In the area of greatest stress cysts form, around which the trabeculae become thickened or sclerotic. The marrow shows vascular congestion.

As the disease progresses, cartilage in peripheral, unstressed areas proliferates and ossifies, producing bony outgrowths (osteophytes). This remodelling process restores a measure of congruity to the increasingly malopposed joint surfaces.

Capsular fibrosis is common and may account for joint stiffness.

The cause of pain is problematic; articular cartilage and synovium have no nerve supply but the capsule is sensitive to stretching and the bone is sensitive to changes in pressure. Pain, therefore, may be due to both capsular fibrosis and vascular congestion of the subarticular bone.

Clinical features

Patients usually present after middle age, although it is likely that cartilage changes start 10 or even 20 years before that. Sometimes – especially in younger patients – there is a history of some preceding joint disorder or injury.

Pain starts insidiously and increases slowly over months or years. It is aggravated by exertion and relieved by rest, although with time relief is less and less complete.

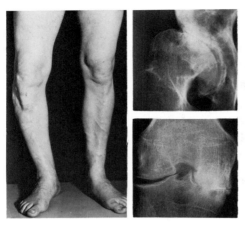

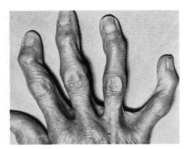

5.4 Heberden's nodes Osteoarthritis of the terminal interphalangeal joints is common. The pain always improves, but the knobbly deformities remain.

5.3 Osteoarthritis – clinical This man had osteoarthritis of the right hip and knee. X-rays show the classical changes: loss of articular space, subchondral sclerosis, bone cysts and osteophytes.

Stiffness, characteristically, is worst after periods of rest. Swelling and deformity are features of advanced disease.

Typically the symptoms of osteoarthritis follow an intermittent course, with periods of remission lasting for months.

In superficial joints swelling and deformity may be obvious; at the hip, deformity is usually masked by postural adjustments of the pelvis and spine. In long-standing cases there is muscle wasting. Local tenderness is common, and in the knee a joint effusion may be demonstrated.

Movement is always restricted and it may be accompanied by crepitus. In the late stages there is progressive instability.

In contrast to inflammatory joint disease, osteoarthritis is unassociated with any systemic manifestations.

X-RAYS The characteristic changes are: (1) narrowing of the joint space; (2) subarticular sclerosis; (3) bone cysts; and (4) osteophytes. Initially the first three features are restricted to the major load-bearing part of the joint, but in late cases the entire joint is affected. Evidence of previous disorders (congenital defects, old fractures, rheumatoid arthritis) may be present.

Nodal osteoarthritis

A nodular arthritis of the distal interphalangeal joints of the fingers (Heberden's nodes) is extremely common in postmenopausal women. Often this is associated with osteoarthritis of the thumb carpometacarpal joint, and sometimes several large joints are involved as well.

TREATMENT OF OA

Conservative
1   Relieve pain
2   Reduce load
3   Improve mobility

Operative
1   Osteotomy
2   Arthrodesis
3   Arthroplasty

Treatment

EARLY There are three principles in the treatment of early osteoarthritis: (1) relieve pain; (2) increase movement; (3) reduce load.

Pain relief is achieved by analgesics and anti-inflammatory agents. Rest periods and modification of activities may be necessary.

Joint mobility can often be improved by physiotherapy; even a small increase in

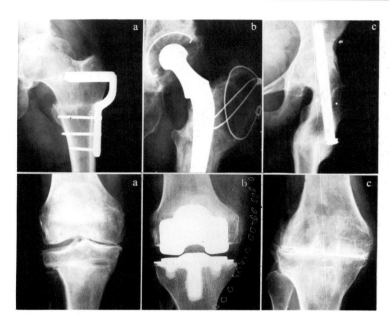

5.5 Operative treatment
The three basic operations: (a) osteotomy, (b) arthroplasty, (c) arthrodesis:

at the hip

at the knee

range and power can reduce pain and improve function.

Load reduction can be achieved by the use of a walking stick, the avoidance of prolonged, stressful activity and by weight reduction.

INTERMEDIATE If symptoms increase despite conservative treatment, *realignment osteotomy* may help. This is particularly applicable to younger patients for whom one wants to avoid an arthroplasty. Pain relief is often dramatic and is ascribed to (1) vascular decompression of the subchondral bone and (2) redistribution of loading forces to less damaged parts of the joint.

LATE The indications for radical surgery are unrelieved pain and progressive disability. For patients over 60, *arthroplasty* is the operation of choice. In younger patients the physical demands are much greater and there is a risk that the arthroplasty might fail after about 10 years.

Arthrodesis is occasionally indicated if stiffness is not a drawback.

Neuropathic arthritis (Charcot's disease)

Neuropathic arthritis is a rapidly progressive degeneration in a joint which lacks position sense and protective pain sensation. In the lower limb it is associated with tabes dorsalis, cauda equina lesions, peripheral neuropathies (especially diabetic) and congenital indifference to pain; in the upper limbs it is usually due to syringomyelia.

Pathology

The joint disorder is a rapidly progressive form of osteoarthritis. There is marked destruction of articular cartilage and the underlying bone, and microscopic spicules of bone become embedded in the synovium. Ligaments and capsule are lax and at the joint periphery there is florid new bone formation.

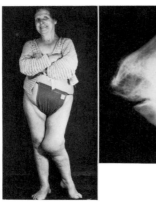
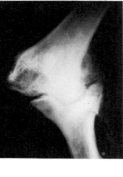

5.6 Charcot's disease The happy expression contrasts sharply with the gross joint destruction. *Moral*: If it's bizarre, do a WR.

Clinical features

The patient complains of instability, swelling and deformity; the symptoms may progress rapidly. The appearance of the joint suggests that movement would be agonizing and yet it is often painless. The paradox is diagnostic.

Swelling and deformity are marked, yet there is no warmth or tenderness. Fluid is greatly increased and bits of bone can be felt everywhere. All movements are increased and the joint is unstable, yet painless.

The underlying neurological disorder should be sought.

X-RAYS The joint may be subluxed or dislocated; gross bone destruction is obvious and there are irregular calcified masses in the capsule.

Treatment

The underlying condition may need treatment, but the affected joints cannot recover. They should, if possible, be stabilized by external splintage (e.g. a caliper). Operation is not advised.

Haemophilic arthropathy

Of the various bleeding disorders, two are associated with recurrent haemarthroses and progressive joint destruction: classic haemophilia, in which there is a deficiency of clotting factor VIII; and Christmas disease, due to deficiency of factor IX. These are rare X-linked recessive disorders manifesting in males but carried by females.

When plasma-clotting factor levels fall below 40 per cent, there is a risk of prolonged bleeding after injury or operation; with levels below 5 per cent, spontaneous bleeding occurs.

ACUTE BLEEDING INTO A JOINT With trivial injury a joint may rapidly fill with blood. Pain, warmth, boggy swelling, tenderness and limited movement are the

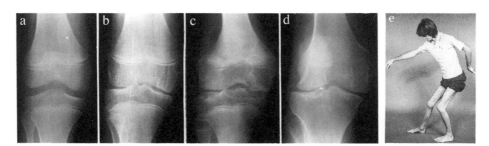

5.7 Haemophilic arthritis   (a) At first there is blood in the joint but the surfaces are intact; (b) later the cartilage is attacked and the joint 'space' narrows; (c) bony erosions appear and eventually the joint becomes deformed and unstable (d). The patient may be disabled by joint contractures (e).

outstanding features. The resemblance to inflammatory arthritis is striking but the history is diagnostic.

The appropriate purified clotting factor must be given intravenously. If this is not available, cryoprecipitate or fresh-frozen plasma will do. Aspiration is avoided unless distension is severe or there is a strong suspicion of infection. A removable splint provides comfort, but once the acute episode has passed movement is encouraged.

ACUTE BLEEDING INTO MUSCLES A painful swelling appears in the arm or leg. There is a danger of a compartment syndrome and Volkmann's ischaemia, but decompression is unwise and ineffectual. The treatment is splintage and early factor replacement, followed by physiotherapy. Later, operation may be needed to correct any resulting joint deformity.

JOINT DEGENERATION This, the sequel to repeated bleeding, usually begins before the age of 15. Chronic synovitis is followed by cartilage degeneration. An affected joint shows wasting and fixed deformity not unlike a tuberculous or rheumatoid joint. X-rays show periarticular osteoporosis and progressive joint erosion.

Treatment

Progressive degeneration is preventable by controlling bleeds, encouraging movement and counteracting joint deformity. Operative treatment (including joint replacement) is feasible but must be covered by factor replacement. It is important to screen patients for hepatitis B virus and HIV antibodies, as their presence demands special precautions during operation.

Osteonecrosis and osteochondritis

Osteonecrosis – bone death – is due either to impaired blood supply or to severe marrow and bone cell damage. *Osteochondritis* is a poorly defined condition in which bone damage and necrosis follow trauma or repetitive stress.

Ischaemic necrosis (avascular necrosis)

Circumscribed bone necrosis occurs in a variety of conditions: Perthes' disease, certain fractures, epiphyseal infection, sickle-cell disease, caisson disease, Gaucher's

---

CAUSES OF BONE NECROSIS

Interruption of arterial supply
Fracture
Dislocation
Infection

Arteriolar occlusion
Sickle-cell disease
Vasculitis
Caisson disease

Capillary compression
Gaucher's disease
Fatty infiltration due to corticosteroids or alcohol abuse

---

disease, alcohol abuse and high-dosage corticosteroid administration. Sites most susceptible are the femoral head, femoral condyles, head of humerus, capitulum, scaphoid, lunate and talus.

Bone ischaemia results from (a) interruption of the arterial inflow (e.g. by trauma to the main vessels or by blockage of the arterioles), or (b) slowing of the venous outflow leading to inadequate perfusion (e.g. by infiltrative lesions that compress the marrow sinusoids).

Pathology

Dead bone is structurally and radiographically indistinguishable from live bone. However, lacking a blood supply, it does not undergo renewal, and after a limited period of repetitive stress it collapses. The changes develop in four overlapping stages.

Stage 1: bone death without structural change Within 24 hours after infarction there is marrow necrosis and cell death. However, for weeks or even months the bone may show no alteration in macroscopic appearance.

Stage 2: repair and early structural failure Some days or weeks after infarction the surrounding, living bone shows a vascular reaction; new bone is laid down upon the dead trabeculae and the increase in bone mass shows on the x-ray as exaggerated density. Despite this active repair, small fractures begin to appear in the dead bone.

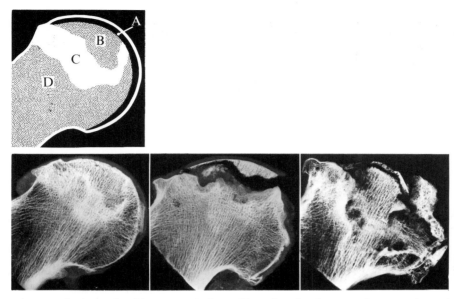

6.1 Avascular necrosis of bone – pathology These fine-detail x-rays of necrotic femoral heads show the progress of osteonecrosis. The articular cartilage (A) remains intact for a long time. The necrotic segment (B) has a texture similar to that of normal bone, but it may develop fine cracks. New bone surrounds the dead trabeculae and causes marked sclerosis (C). Beyond this the bone remains unchanged (D). In the later stages the necrotic bone breaks up and finally the joint surface is destroyed.

Stage 3: major structural failure The necrotic portion starts to crumble and the bone outline becomes distorted.

Stage 4: articular destruction Cartilage, being nourished mainly by synovial fluid, is preserved even in advanced osteonecrosis. However, severe distortion of the surface eventually leads to cartilage breakdown.

Clinical features

By the time the patient presents, the lesion is often well advanced. Pain is the usual complaint; it is felt near a joint and is accompanied by stiffness. Local tenderness may be present and the nearby joint may be swollen. Movements are usually restricted.

IMAGING The earliest changes are seen on MRI. They are due to marrow ischaemia and oedema.

The distinctive x-ray feature of avascular necrosis is increased bone density due to reactive new bone formation in the surrounding living tissue. It appears months or even years after the infarction. Other changes are subarticular fracturing and bone deformation. Radionuclide scanning may show diminished activity in the avascular segment; more often one sees increased activity – due to the vascular reaction in the surrounding bone.

Treatment

If possible, the cause should be eliminated. In stages 1 and 2, bone collapse can sometimes be prevented by a combination of weight-relief, splintage and (in those cases associated with venous stasis and marrow oedema) surgical decompression of the bone. Once bone collapse has occurred (stage 3), a

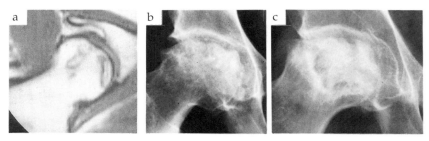

6.2 Avascular necrosis – x-rays   (a) The earliest changes are seen in the MRI. (b,c) Though details may differ, the majority of features are constant: increased bone density and distortion of bone architecture, but an intact joint space.

re-alignment osteotomy, by transferring stress to an undamaged area, may relieve pain and prevent further bone distortion. In stage 4 the treatment is the same as for osteoarthritis. This protocol refers to the lower limb; in the upper limb, often no treatment is needed.

Specific types of avascular necrosis

Post-traumatic

A fracture or dislocation may interrupt the local blood supply. Although bone death is immediate, the diagnosis is usually made only when the x-ray shows increased density in the surrounding bone. The most common sites are (1) the femoral head, (2) the carpal bones and (3) the talus.

TREATMENT   The patient may require no treatment; however, if pain and disability are severe the avascular portion may be replaced or removed, or the adjacent joint may be fused.

Sickle-cell disease

This is a genetic disorder, limited to people of Central and West African Negro descent. Red cells containing abnormal haemoglobin

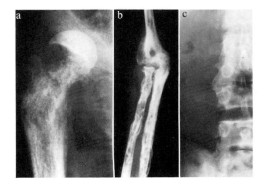

6.3 Sickle-cell disease   (a) Typical changes in the femur due to marrow hyperplasia, with bone infarction and necrosis of the femoral head. (b) Infarctions of tubular bones may resemble osteomyelitis, with sequestra and a marked periosteal reaction (sometimes a true salmonella infection supervenes). (c) The spine also may be involved.

(HbS) become distorted and sickle-shaped; this is especially likely to occur with hypoxia (e.g. under anaesthesia or in extreme cold). Clumping of the sickle-shaped cells causes diminished capillary flow and repeated episodes of pain ('bone crises') or, if more severe, ischaemic necrosis. Almost any bone may be involved and there is a tendency for the infarcts to become infected, sometimes with unusual organisms such as *Salmonella*.

On x-ray the tubular bones (including the phalanges) may show irregular endosteal destruction and medullary sclerosis, together with periosteal new bone formation. Not only does this resemble osteitis, but also true infection is often superimposed on the infarct. In children, femoral head necrosis could be mistaken for Perthes' disease.

Treatment Acute episodes are treated by rest and analgesics, followed by physiotherapy to minimize stiffness. Established necrosis is treated according to the principles on page 43, but with the emphasis on conservatism. Anaesthesia carries serious risks and may even precipitate vascular occlusion in the central nervous system, lungs or kidneys; moreover, the chances of postoperative infection are high.

Caisson disease

Decompression sickness (caisson disease) and osteonecrosis are important causes of disability in deep-sea divers and compressed-air workers building tunnels or underwater structures. Under increased air pressure the blood and other tissues (especially fat) become supersaturated with nitrogen; if decompression is too rapid the gas is released as bubbles, which cause local tissue damage and generalized embolic phenomena. The symptoms of decompression sickness are pain near the joints ('the bends'), breathing difficulty and vertigo ('the staggers'). In the most acute cases there can be circulatory and respiratory collapse, severe neurological changes, coma and death. Bone necrosis may be due to capillary obstruction by gas bubbles and changes in marrow fat.

The patient complains of pain and loss of joint movement, but many lesions remain silent and are found only on routine x-ray examination.

Management The aim is prevention; the incidence of osteonecrosis is proportional to the working pressure, the length of exposure, the rate of decompression and the number of exposures. Strict enforcement of suitable working schedules has reduced the risks considerably. The treatment of established lesions follows the principles already outlined.

Gaucher's disease

This familial disease occurs predominantly in Ashkenazi Jews. Deficiency of the specific enzyme causes an abnormal accumulation of glucocerebroside in the reticuloendothelial system. The effects are seen chiefly in the liver, spleen and bone marrow, where the large, polyhedral 'Gaucher cells' accumulate;

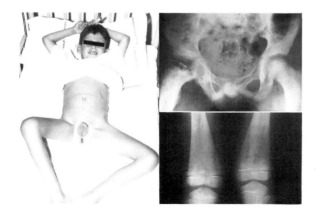

6.4 Gaucher's disease This young boy, whose sister also had Gaucher's disease, developed pain in the right hip; abduction was limited and painful. X-rays show necrosis of the right femoral head and widening of the femoral shafts (the Erlenmeyer flask appearance).

their pressure on the bone sinusoids may be the cause of the bone necrosis.

Bone changes may occur at any age; the femoral head is the most common site. There is a tendency for the Gaucher deposits to become infected and the patient may present with septicaemia. A diagnostic, though inconstant, finding is a raised serum acid phosphatase level.

X-ray A special feature (due to replacement of myeloid tissue by Gaucher cells) is expansion of the tubular bones, especially the distal femur, producing a flask-like appearance. Osteonecrosis of the femoral head is common.

Treatment The general disorder can now be treated by enzyme replacement. Management of the osteonecrosis follows the principles outlined on page 43. If joint replacement is contemplated, antibiotic cover is essential.

Drug-induced necrosis

Corticosteroids in high dosage may give rise to 'spontaneous' osteonecrosis; thus the condition is fairly common in renal transplant patients on immunosuppressive corticosteroids. Alcohol abuse is another potent cause. Both conditions result in widespread fatty changes and marrow infarction, which may be the cause of the bone necrosis.

The sites usually affected are the femoral head, femoral condyles and the head of the humerus.

Pain may be present for many months before x-rays show any abnormality; the earliest signs are a small subarticular fracture and increased bone density. In the late stage there is bone collapse.

Treatment Early on the condition is potentially reversible if the cortisone or alcohol is stopped. Analgesics, weight-relief and physiotherapy are often all that is required. Decompression of the affected bone by drilling may prevent progressive changes. If the joint surface has collapsed, reconstructive surgery is required.

Osteochondritis (osteochondrosis)

The term 'osteochondritis' is applied to a group of conditions in which there is compression, fragmentation or separation of a small segment of bone, usually at the bone end and involving the attached articular surface. The affected portion of bone shows many of the features of ischaemic necrosis, including increased vascularity and reactive sclerosis in the surrounding bone. These conditions occur in children and adolescents, often during phases of rapid growth and increased physical activity. Segmental ischaemia may be caused by trauma or repetitive stress.

Three types of osteochondritis are identified: 'crushing', 'splitting' and 'pulling'.

TYPES OF OSTEOCHONDRITIS

Crushing
Metatarsal head (Freiberg)
Tarsal navicular (Köhler)
Lunate (Kienböck)
Capitulum (Panner)

Splitting (dissecans)
Femoral condyle
Talus
Capitulum

Pulling
Tibial tuberosity (Osgood–Schlatter)
Calcaneum (Sever)

Crushing osteochondritis

This is seen mainly in adolescence. The characteristic feature is an apparently spontaneous necrosis of the ossific nucleus in a long-bone epiphysis or one of the cuboidal bones of the wrist or foot.

Pain and limitation of joint movement are the usual complaints. Tenderness is sharply localized. X-rays show increased density,

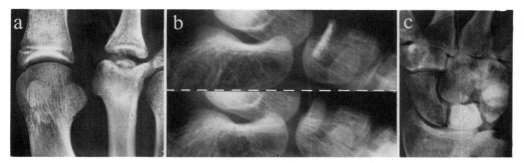

6.5 Crushing osteochondritis (a) Freiberg's disease of the second metatarsal; (b) Köhler's disease of the navicular, compared with the normal side below; (c) Kienböck's disease of the lunate.

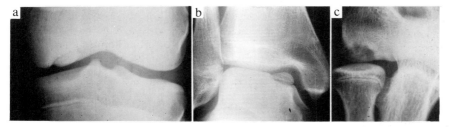

6.6 Splitting osteochondritis The osteochondral fragment usually remains in place at the articular surface. The most common sites are (a) the medial femoral condyle, (b) the talus and (c) the capitulum.

accompanied in the later stages by collapse of the necrotic segment.

The common examples of crushing osteochondritis have, by long tradition, acquired eponymous labels: Freiberg's disease of a metatarsal head; Köhler's disease of the navicular; Kienböck's disease of the carpal lunate; and Panner's disease of the capitulum.

Treatment is usually conservative: analgesics and splintage until the symptoms settle down.

Splitting osteochondritis (dissecans)

A small segment of articular cartilage and the subjacent bone may separate (dissect) as an avascular fragment. The cause is almost certainly repeated minor trauma producing an osteochondral fracture of a convex joint surface.

The condition occurs mainly in young adults, usually male. The knee is much the most common joint to be affected. The patient presents with intermittent pain, swelling and joint effusion. If the necrotic fragment becomes completely detached, it may cause locking or giving way.

X-rays need to show the affected articular surface in tangential projection. The dissecting fragment is defined by a radiolucent line of demarcation. When it separates, the resulting 'crater' may be obvious. So might the loose body in the joint!

If the fragment is in position, treatment consists of weight-relief and restriction of activity. In children complete healing may occur, although it takes up to 2 years. If the fragment becomes detached and causes symptoms, it should be fixed back in position or else completely removed.

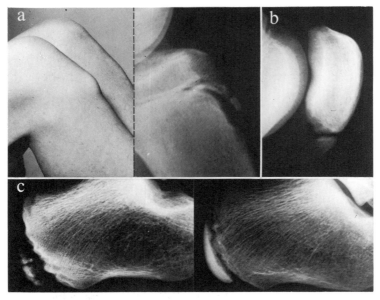

6.7 Pulling osteochondritis   These are merely traction lesions but dignified by eponyms: (a) Osgood–Schlatter's disease involves the apophysis into which the extensor mechanism is inserted; (b) in Johansson–Larsen's disease the calcification is a sequel to the patellar ligament partially pulling away from the bone; (c) Sever's disease, compared with the normal side.

Pulling osteochondritis (traction apophysitis)

Excessive pull by a large tendon may damage the unfused apophysis to which it is attached; this occurs typically at two sites – the tibial tuberosity (Osgood–Schlatter's disease) and the calcaneal apophysis (Sever's disease). The traumatized apophysis becomes painful and tender. With rest the symptoms invariably settle down.

Metabolic and endocrine disorders 7

We think of bones chiefly as forming an articulating framework for the muscles and other soft tissues. And for this purpose their structure is ideal. However, bone as tissue has a more important function: it is a mineral reservoir that helps to regulate the calcium ion concentration of the extracellular fluid and keep it within the limits that are crucial for life. For all its solidity, its microscopic structure is constantly changing in response to alterations in mineral ion concentrations. The metabolic bone disorders are conditions in which generalized skeletal abnormalities result from disruption of this system.

Bone remodelling and ageing

Bone consists of a largely collagenous matrix which is impregnated with mineral salts and populated by cells – osteoclasts (concerned with bone resorption), osteoblasts (for bone formation) and osteocytes (resting bone cells). Alternating resorption and formation proceed throughout life – a process known as remodelling.

During growth the bone increases in size and changes in shape. At the epiphyseal growth plate (physis) new bone is added by endochondral ossification; on the surface, bone is added by subperiosteal appositional ossification; the medullary cavity is expanded by endosteal resorption; bulbous bone ends

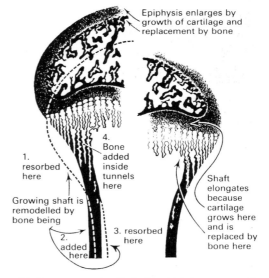

7.1 Bone growth Endochondral bone growth and remodelling. (Reproduced from *Journal of Bone and Joint Surgery* (1952), **34A**, 711 by permission.)

are re-formed and sculpted continuously. *Between 20 and 40 years* of age the haversian canals and intertrabecular spaces are to some extent filled in and the cortices increase in overall thickness; i.e., the bones become heavier and stronger. *From 40 years onwards* there is a slow but steady loss of bone; haversian spaces enlarge, trabeculae become thinner, the endosteal surface is resorbed and the medullary space expands – i.e., year by year the bones become more porous.

Regulation of bone and mineral exchange

Most of the body's calcium and phosphate is tightly packed in bone and can be released only by resorption of the entire tissue – a slow process. The rapidly exchangeable component is in the extracellular fluid where its concentration depends mainly on intestinal absorption and renal excretion; transient alterations in serum levels are accommodated quickly by changes in renal tubular reabsorption.

The control of calcium is much more critical than that of phosphate; thus, in persistent calcium deficiency the extracellular calcium ion concentration is maintained by drawing on bone, whereas phosphate deficiency simply leads to lowered serum phosphate concentration. The regulation of calcium exchange is therefore linked inescapably to that of bone formation and resorption. The complex balance between calcium exchange and bone remodelling is controlled by vitamin D, parathyroid hormone and calcitonin.

Vitamin D

Natural vitamin D_3 (cholecalciferol) is derived either directly from the diet or indirectly by the action of ultraviolet light on precursors in the skin. Vitamin D itself is inactive. Conversion to active metabolites takes place first in the liver to form 25-hydroxycholecalciferol (25-HCC), and then in the kidney to give 1,25-dihydroxycholecalciferol (1,25-DHCC).

The terminal metabolite – and, to a lesser extent, the liver metabolite – stimulates the uptake of calcium by the small intestine and this indirectly promotes mineralization of new-formed bone. At the mineralization front it is also concerned with calcium transport.

The production of 1,25-DHCC is controlled by parathyroid hormone (PTH) and by the serum phosphate concentration: a rise in PTH or a fall in phosphate increases 1,25-DHCC synthesis. (A fall in serum

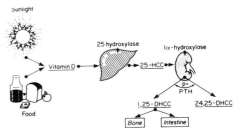

7.2 Vitamin D metabolism Cholecalciferol is derived either from the diet or by conversion of precursors when the skin is exposed to sunlight. This inactive 'vitamin' is hydroxylated, first in the liver and then in the kidney, to form the active metabolite 1,25-dihydroxycholecalciferol.

calcium does the same indirectly, by stimulating PTH production.)

Parathyroid hormone

Parathyroid hormone (PTH) is the fine regulator of calcium exchange: its function is to maintain the extracellular calcium concentration between very narrow limits; production and release are stimulated by a fall and suppressed by a rise in plasma ionized calcium.

The target organs for PTH are kidney and bone. It promotes phosphate excretion by restricting tubular reabsorption and it conserves calcium by increasing its reabsorption. It also stimulates osteoclastic bone resorption, again resulting in a rise in serum calcium.

Calcitonin

Calcitonin, which is secreted by the C cells of the thyroid, does the very opposite of PTH: it suppresses bone resorption and increases renal calcium excretion.

The homoeostatic loop

Under normal circumstances the interaction of these substances ensures calcium

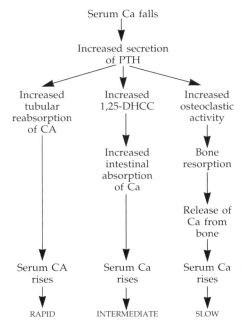

Serum Ca falls

↓

Increased secretion
of PTH

Increased
tubular
reabsorption
of CA

Increased
1,25-DHCC

Increased
osteoclastic
activity

↓

Increased
intestinal
absorption
of Ca

Bone
resorption

↓

Release of
Ca from
bone

↓

Serum CA
rises

Serum Ca
rises

Serum Ca
rises

↓

RAPID INTERMEDIATE SLOW

7.3 Homoeostatic loop Effect of a fall in serum calcium.

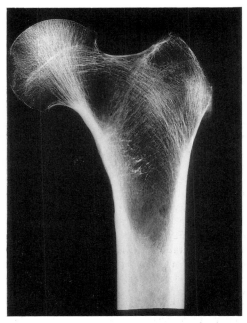

7.4 Wolff's law The elegant trabecular pattern of the upper femur shows how well the anatomical structure conforms to the imposed forces; the thickest trabeculae lie in the lines of the greatest stress.

homoeostasis. If there is a fall in serum calcium, the cascade shown in Figure 7.3 is deployed.

Mechanical stress

It is well known that the direction and thickness of trabeculae in cancellous bone are related to stress trajectories. This is recognized in Wolff's law [1896], which says that the architecture and mass of the skeleton are adjusted to withstand the prevailing forces. Physiological stress is supplied by gravity, loadbearing, muscle action and vascular pulsation. If a bending force is applied, more bone will form on the concave surfaces (where there is compression) and bone will thin down on the convex surfaces (which are under tension). Weightlessness, prolonged bed rest, lack of exercise, muscular weakness and limb immobilization are all associated with osteoporosis.

Rickets

In rickets there is inadequate mineralization of growing bone. This is usually due to a lack of vitamin D or its active metabolites, but it may also be caused by severe calcium deficiency or by hypophosphataemia.

Pathology

The organic matrix of bone (osteoid) is adequately produced but it is incompletely mineralized. In children this is seen mainly at the growth plates where the new juxta-epiphyseal trabeculae are ill-formed and 'softened'.

Clinical features

The infant with rickets may present with tetany or convulsions. The child fails to

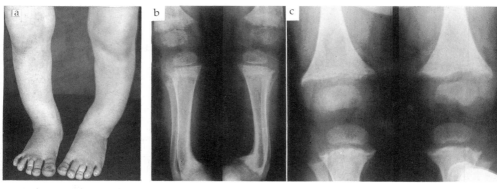

7.5 Rickets   (a) Rickety deformity of the legs; (b, c) x-rays showing overgrowth of the physes and metaphyseal deformity.

thrive and is listless and flaccid. Early bone changes are deformity of the skull (craniotabes), and thickening of the knees, ankles and wrists from physeal overgrowth. Enlargement of the costochondral junctions ('rickety rosary') and lateral indentation of the chest (Harrison's sulcus) may also occur. Once the child stands, lower limb deformities increase; in severe rickets the long bones may fracture.

X-RAYS   The characteristic x-ray change is an increase in depth and width of the physes; the adjacent metaphyses have a 'cupped' appearance. Sometimes the long bones are bowed.

INVESTIGATIONS   Changes common to all types of rickets are diminished serum calcium and increased alkaline phosphatase levels; urinary calcium is also low. Other findings vary according to the type of rickets.

Varieties of rickets

Vitamin D deficiency

Vitamin D deficiency may be due to dietary lack, underexposure to sunlight or both. Affected children are usually between 1 and

2 years old.   Although at one time the common form of rickets, this is not often seen today.

Treatment   There is invariably a rapid response to small doses of calciferol (2000 i.u. a day for 3–6 weeks), and residual deformity is slight.

Familial hypophosphataemia (vitamin D-resistant rickets)

This is the most common type of rickets seen today. It is a genetic disorder starting in infancy and causing diminished growth and severe bony deformity. X-rays show marked epiphyseal changes. Treatment is by large doses of vitamin D (50 000 i.u. or more) and up to 4 g of inorganic phosphate per day (with careful monitoring to prevent overdosage), continued until growth ceases. Bony deformities may require bracing or osteotomy.

Renal tubular rickets

Impaired renal tubular reabsorption of phosphate results in hypophosphataemia; calcium levels are only slightly diminished but there is defective bone mineralization.

Renal glomerular osteodystrophy

In patients with chronic renal disease there may be phosphate retention and a fall in serum calcium which is due partly to the hyperphosphataemia and partly to 1,25-DHCC deficiency. The skeletal changes are due to a combination of severe rickets (or osteomalacia) and secondary hyperparathyroidism; there may also be osteosclerosis and soft-tissue calcification. Biochemical features are low serum calcium, high serum phosphate and elevated alkaline phosphatase levels.

The renal failure, if irreversible, may require haemodialysis or renal transplantation. The osteodystrophy should be treated with large doses of vitamin D (up to 500 000 i.u. daily); in resistant cases, small doses of 1,25-DHCC may be effective.

Osteomalacia

Osteomalacia is the adult counterpart of rickets and may be due to defects anywhere along the metabolic pathway for vitamin D: nutritional lack, underexposure to sunlight, intestinal malabsorption, and defective conversion in the liver or kidney.

Pathology

New bone throughout the skeleton is incompletely calcified so that wide 'seams' of osteoid build up on the older trabeculae and around haversian canals. The weakened bone breaks easily and there may be widespread evidence of poorly healed fractures.

Clinical features

Symptoms usually appear insidiously and are rather vague. Bone pain, backache and muscle weakness may be present for years before the diagnosis is made. Unexplained pain in the hip or one of the long bones may presage a stress fracture. Often the condition

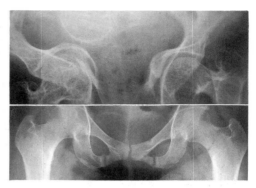

7.6 Osteomalacia Two characteristic features of osteomalacia: above, indentation of the pelvic walls producing the 'trefoil pelvis'; below, Looser's zones in the pubic rami and left femoral neck.

is suspected only when the patient is admitted to hospital with vertebral compression or a long-bone fracture.

X-rays show generalized rarefaction of bone and signs of previous fractures of the vertebrae, ribs, pubic rami or long bones. Almost pathognomic is the Looser zone, a thin transverse band of rarefaction due to a poorly healing stress fracture. There may also be signs of secondary hyperparathyroidism.

Diagnosis

Biochemical changes are often insignificant and biopsy may be needed for diagnosis; excessive amounts of unmineralized osteoid can be demonstrated.

Having made the diagnosis, it is still necessary to establish the type of osteomalacia. Patients should be investigated for malabsorption syndromes, liver disorders and renal disease (which could block conversion to 1,25-DHCC).

Treatment

Osteomalacia due to marked nutritional lack of vitamin D is quickly reversed by an adequate diet and supplements of calciferol and calcium.

Underlying disorders of the gut, liver or kidney will need treatment in their own right.

Hyperparathyroidism

Excessive secretion of parathyroid hormone (PTH) may be primary (usually due to an adenoma) or secondary (due to persistent hypocalcaemia).

The cardinal feature of hyperparathyroidism is a rise in serum calcium: the overproduction of PTH stimulates renal tubular reabsorption of calcium as well as increased bone resorption. The resulting hypercalcaemia increases glomerular filtration of calcium so much that there is hypercalciuria despite the augmented tubular reabsorption. Urinary phosphate also is increased, due to suppressed tubular reabsorption.

The main effects of these changes are seen in the kidney: calcinosis, stone formation, recurrent infection and impaired function.

There may also be calcification of soft tissues.

There is a general loss of bone substance. In more severe cases, osteoclastic hyperactivity produces subperiosteal erosions, endosteal cavitation and replacement of the marrow spaces by vascular granulations and fibrous tissue ('osteitis fibrosa cystica'). Haemorrhage and giant-cell reaction within the fibrous stroma may give rise to brownish, tumour-like masses, whose liquefaction leads to fluid-filled cysts ('brown tumours').

Clinical features

The most common features are due to the hypercalcaemia: anorexia, nausea and depression, abdominal pain, polyuria and recurrent kidney stones.* Bone rarefaction may cause pain, pathological fracture and deformity. Curiously, patients with marked bone disease seldom have renal stones, and vice versa.

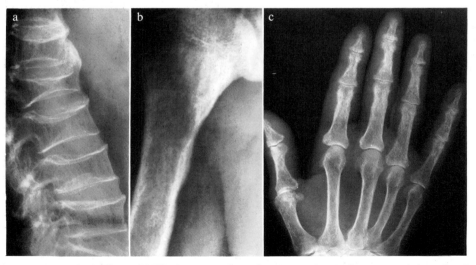

7.7 Hyperparathyroidisr.   (a) This hyperparathyroid patient with spinal osteoporosis later developed pain in the right arm; an x-ray (b) showed cortical erosion of the humerus; he also showed (c) typical erosions of the phalanges.

*Bones, stones, moans and groans.

X-RAYS Generalized osteoporosis is usual but non-specific. The diagnostic sign, when it is present, is subperiosteal bone resorption.

INVESTIGATIONS Hypercalcaemia is common and serum PTH levels may be elevated.

Treatment

Removal of the adenoma or hyperplastic parathyroid tissue is usually indicated. Postoperatively there is a danger of severe hypocalcaemia due to brisk new bone formation (the 'hungry bone syndrome'). This must be treated promptly, with one of the vitamin D metabolites.

Scurvy (vitamin C deficiency)

Vitamin C (ascorbic acid) deficiency causes failure of collagen synthesis and osteoid formation. The result is osteoporosis, which in infants is most marked in the juxtaepiphyseal bone. Spontaneous bleeding is common and may cause subperiosteal haematomas.

The patient is usually an infant. Pain due to subperiosteal haemorrhage may be so intense that the child refuses to move the limb ('pseudoparalysis'). There is swelling and tenderness near the large joints. The gums may be spongy and bleeding.

X-rays show generalized bone rarefaction. The metaphyses may be deformed or fractured. Subperiosteal haematomas show as soft-tissue swellings or periosseous calcification.

Treatment with large doses of vitamin C results in prompt recovery.

Osteoporosis

In osteoporosis the bone is qualitatively normal but there is less of it than would be expected in a person of that age and sex. The bone cortex is thinner than normal and

trabeculae are sparse. Not surprisingly, the bone is also weaker than normal and it fractures relatively easily.

Localized osteoporosis is usually due to disuse (including paralysis) or nearby inflammation.

Generalized osteoporosis may be physiological (age-related), but it is also a feature of many systemic disorders and its precise elucidation can be profoundly difficult.

Age related osteoporosis

Bone mass decreases slowly but steadily from the age of 40 years. Around the menopause this process is accelerated. This is due to oestrogen withdrawal and the same changes occur in younger women after oöphorectomy.

With advancing age there is a further loss of bone; this is a type of involutional change and it affects both men and women over 70

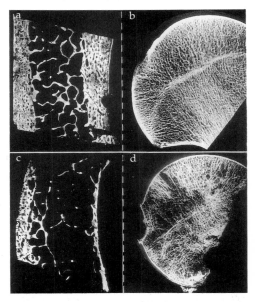

7.8 Osteoporosis Fine-detail x-rays of iliac crest biopsies and femoral head slices, showing the contrast between trabecular density at the age of 40 (a, b) and aged 70 (c, d). No wonder old bones break easily.

years. Furthermore at that age other factors (diminished activity, chronic illness, dietary lack) also take their toll and the bones become lighter and weaker. However, it is only when skeletal failure, or fracture, occurs that osteoporosis presents as a clinical problem – and old people are apt to fall.

Clinical features

Postmenopausal osteoporosis. Women between 55 and 65 may present with acute back pain due to vertebral compression; with repeated minor fractures they develop progressive kyphosis. If they fall they are liable to sustain a Colles' fracture.

Involutional osteoporosis. Over the age of 70 patients (women and men) are more likely to be seen with a fracture of the femoral neck.

Those most at risk of developing severe osteoporosis are women, whites (much more than coloured peoples) and thin individuals (rather than fat or muscular people). Other risk factors are smoking, alcohol and dietary fads.

X-RAYS   show the general reduction in bone density, biconcavity or wedging of one or morevertebrae and perhaps a recent fracture of a long bone.

BIOCHEMICAL TESTS   are normal.

Diagnosis

The diagnosis is usually obvious. What is more difficult is to exclude the many specific causes of osteoporosis.

Many elderly patients with 'osteoporotic' fractures also have osteomalacia. If there are suspicious features (multiple fractures, looser zones, pencil-thin cortices, increased alkaline phosphatase), an iliac crest biopsy is justified.

Patients under 45 need full investigation, including biopsy. An important cause in the fifth decade is multiple myeloma.

SOME CAUSES OF OSTEOPOROSIS

Nutritional	*Malignant*
Scurvy	*disease*
Malnutrition	Carcinomatosis
Malabsorption	Multiple
	myeloma
	Leukaemia
Endocrine disorders	*Inflammatory*
Hyperparathyroidism	*disorders*
Gonadal	Rheumatoid
insufficiency	arthritis
Cushing's	Ankylosing
disease	spondylitis
Thyrotoxicosis	Tuberculosis
Drug-induced	*Miscellaneous*
Corticosteroids	Juvenile
Alcohol	osteoporosis
Heparin	Post-
	menopausal
	osteoporosis
	Disuse

Treatment

Women with multiple risk factors should be encouraged to take a normal diet with adequate calcium (at least 1500 mg per day), to keep up a high level of physical activity and to avoid smoking and excessive consumption of alcohol. In addition, those with oestrogen deficiency (premature or surgically induced menopause) and those with severe bone changes or fractures occurring early in the menopause should receive oestrogen replacement therapy. This has been shown to prevent the accelerated bone loss and to reduce the incidence of further fractures. However, long-term oestrogen therapy is associated with a slight increase in the incidence of breast and uterine cancer.

Fractures may need treatment in their own right; it is important to keep the patient mobile and active.

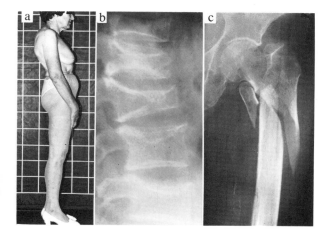

7.9 Osteoporosis (a) This woman noticed that she was becoming more and more 'round-shouldered'; she also had chronic backache and her x-rays (b) show compression of vertebral bodies. Six years after this film was taken she fell in her kitchen and sustained the fracture shown in (c).

Secondary osteoporosis

The most important causes are hypercortisonism, gonadal hormone deficiency, hyperthyroidism, multiple myeloma, chronic alcoholism and immobilization. Patients under 50 years – and older patients with rapidly increasing osteoporosis – should be fully investigated to exclude any potentially reversible disorder.

Paget's disease

Paget's disease is characterized by enlargement and thickening of the bone, but the internal architecture is abnormal and the bone is unusually brittle. The condition is relatively common in Britain, Germany and Australia (more than 3 per cent of people aged over 40), but rare in Asia, Africa and the Middle East. The cause is unknown, although a viral infection has been suggested.

Pathology

Any bone may be affected; in the worst cases many are involved. Cortices are thickened but irregular, at one stage more porous than usual and at another more sclerotic. This is due to alternating phases of rapid bone resorption and formation. While resorption predominates (the 'vascular' stage) the bone is easily deformed; in the late stage the bone becomes increasingly sclerotic and brittle.

Clinical features

Paget's disease affects men and women equally. Only occasionally does it present in patients under 50, but from that age onwards it becomes increasingly common. Often it remains asymptomatic and is discovered accidentally when the patient is x-rayed for some other reason. When pain occurs it is dull

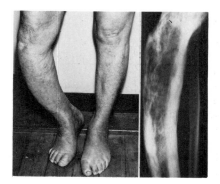

7.10 Paget – localized The typical thick bent tibia.

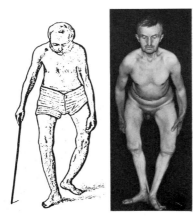

7.11 Paget – generalized   Paget's original case compared with a modern photograph.

and constant, worse at night, but rarely severe unless fracture or sarcoma supervenes.

The bone may be bent and thickened (easily seen and felt in the tibia) and the skin over it is unduly warm, hence the term 'osteitis deformans'. With widespread involvement there may be bowing of the legs and considerable kyphosis, so the patient becomes shorter and ape-like.

A variety of secondary effects can occur: enlargement of the skull and persistent headaches, root pain due to vertebral thickening and deafness due to otosclerosis.

X-RAYS   The bone as a whole is thick and bent; its density in the vascular stage is decreased and in the sclerotic stage increased. The trabeculae are coarse and widely separated, giving a streaky or honeycomb appearance.

INVESTIGATIONS   Plasma alkaline phosphatase and hydroxyproline are high and there is increased excretion of hydroxyproline in the urine.

Complications

Nerve compression and spinal stenosis are sometimes the first abnormalities to be detected.

Fractures   are common, especially in the weight-bearing long bones. In the femur there is a high rate of non-union; for femoral neck fractures prosthetic replacement, and for shaft fractures early internal fixation are recommended.

Bone sarcoma   in the elderly is almost always due to Paget's disease. It should always be suspected if a previously diseased bone becomes more painful, swollen and tender. The prognosis is extremely grave.

Treatment

Most patients with Paget's disease never have symptoms and require no treatment.

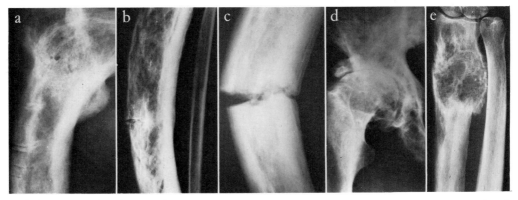

7.12 Paget – complications   (a) Fine cracks (microfractures) on the convex aspect, often associated with pain; (b) incomplete fracture; (c) the characteristic line of a complete fracture; (d) secondary osteoarthritis; (e) sarcoma.

Indeed, there is no specific therapy, but drugs such as calcitonin and diphosphonates can control the disease by suppressing bone turnover. Indications for treatment are: (1) persistent bone pain; (2) repeated fractures; (3) neurological complications; (4) high output cardiac failure; (5) hypercalcaemia due to immobilization; and (6) before and after major bone surgery where there is a risk of excessive haemorrhage.

Endocrine disorders

A number of endocrine disorders are associated with bone disease. Normally there is a fine balance between pituitary growth hormone (which stimulates epiphyseal growth) and gonadal hormone (which promotes growth plate maturation and closure). Thus, at the end of puberty, as gonadal development evolves, growth slows down and the epiphyses fuse. If this balance is disturbed, abnormalities may occur.

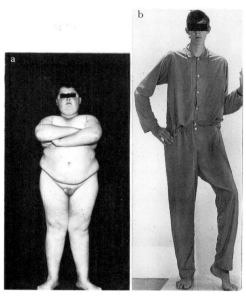

7.13 Endocrine disorders (a) A boy of 12 with the unmistakable build of Frölich's adiposogenital syndrome. (b) This young giant, only 16 years old, suffered from a pituitary adenoma; compare his height with that of the boy in (a).

Hypopituitarism

Growth hormone deficiency produces two distinct disorders: (1) proportionate dwarfism ('Lorain type') due to epiphyseal growth retardation; and (2) delayed skeletal maturation associated with adiposity and hypogonadism (Fröhlich's 'adiposogenital syndrome'). In both, the epiphyses remain unfused and, especially in the adiposogenital syndrome, there is danger of epiphyseal slipping at the hip or knee.

In the acquired types, the disorder may be reversible; e.g. by removing a craniopharyngioma. In others, growth hormone has been used.

Hyperpituitarism

Acidophil cell hypersecretion results in skeletal overgrowth, the effects of which vary according to the age of onset.

Gigantism An acidophil adenoma in childhood stimulates epiphyseal growth. Patients are excessively tall, often with sexual immaturity and mental retardation. Slipping of the upper femoral epiphysis may occur.

Acromegaly Hyperpituitarism starting in adulthood stimulates appositional bone growth and hypertrophy of articular cartilage. The jaw enlarges; together with thickening of the skull this produces a characteristic facies. The hands and feet are big and the long bone ends are markedly thickened; osteoarthritis is common.

Cushing's syndrome

Cushing's syndrome may be due to hypersecretion by the adrenal cortex, but is more often due to corticosteroid therapy. There is a characteristic obesity of the face and trunk, and generalized osteoporosis. With very large doses of steroids there is danger of bone necrosis.

Infantile hypothyroidism (cretinism)

With congenital thyroid deficiency the child is severely dwarfed and mentally retarded. Irregular epiphyseal ossification may be mistaken for avascular necrosis. These changes can be prevented by early treatment with thyroid hormone.

Hyperthyroidism

Hyperthyroidism in adults may give rise to osteoporosis. The investigation of unexplained bone loss should include tests for thyroid function. Treatment of the primary disorder results in improved bone mass.

Genetic disorders, dysplasias and malformations 8

There can be few diseases in which genetic factors do not play some role. Sometimes, however, a genetic defect is the major – or the only – determinant of an abnormality that is either present at birth (i.e. congenital) or inevitably evolves in later years. Such conditions can be broadly divided into three categories:

1. *Chromosome disorders* which are not inherited; these usually have serious effects (e.g. Down's syndrome) and often cause stillbirths.
2. *Single gene disorders*, which are passed on to future generations according to Mendelian principles. The effects may appear as growth disorders or metabolic abnormalities.
3. *Polygenic* or *multifactorial disorders*, which result from the interaction of genetic and environmental factors; congenital hip dislocation and club foot are examples – so is gout, for in someone with familial hyperuricaemia an attack may be provoked by overindulgence or trauma.

Developmental abnormalities may also result from injury to the formed embryo by viral infections (e.g. rubella), certain drugs (e.g. thalidomide) and ionizing radiation.

Patterns of inheritance

Autosomal dominant disorders are inherited even if only one parent is affected. Half the children of both sexes develop the disorder (e.g. hereditary multiple exostosis).

Autosomal recessive disorders appear only when both parents carry the abnormal gene (though they themselves may be clinically normal). An example is one type of osteogenesis imperfecta (brittle bone disease).

X-linked disorders are caused by a faulty gene in the X chromosome. Characteristically, therefore, they never pass directly from father to son because the father's X chromosome inevitably goes to the daughter and the Y chromosome to the son. The best known example is haemophilia: an affected man will have normal children but all his daughters will be carriers and half of their sons will be bleeders.

In-breeding

All types of genetic disease are more likely to occur in the children of consanguineous marriages or in closed communities where many people are related to each other. The rare recessive disorders, in particular, are seen in these circumstances.

Genetic markers

Many common disorders show an unusually close association with certain blood groups, tissue types or other serum proteins that occur with higher than expected frequency in the patients and their relatives. These are referred to as genetic markers. A good example is ankylosing spondylitis: over 90% of patients and 60% of their first-degree relatives are positive for HLA-B27.

Prenatal diagnosis

Many genetic disorders can be diagnosed before birth, thus giving the parents the choice of selective abortion. Ultrasound imaging is harmless and is now done almost routinely. On the other hand, tests that involve amniocentesis or chorionic villus sampling carry a risk of injury to the fetus and are therefore used only when there is reason to suspect some abnormality, e.g. if the mother is over 35 years old or if there is a history of previous chromosomal or genetic abnormalities.

Diagnosis in childhood

Physical abnormalities may be obvious at birth, for example, disproportionately short limbs, club foot or spina bifida.

During infancy the reasons for presentation are failure to grow normally, disproportionate shortness of the limbs, delay in walking or fractures.

Older children are more obviously abnormal, often 'dwarfed' and showing characteristic x-ray signs. However, if the changes do not fit a pattern and there are signs of healing fractures, the battered baby syndrome must be excluded.

The family history is important and may reveal the pattern of inheritance.

Special investigations may be indicated to identify specific enzyme or metabolic abnormalities.

Principles of management

1. *Counselling.* This should include a full explanation of the problem and expert advice about the risks for future children.

2. *Specific treatment.* Treatment is available for certain genetic disorders, e.g. haemophilia and some of the rare enzyme deficiencies. Gene alteration is becoming possible.
3. *Correction of deformities.* Bony deformities, if they interfere with function, should be corrected. Limb lengthening is sometimes performed for short-limbed dwarfs. Joint replacement may be needed in later life.

Classification

There is no completely satisfactory classification of developmental disorders. A practical approach is shown below and some examples are described:

1. *Skeletal dysplasias* – abnormalities of bone growth.
2. *Connective tissue disorders* affecting either soft tissues or bone.
3. *Metabolic disorders.*
4. *Non-heritable chromosome disorders.*
5. *Localized malformations.*

Hereditary multiple exostosis (diaphyseal aclasis)

This, the most common of all skeletal dysplasias is a congenital disorder in which multiple exostoses appear at the metaphyses as the child grows. It is inherited as an autosomal dominant and appears to represent a failure of growth plate modelling.

Each exostosis is covered by a cartilage cap and is, effectively, an osteochondroma; it grows only while the child grows and any enlargement after that (which is rare) may herald malignant change to a chondrosarcoma. The failure of modelling results in deformities of the long bones.

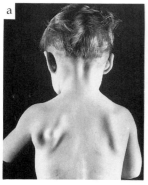
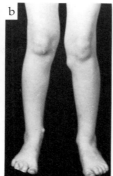
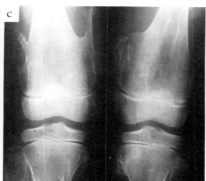

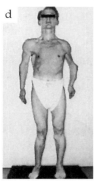

8.1 Hereditary multiple exostoses Presentation at (a) 3 years; (b, c) 6 years; (d) 28 years. In (d) note the numerous small exostoses, the one large tumour near the right shoulder, bowing of the left radius, shortening of the left forearm and valgus deformity of the right knee.

Clinical features

The condition is usually discovered in childhood; hard lumps appear at the ends of the long bones and along the apophyseal borders of the scapula and pelvis. The child may be slightly short, with bowing of the forearms and valgus knees. Occasionally one of the lumps is tender or causes trouble due to pressure on a tendon.

X-rays show the pathognomonic exostoses as well as broadening and lumpiness of the metaphyses.

Management

If an exostosis is troublesome (and certainly if it starts to 'grow' after the parent bone has stopped) it should be removed.

Achondroplasia

This, the commonest form of true dwarfism, is inherited as an autosomal dominant, but because most of the affected individuals do not have children, cases are usually sporadic.

Severe, disproportionate shortening of the limb bones may be diagnosed by x-ray before birth.

Clinical features

The abnormality is obvious in childhood: growth is severely stunted: the limbs are disproportionately short and the skull is quite large with prominent forehead and saddle-shaped nose. The fingers appear stubby and somewhat splayed (trident hands). The trunk seems too long by compar-

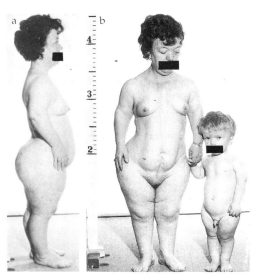

8.2 Achondroplasia   (a) A typical achondroplastic patient with disproportionate shortening of the limbs. (b) Her son has clearly inherited the disorder.

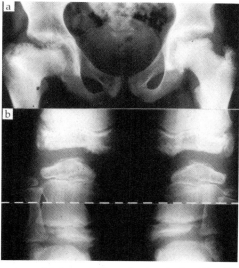

8.3 Multiple epiphyseal dysplasia (a) The grossly abnormal epiphyses led to a mistaken diagnosis of late Perthes' disease. (b) This girl had many epiphyses involved; her sister was similarly affected. Note the characteristic flattening of the femoral condyles.

ison with the limbs, and the posture when standing is typical: the back is excessively lordotic, the buttocks prominent, the hips flexed, the legs bowed and the elbows bent. In infancy there is often a thoracolumbar gibbus, which disappears after a few years.

X-rays show the short bones, anteroposterior narrowing of the pelvis and, sometimes, changes in the spine.

Management

Achondroplastic dwarfs often develop neurological symptoms which may be due to spinal stenosis or progressive spinal deformity. This may need operative treatment.

Leg lengthening is feasible but seldom advisable.

Multiple epiphyseal dysplasia

This is a familial disorder (autosomal dominant) in which the long-bone epiphyses develop abnormally.

Clinical features

Children may present with stunted growth or, occasionally, with joint pain and progressive deformity. The face, skull and spine are normal. In adult life, residual bone defects may lead to joint incongruity and secondary osteoarthritis.

X-ray changes are apparent from early childhood. Epiphyseal ossification is irregular or abnormal in outline. In the growing child the epiphyses are misshapen, and in the hips this may be mistaken for bilateral Perthes' disease. At maturity the femoral heads and femoral condyles are flattened; secondary osteoarthritis may ensue and, if many joints are involved, the patient can be severely crippled.

Spondyloepiphyseal dysplasia is rather similar, but here the vertebrae are deformed as well.

Management

Children may complain of slight pain and limp, but little can (or need) be done about this. At maturity, bony deformities sometimes require corrective osteotomy. In later life, secondary osteoarthritis may call for reconstructive surgery.

Osteogenesis imperfecta

Osteogenesis imperfecta (OI) is one of the commonest of the heritable bone disorders, with an estimated incidence of 1 in 20 000. Because of the marked skeletal abnormalities it is often included among the bone dysplasias. However, it is basically a connective tissue disorder (defective synthesis of type I collagen) with generalized involvement of the bones, teeth, ligaments, sclerae and skin. It is a heterogeneous condition and there are at least four subgroups showing variations in phenotype and pattern of inheritance. What they have in common are (1) osteopenia, (2) proneness to fracture and (3) laxity of ligaments. About two-thirds of patients have (4) blue sclerae and about half have (5) 'crumbling teeth', or dentinogenesis imperfecta.

Clinical features

There are 4 clinical types:

OI type I (mild) This, the commonest variety, is a comparatively mild autosomal dominant disorder. Fractures occur throughout life but deformity is uncommon. Characteristically the sclerae are blue and the joints are hypermobile.

X-rays show osteopenia and thinning of the cortices. Old fractures are usually evident and there may be some bowing of the long bones.

OI type II (lethal) This severe, recessive disorder may be diagnosed before birth by x-ray or ultrasound imaging. Some infants are still-born, and those who survive have

multiple fractures and deformities of the long bones.

OI type III (severe, deforming) This is the classic, though not the commonest, form of OI. It is sometimes diagnosed at birth and by the age of 6 years the child has had numerous fractures and has usually developed severe deformities. It is not as severe as type II, but few of the children survive into adulthood; those who do are markedly dwarfed and disabled.

OI type IV (moderately severe) This autosomal dominant disorder is similar to type I but the sclerae are only a pale blue and they become normal in colour in adult life.

Management

The most severe forms of OI defy treatment and none is indicated apart from sympathetic nursing care. For other types of OI, treatment is aimed at: (1) gentle nursing of infants to prevent fractures as far as possible; (2) prompt splinting when fractures do occur, to prevent unnecessary deformity; (3)

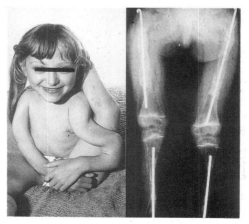

8.4 Osteogenesis imperfecta This patient had severe deformities of both legs; these were corrected by multiple osteotomies and 'rodding'.

mobilization, to prevent further osteoporosis; and (4) correction of deformities, if necessary by multiple osteotomies, bone realignment and intramedullary fixation.

Marfan's syndrome

This is a generalized autosomal dominant disorder affecting the bones, joint ligaments, eyes and cardiovascular structures. It is thought to be due to a cross-linkage defect in collagen and elastin.

Clinical features

Patients are tall, with disproportionately long legs and arms; typically, arm span exceeds height. The digits are unusually long, giving rise to the term 'arachnodactyly' or 'spider fingers'. Spinal abnormalities include spondylolisthesis and scoliosis. There is an increased incidence of slipped upper femoral epiphysis. Generalized joint laxity is usual and patients may develop flat feet or dislocation of the patella or shoulder. Associated abnormalities include a high arched palate, hernias, lens dislocation, retinal detachment, aortic aneurysm and mitral or aortic incompetence.

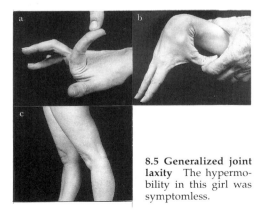

8.5 Generalized joint laxity The hypermobility in this girl was symptomless.

Management

Patients occasionally need treatment for progressive scoliosis or flat feet. The heart should be carefully checked before operation.

Generalized joint laxity

About 5% of people have hypermobile joints. This trait runs in families and is inherited as a mendelian dominant. The condition is not in itself disabling but it may predispose to congenital dislocation of the hip in the newborn or recurrent dislocation of the patella or shoulder in later life. Transient joint pains are common and there is an increased risk of ankle sprains.

Mucopolysaccharidoses

The mucopolysaccharidoses are a group of metabolic disorders in which, because of lack of certain essential degradative enzymes, there is incomplete breakdown and excessive storage of glycosaminoglycans (GAG). Partially degraded GAG's accumulate in the liver, spleen, bones and other tissues and spill over into the blood and urine where they can be detected by suitable biochemical tests. These inborn errors of metabolism are inherited as recessive traits.

Clinical features

Depending on the specific enzyme deficiency and the type of GAG storage, at least six clinical syndromes have been defined. As a group they have certain recognizable features: dwarfism with vertebral deformity, coarse facies, hepatosplenomegaly and (in some cases) mental retardation. X-rays show bone dysplasia affecting the vertebral bodies, epiphyses and metaphyses; typically the bones have a spatulate appearance. The diagnosis can be confirmed by testing for abnormal GAG excretion or demonstrating the enzyme deficiency in blood cells or cultured skin fibroblasts.

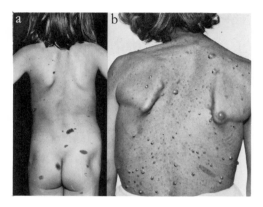

8.6 Neurofibromatosis (a) Café-au-lait spots; (b) multiple neurofibromata, molluscum fibrosum and slight scoliosis.

Management

Specific treatment for these disorders is not yet possible, but enzyme replacement is being developed. Deformities may need correction by osteotomy.

NB: *Growth disorders affecting the spine may cause odontoid hypoplasia and atlanto-axial instability; this calls for special care during anaesthesia.*

Neurofibromatosis

This is a congenital, heritable disorder (autosomal dominant) but clinical features usually do not appear till early childhood. It is characterized by the development of multiple neurofibromata, soft cutaneous fibromata (molluscum fibrosum) and patches of light-brown pigmentation of the skin (café-au-lait spots). Curiously, the patients usually present to the orthopaedic surgeon with scoliosis (why this occurs we do not know); in later life it appears as a cause of nerve root compression due to tumours in the spinal canal. Occasionally it

is found, in infants, in association with pseudarthrosis of the tibia.

Treatment may be necessary for a fracture or to correct bone deformity.

Localized malformations

Localized malformations of the vertebrae or limbs are common. The majority cause no disability and may be discovered incidentally during investigation of some other disorder. Some have a genetic background and similar malformations are seen in association with generalized skeletal dysplasia. Most are sporadic and probably non-genetic – i.e. caused by injury to the developing embryo, especially during the first 3 months of pregnancy. In some cases there is a known teratogenic agent; for example, maternal infection or drug administration. Usually, however, the exact cause is unknown.

Vertebral anomalies

The commonest vertebral anomaly is *spina bifida* (see page 81). Others appear as complete *agenesis, hemivertebrae* or *fused vertebrae*; they may lead to severe deformity (kypho-scoliosis) and paralysis. Operative treatment may be needed for cord compression.

In *Sprengel's deformity* there is elevation of the scapula, with or without vertebral anomalies. Treatment is seldom necessary.

Limb anomalies

These include extra bones, absent bones, hypoplastic bones and fusions. Occasionally a whole limb or part of a limb fails to develop.

These conditions all require specialized reconstructive surgery, often during the first few years of life.

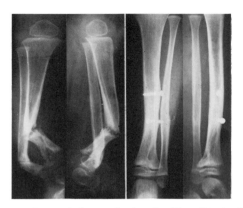

8.7 Congenital pseudarthrosis The tibia is the most common site; in this case bone grafting was successful.

Congenital pseudoarthrosis

A curious anomaly is congenital pseudoarthrosis, usually of the tibia. The baby is born with a fractured lower third of tibia, or with a bent fibula which later breaks. The fracture is resistant to conventional methods of treatment, but specialized techniques, including bone grafting, may be successful.

Tumours 9

All primary bone tumours are rare; by contrast, metastatic deposits in bone, especially in those over the age of 50, are relatively common.

Primary tumours are usually classified by cell type. Some of the benign tumours may become malignant.

Diagnosis

Most tumours cause pain, swelling and local tenderness; occasionally a lesion is discovered accidentally during x-ray examination, or as the result of a pathological fracture.

It is not always easy to tell whether a bone tumour is benign or malignant, but rapid growth, warmth, tenderness and an ill-defined edge suggest malignancy. If treatment is to be rational, we must know the precise diagnosis and also the extent of the lesion, its relationship to perivascular spaces, and the likelihood of distant spread. Therefore, in all cases of suspected malignancy (and sometimes even with unusual benign lesions), investigations should include high-quality radiography, computerized tomography or MRI, bone scanning and a carefully planned biopsy before definitive treatment begins.

Conditions notorious for mimicking bone tumours are *infection* and *stress fractures*.

Principles of treatment

Benign, asymptomatic lesions If the diagnosis is beyond doubt one can temporize: treatment may never be needed. Otherwise a biopsy is advisable, either an excisional biopsy or curettage.

Benign, symptomatic or enlarging tumours Painful lesions, or tumours that continue to enlarge after the end of normal bone growth, require biopsy and confirmation of the diagnosis. Unless they are unusually aggressive, they can generally be removed by local excision.

Suspected malignant tumours If the lesion is thought to be a primary malignant tumour, the patient is admitted for detailed assessment. The various treatment options can then be discussed; they include amputation, limb-sparing operations and different types of adjuvant therapy. The patient must be fully informed about the pros and cons of each.

Table 9.1 A classification of the less rare primary bone tumours

Cell type	Benign	Malignant
Bone	Osteoid osteoma	Osteosarcoma
Cartilage	Chondroma Osteochondroma	Chondrosarcoma
Fibrous tissue	Fibroma	Fibrosarcoma
Marrow	Eosinophilic granuloma	Ewing's sarcoma Myeloma
Vascular	Haemangioma	Angiosarcoma
Uncertain	Giant-cell tumour	Malignant giant-cell tumour

Osteoid osteoma

This is a benign tumour consisting of osteoid and newly formed bone. It is small (usually less than 1 cm in size), round or oval in shape and is encased in dense bone. It is usually seen in patients aged under 30, and over half the cases occur in the femur or tibia. The leading symptom is pain, which is sometimes severe and is usually relieved by aspirin but not by rest.

The important *x-ray* feature is a small radiolucent area surrounded by dense sclerosis. The bone scan shows markedly increased activity. It is sometimes difficult to distinguish an osteoid osteoma from a small Brodie's abscess without biopsy.

Excision of the affected area cures the pain and the tumour does not recur.

9.1 Osteoid osteoma (a) With cortical tumours there is marked bone thickening leaving a small lucent nidus which may have a central speck of ossification. (b) Lesions in cancellous bone produce less periosteal reaction and are easily mistaken for a Brodie's abscess.

Osteochondroma (cartilage-capped exostosis)

This is the most common tumour of bone. It starts, usually in adolescence, as a cartilaginous overgrowth at the edge of the epiphyseal plate, but by the time it is discovered much of it has ossified. The tumour continues to grow as long as the parent bone grows; *any further growth after that is suggestive of malignant change.*

The usual site is the metaphysis of a long bone; lesions may be single or multiple (hereditary multiple exostoses). The patient may complain of pain or disturbed tendon function, but the usual story is that the lump was discovered accidentally. The lump is

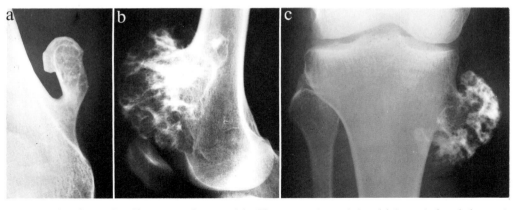

9.2 Osteochondroma (cartilage-capped exostosis)   The two main varieties: (a) is conical and the cartilage does not show on x-ray; (b) and (c) are cauliflower-shaped and the cartilage cap has partly calcified.

bony hard, although sometimes covered by a bursa which may be tender.

On *x-ray* it is well defined; often it looks smaller than it feels, because the cartilage cap is invisible.

If the tumour causes symptoms it should be excised; if, in an adult, it has recently become bigger or painful then operation is urgent – it may be malignant.

Chondroma (enchondroma)

Chondroma is a benign cartilaginous tumour. It may be single or multiple (Ollier's disease) and usually appears in the tubular bones of the hand or foot and in the larger long bones.

The patient presents with pain or a swelling, or with a fracture after trivial injury. *X-ray* shows a well-defined rare area in the medulla, often with characteristic specks of calcification.

The solitary chondroma must be differentiated from a benign cyst (which has no calcification). In patients over 30 it is essential to exclude a chondrosarcoma, especially if the tumour is in a large bone.

The lesion should be excised or curetted and replaced with bone graft.

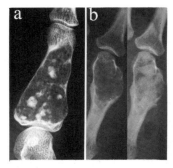

9.3 Cartilaginous tumours (a) Chondroma of a finger. (b) Another digital chondroma, before and after curettage and grafting.

Cysts of bone

Simple (solitary) cyst

This is not strictly a tumour. It usually occurs in the upper humerus, femur or tibia, but other bones may be affected. Solitary cysts are seen in children up to the age of puberty, and after that become increasingly rare. Clinically a cyst presents with local ache or as a pathological fracture.

X-rays show a translucent area on the shaft side of the growth disc. The cortex may be thinned and the bone expanded.

Because cysts are hardly ever seen in adults, it is presumed that many disappear spontaneously. A fracture through a cyst often results in the cyst becoming obliterated. Injecting corticosteroids into the cyst also may lead to its obliteration. If not, it can be evacuated, the wall scraped and the cavity filled with bone chips.

Aneurysmal bone cyst

This tumour-like lesion contains cavities filled with blood. It occurs chiefly in the spine and the metaphysis of long bones, usually affecting young adults. It is an expanding lesion, thinning the cortex.

X-ray shows a well-defined rare area, often trabeculated and eccentrically placed. Radiologically it may resemble a giant-cell tumour, but that tumour extends to the articular surface whereas aneurysmal bone cysts are confined to the metaphyseal side of the growth plate.

Curettage and packing with bone chips gives good results.

Non-ossifying fibroma (fibrous cortical defect)

This is *not* a cyst, but it looks like one on x-ray – because it is filled with translucent fibrous tissue.

It is usually discovered accidentally in a child's x-ray. There is a cyst-like area in the

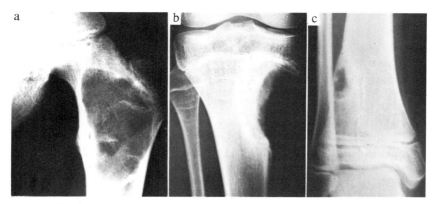

9.4 Cyst-like lesions of bone (a) Solitary bone cyst, (b) aneurysmal bone cyst and (c) fibrous cortical defect (which is not a cyst at all but looks like one because it is radiolucent).

cortex of a long-bone metaphysis; the margin is well defined, even sclerosed.

Most of these defects heal spontaneously, but some may grow, so pathological fracture is a possibility. Unless fracture occurs, they require no treatment.

Giant-cell tumour

Pathology

This tumour derives its name from multi-nucleated giant cells which are seen in large numbers; but these are less significant than the stromal cells, from whose proliferation they probably arise. Macroscopically the tumour is soft and friable, occupying a large excavation in the subarticular cancellous bone. It occurs only in 'mature' bones, i.e. those in which the epiphyses have fused.

The adjective 'benign' was formerly used but is misleading: only about one-third remain truly benign, one-third become locally invasive and one-third metastasize.

Clinical features

Patients are usually between the ages of 20 and 40. They complain of pain near a joint, sometimes with slight swelling. A history of trauma is not uncommon and pathological

fracture occurs in 10 per cent of cases.

On examination, there is a vague swelling of the end of a long bone. The neighbouring joint is often irritated.

X-rays show a rarefied area situated asymmetrically at the very end of a long bone. Often there are trabeculae and a 'soap-bubble' appearance. The cortex is very thin and sometimes ballooned or even perforated.

Treatment

Well-confined, slow-growing lesions with benign histology can be treated by thorough curettage and 'stripping' of the cavity wall with burrs and gouges, followed by packing with bone chips. More aggressive tumours, and recurrent lesions, should be treated by excision followed, if necessary, by bone grafting or prosthetic replacement. Radio-therapy is reserved for surgically inaccessible tumours.

Osteosarcoma

Pathology

Osteosarcoma (formerly called osteogenic sarcoma) implies a primary malignant tumour arising from bone and producing osteoid. It destroys bone and spreads into

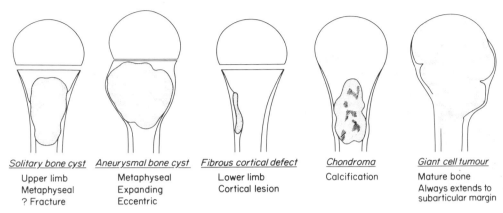

Solitary bone cyst	*Aneurysmal bone cyst*	*Fibrous cortical defect*	*Chondroma*	*Giant cell tumour*
Upper limb Metaphyseal ? Fracture	Metaphyseal Expanding Eccentric	Lower limb Cortical lesion	Calcification	Mature bone Always extends to subarticular margin

9.5 Cysts and cyst-like lesions of bone.

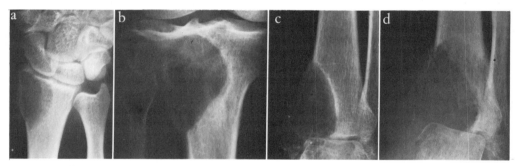

9.6 Giant-cell tumours   (a, b, c) In each of these the tumour abuts against the joint margin, and is asymmetrically placed – these are characteristic features; in (d) malignant change has supervened and the junction of the tumour with the rest of the bone is no longer well defined.

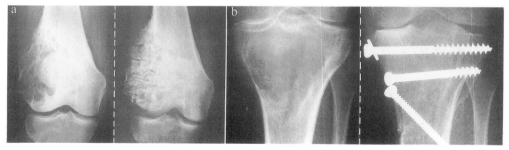

9.7 Giant-cell tumour – treatment   (a) Curettage and bone grafting. (b) Block resection and replacement with a large osteocartilaginous graft.

the surrounding tissues. The histology is variable and may include primitive cartilage or fibrous tissue. Always, however, there will be osteoid or new bone in some part of the lesion. It metastasizes readily, producing secondary deposits in the lungs.

Clinical features

The incidence is highest between the ages of 10 and 20 years, but a second peak occurs after 50 due to malignant change in Paget's disease. The most common site is at the metaphysis of a long bone, especially around the knee and in the proximal humerus.

A history of trauma is present in more than half the cases. Pain is usually the first symptom; it is constant, worse at night and gradually becomes severe. Sometimes the patient presents with a lump.

On examination, the part is swollen and the overlying skin may be shiny and warm. The lump feels tender and lacks a definite edge. The ESR is raised.

IMAGING X-ray appearances are very variable but show a combination of bone destruction and bone formation. The medulla contains areas of rarefaction or density. The cortex is usually perforated and a soft-tissue shadow may be seen. There is subperiosteal new bone formation and streaks of calcification in the adjacent soft tissues – the 'sunray' appearance.

CT, radioisotope scanning and MR imaging are needed to 'stage' the tumour, i.e. to show its full extent. X-ray (and better still CT) of the chest may show pulmonary metastases. Biopsy is essential to establish the diagnosis.

Treatment

The cytotoxic drugs have transformed the outlook for patients with osteosarcoma and 50 per cent now survive 5 years or more. The most certain way of eradicating the primary tumour is by radical amputation. However, with the cytotoxic drugs to take care of metastases, more limited resections and prosthetic replacements are being undertaken. If preoperative investigations show that the tumour is resectable, this may well be the treatment of choice; chemotherapy is started soon after operation and is continued for at least a year.

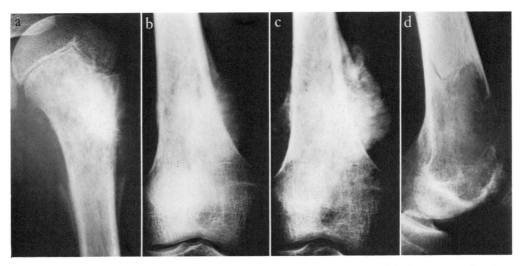

9.8 Osteosarcoma   (a, b) Characteristic appearance with sun-ray spicules and Codman's triangle where the periosteum begins to be lifted away from the shaft; (c) the same patient as (b), after radiotherapy; (d) a predominantly osteolytic tumour.

Inaccessible tumours are treated by radiotherapy combined with chemotherapy.

Chondrosarcoma

Chondrosarcoma occurs in two forms.

First, it may start as a central (medullary) tumour – to all appearances a 'chondroma' – and expand slowly to show its true colours some years later. In this form it is seldom seen under the age of 40, and the patient then presents with pain or with a pathological fracture. *X-rays* show a destructive medullary tumour containing characteristic flecks of calcification.

Secondly, chondrosarcoma may arise by malignant change in the cartilage cap of an osteochondroma. The previously benign tumour starts growing some time after normal bone growth has ceased and it may reach enormous dimensions (especially if it expands into the pelvic basin where it produces no visible swelling) before the patient seeks attention. Here the *x-ray* shows a large exostosis surmounted by flecks of calcification in the cartilage cap.

As with other malignant bone tumours, investigations should include CT, MRI and radioisotope scanning to establish the full extent of the lesion before embarking on treatment.

Chondrosarcomas tend to metastasize late, and at least one attempt at wide local excision is justified. Where neither excision nor amputation is practicable, radiotherapy may be tried.

Ewing's tumour

This is a rare malignant tumour arising from vascular endothelium in the bone marrow. It usually occurs in the diaphysis of a long bone and gives rise to a florid periosteal reaction. Metastases may be widespread.

The tumour occurs most commonly between the ages of 10 and 20 years, usually in a long bone.

Pain and swelling are the chief presenting features. The lump is warm and tender, with an ill-defined edge. The clinical features may resemble those of osteomyelitis.

X-rays show bone destruction with overlying 'onion-skin' layers of periosteal new bone. Radioisotope scanning shows marked activity.

A solitary lesion may be treated by either amputation or radiotherapy, together with chemotherapy.

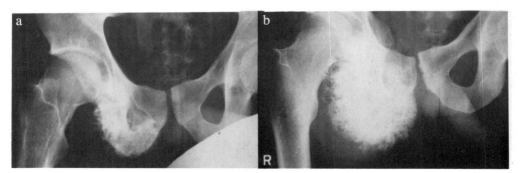

9.9 Chondrosarcoma   At the age of 20 this young man complained of pain in the right groin; x-ray showed an osteochondroma of the right inferior pubic ramus (a). A biopsy showed 'benign cartilage' but a year later the tumour had doubled its size (b), a clear sign that it was a chondrosarcoma.

Multiple myeloma

Myelomas are said to arise from plasma cells of the marrow and they are found wherever red marrow occurs. They are usually multiple from the start but occasionally a large tumour presents as a solitary bone lesion – a 'plasmacytoma'.

Clinical features

The patient, aged 45–65, presents with weakness, bone pain or a pathological fracture. The pain is constant and backache in particular is common, sometimes with root pain and occasionally paraplegia. Anaemia, cachexia and chronic nephritis all contribute to the general ill-health. There is almost invariably a high ESR*. The usual cause of death is renal failure.

X-rays may show nothing more than overall reduction of density; however, there may be multiple punched-out defects in more than one bone. Vertebral involvement may cause compression fractures.

Investigations of importance in establishing a diagnosis are: urinalysis, which in over half the cases shows Bence-Jones protein; electrophoretic analysis of plasma and urine proteins, which shows a characteristic pattern; and sternal marrow puncture, which reveals the typical myeloma cells.

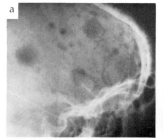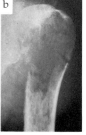

9.10 Myelomatosis Punched-out lesions in the skull (a) and an osteolytic deposit in the humerus (b).

Treatment

Radiotherapy and chemotherapy relieve pain and pressure effects for a time, and may prolong survival. Pathological fractures in the limbs are best treated by internal fixation. Spinal fractures are treated with a brace; unrelieved cord pressure may need decompression.

Metastatic tumours in bone

Metastatic deposits are commoner than all primary malignant bone tumours put together; two-thirds arise from carcinoma of the breast or prostate and the remainder mainly from carcinoma of the thyroid, kidney, lung and gastrointestinal tract. Sometimes no primary tumour can be found.

Metastases usually appear in areas containing red marrow. They destroy and replace bone, partly by their own expansion and partly by stimulating active bone resorption.

Clinical features

A patient of 50–70 years may present with bone pain – perhaps in the spine, or the pelvis or the ends of the long bones. Often nothing is suspected until a pathological fracture occurs (see page 263).

The primary tumour may be obvious but sometimes even a meticulous search fails to reveal it. The neck, breasts, axillae, lungs, abdomen and genitalia should be examined, and rectal or vaginal examination is usually necessary. Investigations which may be required include: x-rays of the chest and urogenital tract; blood count, sedimentation rate, protein electrophoresis and estimation of the serum phosphatases; and isotope scans to reveal other lesions.

X-ray appearances

The usual picture is of purely destructive (osteolytic) lesions, which gives the bone a moth-eaten appearance. Less often (mainly in cases of prostatic carcinoma) there are

*Osteoporosis + a high ESR = myelomatosis until proved otherwise.

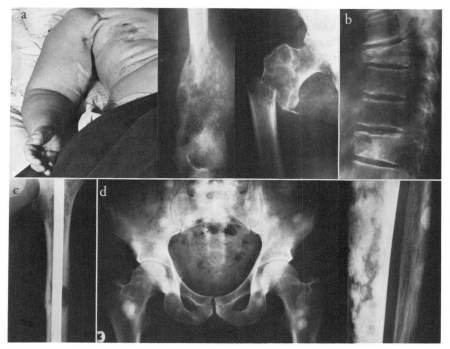

9.11 Secondary deposits   (a) This patient has had a mastectomy for carcinoma; (b) spinal secondaries; (c) osteolytic deposits are liable to fracture and invite internal fixation; (d) osteoblastic deposits in the pelvis and tibia, from prostatic carcinoma.

sclerotic (osteoblastic) deposits. Generalized osteoporosis is common and chest x-rays may reveal lung metastases. Bone scans show increased activity and sometimes they reveal unsuspected lesions.

Treatment

By the time the patient has developed secondary deposits the prognosis is obviously poor and treatment is mainly palliative. Yet the quality of life may be immeasurably improved during the remaining months or years by careful management, which may include radiotherapy and chemotherapy.

Pathological fractures (and even large lytic secondaries that have not fractured) need internal fixation. Vertebral lesions with deteriorating neurological signs need urgent treatment if paraplegia is to be prevented; this usually means radiotherapy but surgical decompression and fusion may be required as well.

Neurological disorders

Of the vast range of neurological disorders, several produce characteristic defects in musculoskeletal function. The commonest of these conditions are:

1. *Cerebral palsy and other upper motor neuron (spastic) disorders.*
2. *Compressive lesions of the spinal cord.*
3. *Neural tube defects (spina bifida).*
4. *Anterior poliomyelitis.*
5. *Peripheral neuropathies.*

Clinical assessment

Cerebral palsy and spina bifida present during infancy; poliomyelitis usually occurs in childhood; spinal cord lesions and peripheral neuropathies are more common in adults. However, the residual effects of neurological disease may present throughout life.

Examination should include a complete neurological assessment and examination of the back.

GAIT AND POSTURE   Typical patterns of walking can often be recognized:

A *spastic gait* is stiff and jerky, often with the feet in equinus, the knees somewhat flexed and the hips adducted ('scissoring').

A *high-stepping gait* signifies either a problem with proprioception and balance or foot drop.

A *drop foot gait* is due to peripheral neuropathy or injury of the nerves supplying the dorsiflexors of the ankle. During the swing phase the foot falls into equinus ('drops') and if it were not lifted higher than usual the toes would drag along the ground.

A *waddling gait* in which the trunk is thrown from side to side with each step, may be due to dislocation of the hips or to weakness of the abductor muscles.

Ataxia produces a more obvious and irregular loss of balance, which is compensated for by a broad-based gait, or sometimes uncontrollable staggering.

DEFORMITY   When all muscle groups are equally weak (balanced paralysis) the joint simply assumes the position imposed on it by gravity. It is unstable and the limb feels floppy or flail. Deformity occurs when one group of muscles is too weak to balance the pull of antagonists (unbalanced paralysis). At first it can be corrected passively but with time it becomes fixed. In children, paralysis may affect bone growth.

MUSCLE WEAKNESS   This may be due to upper motor neuron lesions (spastic paresis), lower motor neuron lesions (flaccid paresis) or muscle disorders. Weakness is graded as shown in the box:

GRADES OF MUSCLE POWER

0 total paralysis
1 barely detectable contraction
2 not enough power to act against gravity
3 strong enough to act against gravity
4 still stronger but less than normal
5 full power

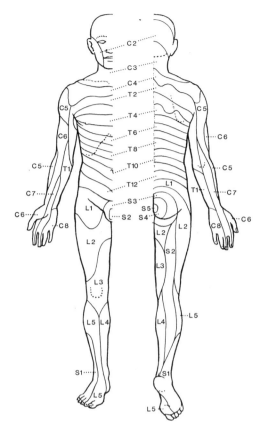

10.1 Examination Skin areas (dermatomes) supplied by the spinal nerve roots.

SENSORY CHANGES Numbness and paraesthesia may be the main complaints. It is important to establish their exact distribution as this will help to localize the lesion.

Investigations

Imaging Plain x-rays of the skull or spine are routine for all disorders of the central nervous system. Specialized imaging of the brain and spinal cord may be necessary to reveal degenerative or space-occupying lesions.

Electrodiagnosis Electromyography and nerve conduction studies are helpful in establishing (1) whether weakness is due to nerve or muscle disorder, and (2) whether (and where) a peripheral nerve is compressed or damaged.

Muscle biopsy A biopsy may yield valuable diagnostic information.

Cerebral palsy

The term 'cerebral palsy' includes a group of disorders which result from non-progressive brain damage during early development. The incidence is about 2 per 1000 live births. Known causal factors are prematurity, perinatal anoxia, birth injury, kernicterus and postnatal brain infections or injury. The main consequence is the development of neuromuscular incoordination, weakness and spasticity; in addition there may be convulsions, perceptual problems, speech disorder and mental retardation.

Early diagnosis

A history of perinatal difficulties may suggest the diagnosis, but at birth the disease is rarely recognized. Early symptoms include difficulty in sucking and swallowing, with dribbling at the mouth; the mother may notice that the baby feels stiff or wriggles awkwardly. Gradually it becomes apparent that the milestones are delayed (the normal child usually holds up its head at 3 months, sits up at 6 months and begins walking at about 1 year). Neonatal reflexes may be delayed.

Late diagnosis

The clinical picture emerges slowly and varies considerably from case to case. Some patients have severe athetosis; others are ataxic; but by far the majority have a *spastic paresis*. As the name implies, there is both spasticity and weakness, although the former may make it difficult to assess the latter.

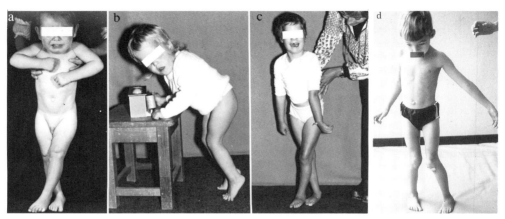

10.2 Cerebral palsy – late diagnosis (a) Scissors stance; (b) flexion deformity of hips and knees with equinus of the feet; (c) characteristic posture and limb deformities; (d) ataxic type of palsy.

Tendon reflexes are brisk and plantar responses extensor. Muscle imbalance gives rise to characteristic deformities: flexion of the elbows and wrists, flexion and adduction of the hips, flexion of the knees and plantarflexion (equinus) of the ankles. The abnormal posture is exaggerated when the child attempts to stand or walk.

The children are often emotionally unstable and sometimes suffer from fits. Intelligence may be impaired.

Treatment

Treatment is best carried out in special centres where the child can have the benefit of combined physiotherapy, occupational therapy, speech therapy and remedial education.

Medication may be needed to control fits and reduce hyperactivity. *Physical therapy* is started during the first year of life, before abnormal motor patterns have become established; it may be continued into adolescence. *Splintage* is often necessary to counteract spastic deformities. If deformities persist or progress in spite of conservative treatment, *corrective surgery* may be employed to restore muscle balance; postoperative physiotherapy is a *sine qua non*. Low intelligence does not preclude

surgery, as long as the child has sufficient motivation.

Operations are of two types: (1) soft-tissue procedures to improve muscle balance by rerouting or dividing tendons or muscles; and (2) bone operations to correct position and stabilize joints.

For a regional survey of operative treatment the reader is referred to *Apley's System of Orthopaedic and Fractures, 7th edition.*

Stroke

Cerebral damage following a stroke may cause persistent spastic paresis in the adult; disturbance of proprioception and stereognosis may coexist. In the early recuperative stage, physiotherapy and splintage are important in preventing fixed contractures; all affected joints should be put through a full range of movement every day, and deformities should be corrected and splinted until controlled muscle power returns. Proprioception and co-ordination can be improved by occupational therapy. Once maximal motor recovery has been achieved – usually by 9 months – residual deformity or joint instability may need surgical correction or permanent splinting.

Table 10.1   Spastic paresis – treatment of the principal deformities of the limbs

	Deformity	Splintage	Surgery
Foot	Equinus	Spring-loaded dorsiflexion	Lengthen tendo Achillis
	Equinovarus	Bracing in eversion and dorsiflexion	Lengthen tendo Achillis and transfer lateral half of tibialis anterior to cuboid
Knee	Flexion	Long caliper	Hamstring release
Hip	Adduction	–	Adductor muscle release
Shoulder	Adduction	–	Subscapularis release
Elbow	Flexion	–	Release elbow flexors
Wrist	Flexion	Wrist splint	Lengthen or release wrist flexors

Lesions of the spinal cord

With lesions of the spinal cord, patients complain of muscle weakness, numbness or loss of balance; bladder and bowel control may be impaired and men may complain of impotence. Examination reveals a spastic (upper motor neuron) paresis, with exaggerated reflexes and a Babinski response; there may be a fairly precise boundary of sensory change, suggesting the level of cord involvement.

Diagnosis

The more common causes of spinal cord dysfunction are listed in Table 10.2. Traumatic and compressive lesions are the ones most likely to be seen by orthopaedic surgeons. Plain x-rays will show structural abnormalities of the spine; cord compression can be visualized by myelography, alone or combined with CT. Intrinsic lesions of the cord require further investigation by blood tests, CSF examination and MRI.

Management

Acute compressive lesions require urgent diagnosis and treatment if permanent damage is to be prevented. Bladder dysfunction is ominous: whereas motor and sensory signs may improve after decompression, *loss of bladder control, if present for more than 24 hours, is usually irreversible.*

Table 10.2   Causes of spinal cord dysfunction

Acute injury
Infection (e.g. tuberculosis)
Intervertebral disc prolapse
Vertebral bone disease (e.g. metastases)
Spinal cord tumours
Intrinsic cord lesions (e.g. syringomyelia)

With chronic lesions one can afford to temporise. Once the diagnosis is certain, appropriate treatment can be applied.

Spina bifida

Spina bifida is a congenital disorder in which the two halves of the posterior vertebral arch (or several arches) have failed to fuse. This is often associated with maldevelopment of the neural tube and the overlying skin; the combination of faults is called *dysraphism*. It usually occurs in the lumbar or lumbo-sacral region. If neural elements are involved there may be paralysis and loss of sensation and sphincter control.

Spina bifida occulta   In the mildest forms of dysraphism there is a midline defect between the laminae and nothing more; hence the term 'occulta' (meaning 'secret'). However, there may be telltale defects in the overlying skin: a dimple, a pit or a tuft of hair.

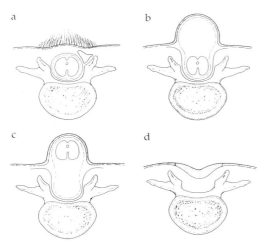

10.3 Dysraphism (a) Spina bifida occulta. (b) Meningocele. (c) Myelomeningocele. (d) Open myelomeningocele.

Spina bifida cystica In severe forms of dysraphism the vertebral laminae are missing and the contents of the vertebral canal prolapse through the defect – either as a CSF-filled meningeal sac or *meningocele* or as a sac containing part of the spinal cord and nerve roots, a *myelomeningocele*. The cord may be in its primitive state, the unfolded neural plate forming part of the roof of the sac; this is an *'open' myelomeningocele* or *rachischisis*. In a *'closed' myelomeningocele* the neural tube is fully formed and covered by membrane and skin.

Hydrocephalus Distal tethering of the cord may cause herniation of the cerebellum and brainstem through the foramen magnum, resulting in obstruction to CSF circulation and hydrocephalus. The ventricles dilate and the skull enlarges by separation of the cranial sutures. Persistently raised intracranial pressure may cause cerebral atrophy and mental retardation.

Neurological dysfunction Myelomeningocele is always associated with neurological deficit below the level of the lesion. This may also occur – though less frequently and much less severely – in spina bifida occulta.

Incidence and screening

Isolated laminar defects are seen in over 5% of lumbar spine x-rays. By comparison, cystic spina bifida is rare at 2–3 per 1000 live births, but if one child is affected the risk for the next child is ten times greater.

Neural-type defects are associated with high levels of alpha-fetoprotein in the amniotic fluid and serum. This offers an effective method of antenatal screening.

Clinical features

Spina bifida occulta Isolated laminar defects are often seen in normal people and usually they can be ignored. However, a posterior midline dimple, a tuft of hair or a pigmented naevus is more serious; patients may present at any age with neurological symptoms and signs.

Spina bifida cystica The saccular lesion over the lumbosacral spine is obvious at birth. It may be covered only with membrane, or with membrane and skin. In open myelomeningoceles the neural elements form the roof of the cyst. Hydrocephalus is common.

The baby's posture may suggest the type of paralysis and sometimes indicates its neurological level. There is generally a flaccid weakness of muscle groups in the lower limbs; sensibility is impaired and there may be urinary and bowel incontinence. The precise neurological deficit varies according to the level of the lesion.

Deformities such as hip dislocation, genu recurvatum and talipes may be present at birth, or they may develop later due to muscle imbalance.

Treatment

Selection of patients for operative closure of the spinal lesion is ethically controversial. Most centres avoid urgent operation if the neurological level is high (above L1), if spinal deformities are severe or if there is marked hydrocephalus. In the remainder (about half) the skin lesion is closed within 48 hours.

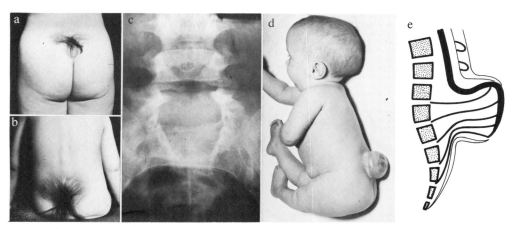

10.4 Spina bifida (a, b) Examples of the hairy patches which suggest a bony defect such as that in (c). (d, e) Myelomeningocele: the diagram shows the neural plaque on the surface, and also why traction lesions of the nerve roots develop with growth.

Subsequent management may involve neuro-surgery (for hydrocephalus), urological surgery (for bladder incontinence) and orthopaedic surgery (for muscle imbalance and joint deformity). Surgical treatment must however always be backed up by prolonged and skilled physiotherapy and splintage, preferably carried out in a specialized centre.

For a regional survey of operative treatment the reader is referred to *Apley's System of Orthopaedics and Fractures, 7th edition.*

Poliomyelitis

Poliomyelitis is a viral infection of the anterior horn cells of the spinal cord which may lead to permanent paralysis of isolated groups of muscles.

Following a trivial and often unrecognized minor illness (a sore throat or diarrhoea), the patient develops meningitis. Two or three days afterwards, paralysis may follow and the muscles are both weak and painful. If the patient does not succumb from respiratory paralysis, pain and pyrexia subside – the convalescent stage has been reached.

Some anterior horn cells will have been destroyed by the virus; others, merely damaged by oedema, survive, and the muscles they supply can regain their lost power. Such recovery may continue for about 2 years but after that any residual weakness is permanent. The clinical features of this stage will be described.

Clinical features

The patient is fit (except for residual paralysis) although, if the trunk muscles were involved, he may have respiratory difficulty and he may have scoliosis. An affected limb often looks bluish, wasted and deformed; there are frequently extensive chilblains and the skin feels cold. Paralysis may be obvious, but lesser degrees of weakness are only discovered by systematic examination. Sensation is unaffected. When a badly paralysed limb is picked up it has a floppy feel which, in the presence of normal sensation, is characteristic. If the disease occurred in childhood there may also be shortening.

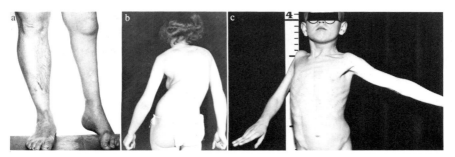

10.5 Polio   (a) Shortening and wasting of the left leg, with equinus of the ankle. (b) This long curve is typical of a paralytic scoliosis. (c) This boy is trying to abduct both arms, but the right deltoid and supraspinatus are paralysed.

Prevention

In some countries immunization has been so successful that poliomyelitis has become a rare disease. However, the victims of earlier epidemics continue to pose challenging problems.

Treatment

During the acute stage bed rest and sedation are all that can be offered. When paralysis occurs, supportive treatment becomes increasingly important. Respiratory paralysis calls for artificial respiration and the painful limb muscles need warmth and gentle physiotherapy.

During the long period of recovery, physiotherapy is stepped up and every effort is made to regain maximum power; because of the associated trophic changes, hydrotherapy also is useful. Between exercise periods splintage may be necessary to prevent fixed deformities.

Later, during the stage of residual paralysis, there are four types of problem that may require treatment.

1. Isolated muscle weakness without deformity Quadriceps paralysis may make walking impossible; it is best managed with a splint (or caliper) which holds the knee straight. Elsewhere isolated weakness (e.g. of thumb opposition) may be treated by tendon transfer.

2. Deformity Unbalanced paralysis may lead to deformity. At first this is passively correctable and can be counteracted by a splint (e.g. a below-knee caliper with corrective strap to control valgus or varus of the foot). However, an appropriate tendon transfer may solve the problem permanently.

Fixed deformity cannot be corrected by either splintage or tendon transfer alone; it is also necessary to restore alignment operatively, and to stabilize the joint (if necessary, by arthrodesis). This is especially applicable to fixed deformities of the ankle and foot, but the same principle applies in treating paralytic scoliosis.

Occasionally fixed deformity is an advantage. Thus, an equinus foot may help to compensate mechanically for quadriceps weakness and, if so, it should not be corrected.

3. Flail joint Balanced paralysis, because it causes no deformity, may need no treatment. However, if the joint is unstable or flail it must be stabilized, either by permanent splintage or by arthrodesis.

4. Shortening Leg length inequality of up to 3 cm can be compensated for by building up the shoe. Anything more is unsightly and operative lengthening of the femur or tibia (or shortening of the opposite limb) might be preferable (see page 98).

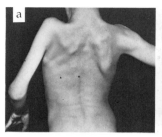 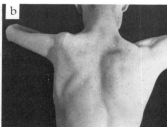

10.6 Polio-treatment (a) This patient had paralysis of the left deltoid; after arthrodesis he could lift his arm by using his scapular muscles (b).

Peripheral neuropathy

The peripheral neuropathies are disorders in which axonal degeneration and demyelination result in loss of motor and/or sensory function, usually in the limbs.

The clinical disorders are divided into:

1. *Mononeuropathy* – involvement of a single nerve (e.g. nerve entrapment)
2. *Multiple mononeuropathy* – involvement of several isolated nerves (e.g. leprosy)
3. *Polyneuropathy* – widespread symmetrical dysfunction (e.g. diabetic neuropathy and hereditary neuropathies)

Clinical features

Patients usually complain of 'pins and needles' or numbness. They may also notice weakness or loss of balance in walking. Occasionally (in the predominantly motor neuropathies) the main complaint is of progressive deformity; for example, claw hand or cavus foot.

The onset may be rapid (over a few days) or very gradual (over weeks or months). Sometimes there is a history of injury, infection, a known disease such as diabetes or malignancy, alcohol abuse or nutritional deficiency.

Examination may reveal weakness in a particular muscle group. In the polyneuropathies the limbs are involved symmetrically, usually legs before arms and distal before proximal parts. In mononeuropathy, sensory loss follows the 'map' of the affected nerve. Trophic skin changes may be present. Deep sensation is also affected and some

patients develop ataxia. If pain sensibility and proprioception are depressed there may be joint instability or breakdown of the articular surfaces (Charcot joints). It is important always to exclude diabetes.

The *mononeuropathies* – mainly nerve injuries and entrapment syndromes – are dealt with in Chapter 11. Of the *polyneuropathies*, two – though uncommon – are liable to cause troublesome foot deformities.

Peroneal muscular atrophy (Charcot–Marie–Tooth) is a familial disorder in which the peripheral nerves, motor nerve roots and the spinal cord degenerate. The typical deformities are pes cavus, peroneal wasting and claw hand. The worst cases begin in early childhood and progress to complete disability. Milder cases present in adolescence, usually with pes cavus and may need nothing more than operation to correct the deformity.

Friedreich's ataxia is also inherited. There is degeneration of the posterolateral columns of the spinal cord and part of the cerebellum. Patients present at the age of 5 or 6 with clumsy gait, ataxia and cavovarus deformities of the feet. The most severe cases end in a wheelchair before the age of 20; in milder cases operative correction of the foot deformities is worthwhile.

Muscular dystrophy

The muscular dystrophies are extremely rare and only one of them will be considered. Pseudohypertrophic muscular dystrophy (Duchenne dystrophy) is a progressive

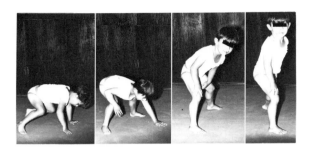

10.7 Muscle dystrophy This boy, with a Duchenne type of dystrophy, has to climb up his legs in order to achieve the upright position.

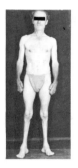 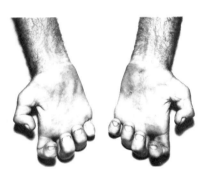

10.8 Peroneal muscular atrophy The most peripheral muscles are the most severely affected, producing cavus feet, claw toes and claw hands. This man could ride a bicycle, but scarcely walk – until his feet were straightened surgically. His hands were left untreated – it seems incredible, but he made beautiful model ships as a hobby.

disorder of sex-linked recessive inheritance. It is usually unsuspected until the child, always a boy, starts to walk. He has difficulty standing and falls frequently. The muscle bulk (pseudohypertrophy) is due to fat and belies the weakness, which is progressive and generalized. By 10 years of age the child is unable to walk and he rarely survives into adult life. Manipulation, splintage or even tendon operations may help to prevent and correct deformities and to keep the child mobile.

Peripheral nerve lesions 11

Nerves may be damaged by laceration, traction, pressure or prolonged ischaemia. According to its severity, the lesion is referred to as a neurapraxia, axonotmesis or neurotmesis.

NEURAPRAXIA Damage is minimal. The axons remain intact but conduction ceases due to segmental demyelination. It is a transient lesion with spontaneous recovery in a few days or weeks.

AXONOTMESIS This means, literally, axonal separation. The axons are severely damaged – usually by compression or traction – and the distal portions degenerate. However, the investing sheaths (endoneurial tubes) remain intact and recovery, though delayed, is likely.

NEUROTMESIS The nerve is completely divided and spontaneous recovery cannot occur.

Nerve recovery

Damaged axons regenerate, but the growing fibrils need to be guided accurately to their original peripheral targets; *this can happen only if the investing sheaths remain intact or are repaired*. In axonotmesis this is the rule but in neurotmesis it cannot occur. Instead, the growing fibrils may bunch up to form a painful neuroma at the site of injury.

Axonal regeneration proceeds at the rate of 1 mm a day. It may be measured by noting the progress of nerve sensitivity at successive visits.

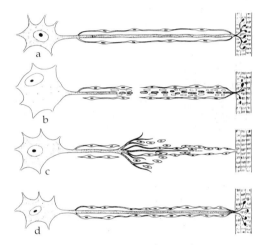

11.1 Nerve injury and repair (a) Normal axon and target organ (striated muscle). (b) Following nerve injury the distal part of the axon disintegrates and the myelin sheath breaks up. The nerve cell nucleus becomes eccentric and Nissl bodies are sparse. (c) New axonal tendrils grow into the mass of proliferating Schwann cells. One of the tendrils will find its way into the old endoneurial tube and (d) the axon will slowly regenerate.

Clinical features

Nerve injuries are easily missed. Following any kind of trauma, patients should be questioned about numbness, any change of feeling or weakness without waiting for them to complain.

On examination the skin may look smooth and shiny; muscle wasting is apparent and the attitude of the limb may be characteristic. Certain active movements are weak or absent and sensation is blunted. Tapping the nerve may cause tingling (Tinel's sign). Skin over the fingers feels dry due to loss of autonomic function.

Electromyography and nerve conduction tests may help to establish the level and severity of the lesion.

DIAGNOSIS

Is a nerve lesion present?
At what level?
Of which type?
Is it recovering?

Treatment

Open injuries   Nerve lesions associated with an open injury should always be explored at the primary operation. If the nerve is cleanly divided it may be repaired immediately. If it is crushed or torn it should be left alone (or the ends lightly tacked together) and re-explored 2 or 3 weeks later; at that stage it will be clear how much scar tissue needs to be removed before suturing.

Closed injuries   With closed nerve lesions it is more difficult to decide what to do, especially during the first few weeks after injury. In most cases the nerve sheath is intact (axonotmesis or neurapraxia), so one can afford to wait at least until the muscle whose nerve branch arises just below the injury should have recovered (allowing for a rate of regeneration of 1 mm a day). If at that time there is still no sign of recovery, the nerve should be explored. Scar tissue is excised and the clean-cut ends are sutured.

Sometimes the gap between the nerve stumps is too large to permit end-to-end suture. A little slack can be gained by mobilizing the nerve, but if it is still difficult to suture the ends without tension, nerve grafts can be used to span the gap.

The limb is then splinted in a position to ensure minimal tension on the nerve. The splint is retained for 3–6 weeks and thereafter physiotherapy is encouraged. If there is sensory loss the skin should be protected from injury.

Brachial plexus injuries

The commonest cause is severe traction with the arm in abduction (usually after a motor cycle accident). Shoulder dislocation may give a partial paralysis, but it usually recovers. Direct injury may result from a stab or gunshot wound.

Clinical features

The pattern of paralysis and sensory loss will be determined by the level of the lesion. In the *upper arm type* of lesion (C5 and C6) the shoulder abductors and external rotators are paralysed, so the arm hangs close to the body and internally rotated; sensation is lost along the outer aspect of the arm. *In the lower arm type* (much rarer) the intrinsic muscles of the hand are paralysed, resulting in a claw hand, and sensation is lost in the ulnar part of the hand and forearm. If the *entire plexus* is damaged, the whole limb is paralysed and numb.

Prognosis

The closer the lesion to the cord, the worse the outlook. If nerve roots have been avulsed from the cord, recovery is impossible; with more distal lesions there is at least a chance of regaining some function and attempts at repair are therefore justified. Cervical myelography combined with CT, and special tests for nerve function, help to pinpoint the level of the lesion.

Treatment

Early   When the patient is first seen fractures and other acute injuries will be given priority. However, open injuries (including stab wounds) should be explored

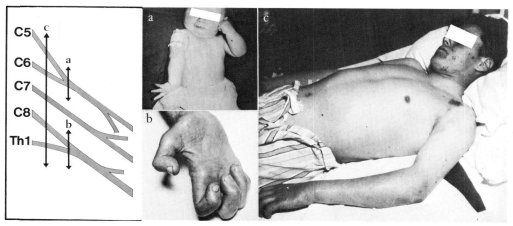

11.2 Brachial plexus Site of the lesions and clinical appearance of brachial plexus injuries: (a) upper arm type (Erb's palsy); (b) lower arm type (Klumpke); (c) tell-tale abrasions on the face and shoulder show how this motorcyclist pulled his entire plexus apart.

without delay and clean-cut nerves repaired or grafted.

Late The limb should be maintained in good condition because, with incomplete lesions, a useful amount of recovery sometimes occurs. With complete lesions, the only hope of recovery lies in painstaking microsurgery.

When the lower trunk is spared, the hand remains useful. It is then sometimes worth while arthrodesing the shoulder so that the arm can be abducted by the scapular muscles.

If there has been a preganglionic avulsion of all the nerve roots, leaving a flail insensitive limb, the best treatment is probably amputation.

BIRTH INJURIES

A traction injury during difficult labour may damage the brachial plexus. The most common is the *upper arm lesion* (Erb's palsy). The arm is held to the side and medially rotated; if recovery does not occur, contractures develop. Most cases recover without treatment, but while waiting the mother should maintain

passive movement so that deformities do not become fixed. If fixed deformities have been allowed to develop, they may require operative correction.

The *lower arm lesion* (Klumpke's palsy) is rare. Here the muscles of the hand and the fingers are paralysed. The fingers should be kept supple in the hope of recovery, which is a slender one.

If there is no recovery by 3 months, specialized nerve grafting should be considered.

Long thoracic nerve

The nerve to serratus anterior (C5, 6, 7) may be damaged in shoulder or neck injuries. Serratus anterior palsy is also seen after carrying loads on the shoulder, viral illnesses or toxoid injections.

Damage leads to winging of the scapula. This is displayed by asking the patient to push forwards against a wall.

Except after direct injury or division, the nerve usually recovers spontaneously, though this may take a year or longer.

Spinal accessory nerve

The spinal accessory nerve (C3, 4) supplies the sternomastoid muscle and then runs obliquely across the posterior triangle of the neck to innervate the upper half of the trapezius. Because of its superficial course, it is easily injured in stab wounds and operations in the posterior triangle of the neck.

The patient complains of pain in the shoulder and weakness on abduction of the arm. There is mild winging of the scapula on active abduction against resistance. In late cases there may be wasting of the trapezius and drooping of the shoulder.

Stab injuries should be explored immediately and the nerve repaired. If the exact cause of injury is uncertain, it is prudent to wait for 6 weeks for signs of recovery. If this does not occur, the nerve should be repaired or grafted.

Axillary nerve

The nerve is sometimes injured during shoulder dislocation or fractures of the humeral neck. The patient cannot abduct the shoulder (even when pain subsides) due to deltoid weakness. There may be a small patch of numbness over the deltoid. Spontaneous recovery is the rule.

Radial nerve

The radial nerve may be injured at the elbow, in the upper arm or in the axilla.

Low lesions are usually due to fractures or dislocations at the elbow, or to a local wound (or operation). The patient cannot extend the metacarpophalangeal joints.

High lesions occur with fractures of the humerus or after prolonged tourniquet pressure. They are also seen in patients who fall asleep with the arm dangling over the back of a chair (Saturday night palsy). There is an obvious wrist drop due to weakness of the wrist extensors and a small patch of sensory loss on the back of the hand at the base of the thumb.

Very high lesions are usually due to pressure in the axilla ('crutch palsy'). The triceps muscle is wasted and paralysed. Spontaneous recovery is the rule.

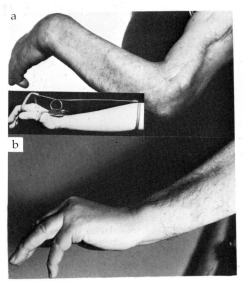
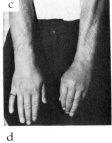
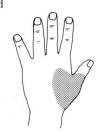

11.3 Radial nerve lesions (a) Complete division with drop wrist (*inset*: Brian Thomas' splint); (b) this patient demonstrates the inability to extend the fingers at the knuckle joints, but he can straighten the interphalangeal joints with his intrinsic muscles; (c) wasting; (d) sensory loss.

Open wounds should be explored and the nerve repaired or grafted as soon as possible.

The lesion associated with a fractured humerus is usually an axonotmesis and function eventually returns. One can therefore afford to wait. However, if there is no sign of recovery by 6 weeks it may be wise to explore the area – if only to confirm that the nerve is intact.

In radial nerve lesions that do not recover, the disability can be largely overcome by suitable tendon transfers.

Ulnar nerve

Injuries of the ulnar nerve are usually either near the wrist or near the elbow, although open wounds may damage it at any level.

Low lesions may be caused by pressure (e.g. from a deep ganglion) or a laceration at the wrist. There is hypothenar wasting and the hand is clawed due to paralysis of the intrinsic muscles. Finger abduction is weak, and the loss of thumb adduction makes pinch difficult. Sensation is lost over the ulnar one and a half fingers.

High lesions occur with elbow fractures; they are also seen (much later) if malunion produces marked cubitus valgus with tension on the nerve where it skirts the medial epicondyle. 'Ulnar neuritis' sometimes occurs without any elbow deformity, due to nerve entrapment in the cubital tunnel. Curiously, the visible deformity is not marked, because the ulnar half of flexor digitorum profundus is paralysed and the fingers are therefore less 'clawed'. Otherwise motor and sensory loss are the same as in low lesions.

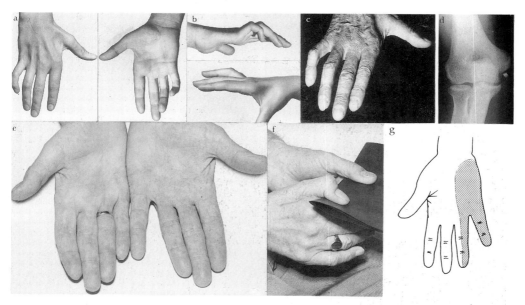

11.4 Ulnar nerve lesions   (a, b) Low ulnar palsy: intrinsic muscle wasting; in the ring and little fingers the knuckle joints are hyperextended (paralysed lumbricals) and the interphalangeal joints are flexed (paralysed interossei). (c) High ulnar palsy: profundus action is lost, so the terminal interphalangeal joints are not flexed (ulnar paradox). He had cut his elbow on some glass; (d) the x-ray shows the glass fragment. (e) When the patient tries to push his little fingers apart, weakness of one abductor digiti minimi is displayed. (f) Froment's sign – because adductor pollicis is weak, the flexor pollicis longus is being used. (g) Sensory loss.

Exploration and suture of a divided ulnar nerve is rewarding; large gaps can be bridged because one can always gain length by transposing the nerve to the front of the elbow. If recovery does not occur, tendon transfers can restore a useful measure of function to the hand.

Nerve entrapment may need decompression by splitting of the aponeurosis between the humeral and ulnar heads of the flexor carpi ulnaris.

Median nerve

The median nerve is commonly injured near the wrist or high up in the forearm.

Low lesions may be caused by cuts in front of the wrist or by carpal dislocations. The thenar eminence is wasted and thumb abduction and opposition are weak. Sensation is lost over the radial three and a half digits and trophic changes may be seen.

Nerve entrapment in the carpal tunnel is common (see Chapter 15).

High lesions are generally due to forearm fractures or elbow dislocation, but stabs and gunshot wounds may damage the nerve at any level. The signs are the same as those of low lesions but, in addition, the long flexors to the thumb, index and middle fingers are paralysed.

If the nerve is divided, suture should always be attempted; if this cannot be done without producing tension, nerve grafts can be placed in the gap. If no recovery occurs, disability is severe – mainly because of sensory loss. If there is some sensation a tendon transfer can be done to restore thumb opposition.

Nerve entrapment at the wrist is treated by slitting the transverse carpal ligament to decompress the carpal tunnel.

Lumbosacral plexus

Any part of the plexus may be injured by fractures of the sacrum. These lesions are usually incomplete and often missed; the patient may complain of no more than patchy muscle weakness and some difficulty with micturition. Sensation is diminished in the perineum or in one or more of the lower limb dermatomes. *Plexus injuries should always be looked for in patients with fractures of the pelvis.*

Recovery is usually quite good and no purpose is served by operative exploration.

INDIVIDUAL ROOTS may be compressed by a tumour, by a prolapsed intervertebral disc or by narrowing of the spinal canal. Pressure on L3 and L4 roots causes weakness of knee extension, depression of the knee reflex and loss of sensation over the

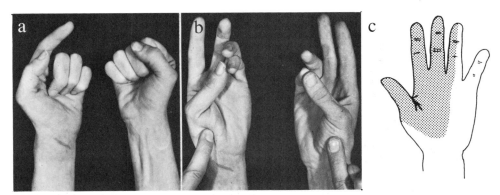

11.5 Cut median nerve   (a) the pointing index when trying to clench the hand; (b) opponens wasting; (c) sensory loss.

anterior thigh and medial side of the leg. Pressure on L5 causes weakness of big toe extension and altered sensation over the front of the leg and foot. Pressure on S1 causes weakness of plantarflexion, a depressed ankle jerk and altered sensation along the sole of the foot. X-ray of the spine, contrast myelography and computed tomography may be needed to pinpoint the lesion. The indications for operation and nerve root decompression are pain, progressive muscle weakness or sphincter dysfunction.

Femoral nerve

The femoral nerve may be injured by a gunshot wound, by traction during an operation or by bleeding into the thigh. There is weakness of knee extension (quadriceps) and numbness of the anterior thigh and medial aspect of the leg. The knee jerk is depressed.

This is a fairly disabling lesion and, where possible, counter-measures should be undertaken. A thigh haematoma may need to be evacuated. A clean cut of the nerve may be treated successfully by careful suturing or grafting.

Sciatic nerve

Division of the main sciatic nerve is rare except in gunshot wounds. Traction lesions are more common and occur with traumatic hip dislocations.

The patient walks with a drop foot, and the calf is wasted. All muscles below the knee are paralysed, and sensation is absent in most of the leg.

Suture should be performed if possible. While recovery is awaited, a drop-foot splint must be worn.

If recovery fails and sores develop, a below-knee amputation may be necessary.

Iatrogenic lesions (usually of the common peroneal division) are sometimes discovered after total hip replacement. The patient complains of numbness or paraesthesia over the lateral part of the foot and, on testing, is unable to dorsiflex or evert the foot. The lesion is due either to direct trauma or traction on the nerve. If direct injury is suspected (excessive pain or paraesthesia) the nerve should be explored. 'Silent' injuries usually recover spontaneously. In all cases the foot should be splinted to prevent a permanent equinus deformity.

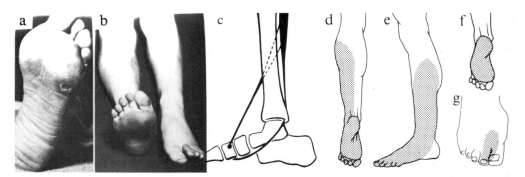

11.6 Sciatic nerve Two problems in sciatic lesions are: (a) sensory loss, which may lead to trophic ulcer; and (b) foot drop, which can be treated with a drop-foot splint, or by rerouting tibialis posterior to the front (c). The remaining diagrams show the areas of sensory loss following division of (d) complete sciatic nerve, (e) common peroneal nerve, (f) posterior tibial nerve, and (g) anterior tibial (deep peroneal) nerve.

Peroneal nerves

The *common peroneal nerve* may be damaged in lateral ligament injuries when the knee is forced into varus, or by pressure from a splint or a plaster cast, or from lying with the leg externally rotated. The patient has a drop foot, and both dorsiflexion and eversion of the foot are weak. Sensation is lost over the front and outer half of the leg and the dorsum of the foot.

If only the *superficial branch* is involved, the peroneal muscles are paralysed and eversion is lost, but dorsiflexion is intact. There is loss of sensation over the outer side of the leg and foot.

The *deep branch* may be threatened in an anterior compartment syndrome (see page 257). There is weakness of dorsiflexion and a small area of sensory loss around the first web space on the dorsum of the foot.

Where indicated, the nerve is sutured. While recovery is awaited, a splint should be worn to control the drop foot; the skin must be protected against ulceration. If recovery does not occur, any disability can be minimized by tendon transfers or foot stabilization.

A threatened compartment syndrome must be treated as an emergency by immediate decompression.

Nerve entrapment

Wherever peripheral nerves traverse fibro-osseous tunnels they are at risk of compression, especially if the soft tissues increase in bulk, as they may in pregnancy, myxoedema or with rheumatoid synovitis. Damage is due to a combination of nerve compression and ischaemia.

Common sites are the *carpal tunnel* (median nerve) and the *epicondylar tunnel* at the elbow (ulnar nerve); less common sites are the *tarsal tunnel* (posterior tibial nerve) and the *inguinal ligament* (lateral cutaneous nerve of the thigh – meralgia paraesthetica).

The patient complains of unpleasant tingling or pain or numbness. Typically symptoms occur at night when the related joint is held still for several hours; relief is obtained by moving the hand or foot 'to get the circulation going'. Symptoms can sometimes be reproduced by proximal compression (e.g. with a sphygmomanometer cuff). Nerve conduction is slowed.

Tunnel syndromes can usually be cured by operative decompression.

Reflex sympathetic dystrophy

This is the preferred name for *Sudeck's atrophy* and *algodystrophy*. The main features are pain, trophic skin changes, vasomotor instability and osteoporosis. Precipitating causes may be trauma, a peripheral nerve lesion, myocardial infarction or a stroke. The mechanism is unknown but peripheral sympathetic overactivity is an important component.

Clinical features

Following some precipitating event, the patient complains of persistent pain in the affected area – usually the hand or foot, sometimes the knee, hip or shoulder. In the mild or early case there may be no more than slight swelling, with tenderness and stiffness of the nearby joints. More suspicious are local redness and warmth, sometimes changing to cyanosis with a blotchy, cold and sweaty skin. X-rays are usually normal but radionuclide scanning at this stage shows increased activity.

Later, or in more severe cases, trophic changes become apparent: a smooth shiny skin with scanty hair and atrophic brittle nails. Swelling and tenderness persist and there may be marked loss of movement. X-rays now show patchy osteoporosis, which may be quite diffuse. In the most advanced stage, there may be severe joint stiffness and fixed deformities. The acute symptoms may subside after a year or 18 months, but some degree of pain often persists indefinitely.

Treatment

Treatment should be started as soon as the diagnosis is suspected. Analgesics, anti-inflammatory drugs, ice-packs and active exercises may help. Specific measures include: (1) 'chemical sympathectomy' – intravenous injection of guanethidine diluted with saline; and (2) sympathetic interruption by injection or operation.

Orthopaedic procedures and appliances   12

Orthopaedic operations

To operate on bone requires the tools of a carpenter, yet orthopaedic surgery is not carpentry; biological imperatives ensure that it never can be. The art and skill of orthopaedic surgery is directed not to constructing a particular arrangement of parts, but to restoring function to the whole.

Preparation

PLANNING Operations must be carefully planned in advance, when accurate measurements can be made and bones can be compared for symmetry with those of the opposite limb.

STERILITY The need for sterility is even greater in bone surgery than in soft-tissue surgery; any wound infection represents a setback, but bone infection can be a disaster. For major operations, prophylactic antibiotics and special clean-air theatres are desirable.

EQUIPMENT Basic orthopaedic instruments include drills (for boring holes), osteotomes (for cutting cancellous bone), saws (for cutting cortical bone), chisels (for shaping bone), gouges (for scooping out bone) and implants (for fixing bone). Operations such as joint replacement, spinal fusion and the various types of internal fixation require special instruments to ensure that the implants are correctly aligned and fixed.

THE 'BLOODLESS FIELD' Many operations on limbs can be done more rapidly and accurately if bleeding is prevented by a tourniquet. This should always be a pneumatic cuff, applied over bulky soft tissues to prevent nerve pressure, inflated to not more than 100 mmHg above the systolic pressure and removed within 2 hours; whenever practicable it should be removed before the wound is closed, so that bleeding can be controlled and a 'silent' postoperative haematoma avoided. Excessive or prolonged pressure can cause permanent nerve or muscle damage.

Basic procedures

DRILLING Drilling may be necessary simply to evacuate a bone abscess; most commonly, however, the drill is used to prepare seat-holes for screws.

CUTTING Cancellous bone can be cut with an osteotome; the tapered edge cleaves soft bone, but may shatter cortical bone. The tubular shaft, therefore, is cut with a motorized saw.

MODELLING The bone surface can be shaped with a chisel; concave surfaces are more easily worked with a gouge.

REAMING To ream means (literally) to widen. A joint socket, or the medullary cavity of a tubular bone, may need reaming before it will accept a prosthesis or a nail of suitable size.

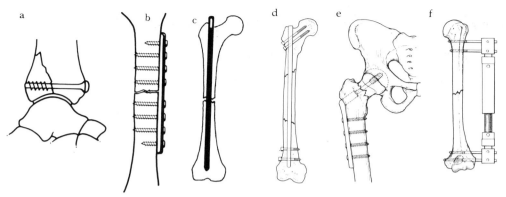

12.1 Some ways of fixing bone   (a) With a single screw – this is a lag screw (threaded only distally) and therefore achieving interfragmentary compression. (b) Plate and screws. (c) Intramedullary nail. (d) Locked intramedullary nail. (e) Dynamic hip screw. (f) External fixator.

FIXING   Bone fragments can be firmly joined by simple *screwing* (especially if a small piece has to be fixed back in position), by attaching a *bridging plate* to the bone with a row of screws, by passing a *long nail* down the medullary canal, by using an *external fixator*, by transfixing the fragments with *pins*, by securing the pieces with *malleable wire*, or by a combination of these methods. All these will eventually loosen or break unless natural union occurs.

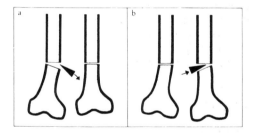

12.2 Osteotomy   A bent bone can be straightened (a) by removing a wedge of bone, or (b) by inserting one: (a) is sometimes called a 'closing wedge osteotomy' – it is easier but leaves the bone shorter; (b) is an 'opening wedge' – it maintains length but may be more difficult to do.

Operations on bones

Osteotomy

Osteotomy may be used to correct deformity, to change the shape of the bone or to relieve pain in arthritis. Preoperative planning is essential, with precise measurements of the patient and the x-rays. To correct an angular deformity a wedge of bone may have to be removed ('closing wedge') or inserted ('opening wedge'). The size of the wedge should be calculated accurately and reproduced on a template for use during the operation. After the bone is divided, it is fixed in its new position, usually with a plate and screws.

Bone grafts

Bone grafts serve two purposes: (1) they can replace missing bone and (2) they can stimulate osteogenesis and are therefore useful in treating ununited fractures.

Autografts   Bone taken from the patient himself has the best chance of survival and incorporation. Most of the transplanted bone dies, but it stimulates new bone ingrowth (osteoinduction) and acts as a scaffold upon which new bone is laid down (osteoconduction). Cancellous bone is more readily incorporated than cortical bone. In certain sites

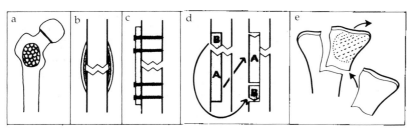

12.3 Bone grafts   (a) Chip grafts to fill a cavity; (b) onlay strips of cancellous bone (Phemister technique); (c) onlay cortical graft; (d) sliding graft; (e) cadaveric osteo-cartilaginous graft.

the graft may be transferred with its blood supply intact; the small vessels are anastomosed by microsurgical techniques.

Allografts (homografts)   Bone transferred from one individual to another of the same species is immunologically less than ideal. The advantage is that allografts are plentiful and can be stored. Osteocartilaginous grafts from fresh cadavers can be used to replace segments of bone after local resection of tumours.

Antigenicity can be reduced by freezing or demineralization and osteoinduction can be enhanced by impregnating the graft with host marrow. The biggest problem is sterility and especially the effort to exclude HIV in the donor material.

APPLICATIONS   Cancellous grafts are used for filling cavities, augmenting fracture healing and promoting arthrodesis. Cortical grafts – preferably on a vascular pedicle – are used where stability is important or to replace missing segments of bone.

Fixation of fractures

INTERNAL FIXATION with screws, plates or intramedullary nails enables a reduced fracture to be held so securely that activity (although not necessarily weight-bearing) can begin immediately. It is particularly useful for fractures in elderly patients, those with multiple injuries or who are difficult to nurse, and for fractures (e.g. of the

ankle and forearm in adults) which are prone to malunion. Scrupulous asepsis and meticulous technique are imperative.

EXTERNAL FIXATION is used for fractures associated with severe soft-tissue injuries and for the treatment of non-union. The principles are straightforward: metal pins are driven through the bone above and below the fracture; the fracture is reduced and the pins are attached to bars which hold the bone rigid while leaving the soft tissues exposed and accessible for treatment (see Figure 12.1(f)). In practice there are numerous variations in pin and frame configuration, aiming to provide the best mechanical system for the particular fracture. Modifications in design have extended the use of external fixation to the management of non-union, bone elongation, repair of bone defects and correction of deformities.

Leg equalization

Inequality of leg length amounting to more than 2.5 cm needs treatment. There are two possibilities:

1. LENGTHENING THE SHORTER LEG
The simplest and safest method is a raised shoe. The alternative is operation, by which 10 cm of length can be gained in the tibia or femur. Two methods are used:

Callotasis   The bone is osteotomized and, as callus forms, the fragments are slowly

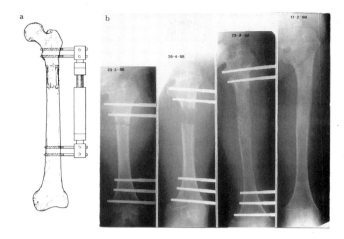

12.4 Leg length equalization – callotasis   At any age, lengthening can be achieved by callotasis (callus 'stretching') after osteotomy. (a) Shows one technique. (b) 10 cm was gained in this achondroplastic patient. (Courtesy of Mr M. Saleh.)

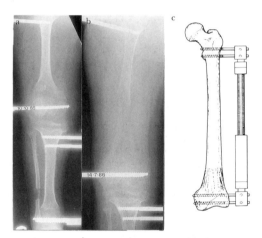

12.5 Leg length equalization – chondrodiatasis The shorter leg can, in a child, be lengthened by (a, b) chondrodiatasis; the interval between the two films is 9 months. (Courtesy of Mr M. Saleh.) The drawing (c) shows where the growth plate has been 'stretched'.

Chondrodiatasis   In children an external fixator can be used to distract the growth plate. Ossification follows in the elongated segment. The principles are the same as for callotasis.

2. SHORTENING THE LONGER LEG
In children, growth in the normal leg can be stopped by arresting the activity of the epiphyseal plate; this can be temporary, using staples, or permanent, using bone grafts. In adults a piece of bone can be excised and the approximated ends held by internal fixation. The drawback with this approach is that the normal leg is placed at risk; should serious complications ensue, the patient may literally not 'have a leg to stand on'.

distracted by skeletal pins in an external fixator. Distraction must be gradual (not more than 1 mm a day) to avoid non-union or damage to nerves and vessels. When the desired length is reached, the fixator is left undisturbed for a further 3 or 4 weeks, after which weightbearing is permitted. When the bone looks solid on x-ray, the fixator is removed.

Operations on joints

Arthroscopy

The interior of a joint can be visualized by inserting an endoscope through a minute incision. In addition, certain operative procedures can be performed by introducing special instruments through separate portals.

Arthrotomy

Arthrotomy (opening a joint) may be indicated: (1) to inspect the interior or perform a synovial biopsy; (2) to drain a haematoma or an abscess; (3) to remove a loose body or damaged structure (e.g. a torn meniscus), and (4) to excise inflamed synovium (synovectomy).

Realignment osteotomy

This is a useful way of treating painful osteoarthritis of the hip or knee when the disease is too mild or the patient too young to consider total joint replacement. The bone is osteotomized close to the affected joint and the articular surface is realigned so that a less damaged segment is exposed to weightbearing. Often there is immediate pain relief, which can be explained only by postulating that bone transection causes a reduction in intraosseous pressure.

An important part of the procedure is the preoperative planning – working out, from x-rays, the precise angles and wedges that will have to be cut in order to achieve the desired position of the joint surfaces.

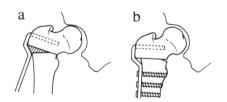

12.6 Joint realignment   (a) The joint space is not congruent; (b) an osteotomy has realigned it – now it is nearly equal throughout.

After the bone is divided and repositioned, the fragments are held with internal fixation. Bone union usually occurs within 3 months.

Arthrodesis

The most reliable operation for a painful or unstable joint is arthrodesis; where stiffness does not seriously affect function, this is often the treatment of choice (e.g. in the spine, the tarsus, the ankle and the wrist). Arthrodesis is useful also for a knee which is already stiff but painful (provided the other knee has good movement) and for a flail shoulder. More controversial is arthrodesis of the hip. It is difficult to convey to the patient that a fused hip can still 'move' by virtue of pelvic tilting and rotation: the best approach is to introduce the patient to someone who has had a successful arthrodesis.

The principles of the operation are straightforward: (1) both joint surfaces are denuded of cartilage; (2) they are apposed in the optimum position and held by some form of fixation; (3) bone grafts are added in the larger joints to promote osseous bridging; and (4) the limb is usually splinted until union is complete (3–6 months).

Arthroplasty

Arthroplasty aims to relieve pain and to retain or restore movement. The following are the main varieties.

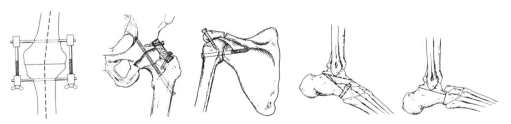

12.7 Arthrodesis   Methods used for the knee, hip, shoulder and foot.

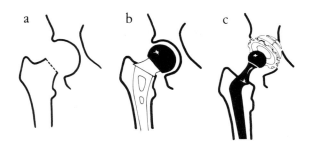

12.8 Arthroplasty The main varieties as applied to the hip joint: (a) excision arthroplasty (Girdlestone); (b) partial replacement – an Austin Moore prosthesis has been inserted after removing the femoral head; (c) total replacement.

EXCISION ARTHROPLASTY Sufficient bone is excised to create a gap at which movement can occur (e.g. Girdlestone's hip arthroplasty).

PARTIAL REPLACEMENT Only one articular surface (or part of the surface) is replaced by a prosthesis (e.g. Moore's prosthesis for a fractured femoral neck). The prosthesis is kept in position either by acrylic cement or by a cementless fit between implant and bone.

TOTAL REPLACEMENT Both articular surfaces are replaced by prosthetic implants; for mechanical reasons, the convex component is usually of metal or ceramic and the concave of high-density polyethylene. They are fixed to the host bone either with acrylic cement or by a cementless press-fit technique.

Total replacement has been spectacularly successful at the hip and the knee. However, the dangers of loosening and infection, and the problems of redoing the operation successfully, dictate that total joint replacement be reserved for patients over 60 and those whose other disabilities ensure that they will not overstress the prostheses.

Amputations

Indications

Colloquially the indications are three Ds – the limb is Dead, Dangerous or a Damn nuisance.

DEAD (OR DYING) usually from *peripheral vascular disease*, but sometimes following *severe trauma, burns* or *frostbite*.

DANGEROUS because it harbours a *malignant tumour*, or *potentially lethal sepsis* (especially gas gangrene), or because of a *crush injury*, where releasing the compression may result in renal failure (the crush syndrome).

DAMN NUISANCE or worse than no limb at all – because of *pain, gross malformation, recurrent sepsis* or *severe loss of function*.

Site of amputation

Most lower limb amputations are for ischaemic disease and are performed through the site of election below the most distal palpable pulse. The 'sites of election' are determined by the demands of prosthetic design and local function. Too short a stump may tend to slip out of the prosthesis. Too long a stump may have inadequate circulation and can become painful, or ulcerate; moreover, it complicates the incorporation of a joint in the prosthesis. For all that, the skill of the modern prosthetist has made it possible to amputate at almost any site.

Prostheses

All prostheses must fit comfortably; they should also function well and look presentable. The patient accepts and uses a prosthesis much better if it is fitted soon after operation.

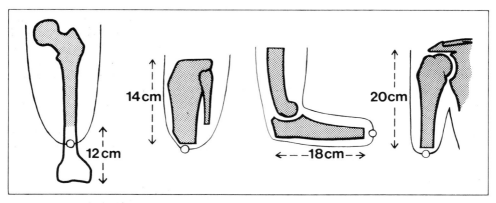

12.9 Amputations (1)   The traditional sites of election; the scar is made terminal because these are not end-bearing stumps.

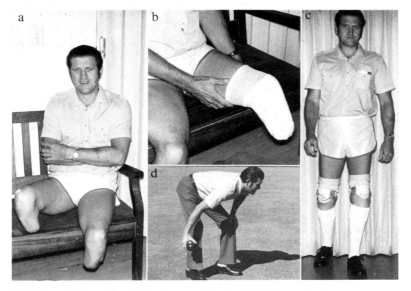

12.10 Amputations (2) – fitting the prosthesis   (a) This man had severe congenital deformities which necessitated bilateral below-knee amputations. (b) A cast was made of each stump, and from this the stump socket was fashioned and fitted into a prosthesis. (c) The prosthesis (held on in this case by straps above the knee) is called 'patellar-tendon-bearing', but most of the weight is taken on the femoral condyles. (d) After rehabilitation he has excellent balance and resumes a near-normal life.

In the upper limb, the distal portion of the prosthesis is detachable and can be replaced by a 'dress hand' or by a variety of useful gadgets.

In the lower limb, weight can be transmitted through the ischial tuberosity, the patellar tendon, the upper tibia or the soft tissues. The prosthesis is held on by braces, or a belt or a tight thigh corset; for above-knee stumps a suction socket is available.

Early complications

In addition to the complications of any operation, there are two special hazards.

1. Breakdown of skin flaps This may be due to ischaemia or to suturing under excessive tension.

2. Gas gangrene *Clostridia* and spores from the perineum may infect a high above-knee amputation, especially if performed through ischaemic tissue.

Late complications

ARTERY Poor circulation gives a cold, blue stump which is liable to ulcerate. This problem chiefly arises with below-knee amputations and often reamputation is necessary.

NERVE A cut nerve always forms a bulb and occasionally this is painful and tender. The treatment is either to excise 3 cm of the nerve well above the bulb or to free the nerve sheath and seal it with a tissue adhesive.

'Phantom limb' is the term used to describe the feeling that the amputated limb is still present. The patient should be warned of the possibility; eventually the feeling recedes or disappears.

Postoperative complications

The important general complications of orthopaedic operations are discussed below. Complications related to particular operations are more properly dealt with in specialized texts on operative surgery.

Soft-tissue swelling

Swelling is common after operations on the limbs and its effects are often aggravated by tight dressings or plaster casts. This may prove a threat to wound healing and will delay the recovery of joint movement. In the worst cases it may interfere with vascular perfusion and give rise to an ischaemic compartment syndrome (see page 257). Prevention is all important: 1. Dressings should be snug but not tight. 2. The limb should be elevated. 3. Movements should be encouraged. 4. If a cast is used, it should be well padded or split.

Haematoma formation

Postoperative bleeding or oozing from cut surfaces may be considerable. Haematoma formation is reduced by adequate suction drainage; however, this should not be too vigorous or prolonged, lest it encourages further bleeding.

Delayed wound healing

Poor peripheral circulation may cause delayed healing or breakdown of the wound. The circulation should always be checked before any operation is undertaken.

Infection

Postoperative infection is always a nuisance; in joint replacement surgery it may be a disaster. The subject is dealt with on page 16.

Thromboembolism

The incidence of postoperative deep vein thrombosis (DVT) is at least 20%; 2% of patients (mainly those with femoral or pelvic vein thrombosis) will develop pulmonary embolism and 0.2% will die of this. The highest incidence is seen after hip surgery, where these figures are more than doubled. Other high risk factors are advanced age, prolonged illness, cardiovascular disease and a previous history of venous problems.

The patient may complain of pain in the calf or thigh. However, thrombosis is usually 'silent', so following an operation (or trauma) even those who do not complain should be examined for swelling, soft-tissue tenderness and a sudden slight increase in temperature and pulse rate; in calf vein thrombosis there may be increased pain on dorsiflexion of the foot (Homan's sign). The diagnosis can be confirmed by ascending venography. Duplex ultrasound scanning is highly accurate for proximal DVT, the usual prelude to pulmonary embolism.

Most patients with pulmonary embolism have no symptoms. A minority have chest pain, dyspnoea or haemoptysis; occasionally this leads rapidly to cardiovascular collapse and death. If there are warning symptoms, and in all cases of thigh thrombosis, the chest should be examined. The diagnosis is readily confirmed by advanced scintigraphic techniques.

Prevention

The risk of DVT can be reduced by physical measures such as elevation of the foot of the bed, elastic or graduated compression stockings, and above all early exercises and mobilization. Prophylactic anticoagulation with fractionated heparin is effective, but it causes increased bleeding and is therefore not used as widely as it might be.

Treatment

Calf vein DVT can be treated simply by applying elastic stockings and giving low-dose subcutaneous heparin (5000 units three times a day) until the patient is fully mobile; there is only a small risk of pulmonary embolism. Thigh vein thrombosis is much more ominous and calls for immediate full anticoagulation, first with heparin (for 5–7 days) and thereafter with warfarin for at least 3 months. Confirmed pulmonary embolism demands cardiorespiratory resuscitation, vasopressors for shock, oxygen and large doses of heparin. Streptokinase can be used to prevent further embolization and antibiotics are given to forestall lung infection.

Physiotherapy

Physiotherapy has a valued place in the management of orthopaedic disorders. It is employed to reduce pain, increase mobility, strengthen muscles and restore function.

Heat

The time-honoured method of alleviating pain and muscle spasm is by applying heat directly to the skin (hot packs, heat pads or simple radiation). The deeper tissues can be reached effectively by short wave diathermy or ultrasonic vibration.

Cold

Ice packs can relieve pain and reduce swelling. They are especially useful in managing shoulder, hand and ankle injuries.

Transcutaneous nerve stimulation (TNS)

Electrical stimulation over a painful area may provide unexpected relief. It is sometimes employed when simpler methods fail. Patients can treat themselves at home using small portable sets.

Traction

Intermittent spinal traction is sometimes helpful in relieving neck or low back pain. This implies that relatively small degrees of distraction may significantly alter the mechanics (and the pain responses) in abnormal spinal segments.

Manipulation

Physiotherapists have become very skilled at moving or manipulating small segments of the vertebral column. This is a useful technique for the treatment of painful instability and facet joint dysfunction. Mobilization is also employed for painful peripheral joints.

Continuous passive movement (CPM)

Passive mobilization can be applied by machines that control precisely the speed and range of movement throughout the day. CPM machines are used especially after injuries or operations on joints, where stiffness is likely to be a problem (e.g. following a tibial plateau fracture or total knee replacement).

Electrical stimulation and exercises

Where there is obvious muscle weakness, electrical stimulation can restore muscle bulk and power; active exercises are, however, more effective. These techniques are also useful for strengthening normal muscle groups in situations where extra stability is required – e.g. in lumbar spine dysfunction or knee instability. Special techniques, such as proprioceptive neuromuscular facilitation, are valuable in the treatment of cerebral palsy.

Ergonomic training

'Hands-on' alone is not enough. Patients have to be trained to use their bodies in ways that are ergonomically efficient and protective of the underlying pathology. Posture, movements and lifting techniques may have to be modified to suit individual patients.

Occupational therapy

Physiotherapy aims to restore movement and power to a particular part; occupational therapy translates that movement into useful function as part of the individual's daily activity.

Occupational therapy may be purely diversional – keeping the patient happily occupied is a form of psychological rehabilitation. More important, though, is the retraining that permits the patient to use the injured or operated limb for specific tasks in personal care, household activities, work and recreation. This means that, ideally, the occupational therapy department should be equipped to simulate all these activities in a 'real life' manner.

Injections

It is often necessary to enter a joint with a sterile needle, either to aspirate fluid or to instill something into the joint. *Aspiration* may be purely diagnostic (e.g. in the management of suspected joint infection) or partly therapeutic (e.g. relief of a tense haemarthrosis). *Injection*, too, may be used for diagnostic purposes (e.g. in performing arthrography); usually, though, it means instillation of an antibiotic or corticosteroid preparation into an infected or inflamed joint. Corticosteroid injections should be used only for the treatment of painful synovitis and should not be repeated more than three times over a period of 6 months. Although the injected preparation is called a 'depot steroid', some of it is absorbed and systemic effects are usual. All injections should be performed with full aseptic precautions.

Injections of corticosteroids into bursae (e.g. for subacromial bursitis) and into the soft tissues (e.g. for tennis elbow) are often helpful.

Functional aids

The *walking stick* or cane is the prototypical, universal functional aid. It doesn't take a degree in biomechanics to know instinctively that leaning on a stick will reduce the load on one side of the body and so diminish pain associated with weightbearing. What is more difficult to recognize (and even doctors often miss the point) is that with hip disorders the stick must be used on the side opposite to the painful limb. *Crutches* provide even greater load reduction, and *walking frames* have the added advantage of stability.

Upper limb aids, limited in variety only by the ingenuity of their inventors, are available: handles that make cutlery, taps and door-knobs more manageable; extending 'slip-ons' that help with putting on socks and shoes; long pincers that can reach the floor for those who cannot bend down; and many more.

Appliances

Gone are the days when struts, corsets and braces were the mainstay of orthopaedic treatment. Paralysed limbs are less common than before, and deformed or unstable joints can be managed by reconstructive surgery. Yet appliances are still useful where more radical methods are contraindicated, and in some parts of the world they are the *only* methods available.

Appliances are prescribed for 4 purposes: (1) protection, (2) lengthening, (3) splintage and (4) stabilization. Usually they are employed as stand-ins while recovery or more definitive treatment is awaited. Often, though, they prove so useful that patients prefer them to operation. The most common examples are described below.

Collars

Collars are used to provide rest or partial splintage of a painful neck. With soft-tissue sprains, or even disc lesions, a soft collar is usually sufficient. For more severe injuries (including stable fractures), a rigid brace is preferable; it is usually worn for 6–8 weeks.

Spinal supports

A rigid spinal brace may be used to alleviate pain and prevent deformity after stable vertebral injuries, in the management of infection or metastatic disease, or after spinal fusion. Specialized braces are also used in the management of scoliosis. Soft supports (corsets) are sometimes prescribed for disc lesions or non-specific low back pain; they obviously cannot immobilize the spine but they restrict movement by compressing the soft tissues into a less flexible tube. All of these should be regarded as temporary measures; if continued for too long they weaken the muscles, reduce mobility and predispose to vertebral osteoporosis.

Footwear

Custom-made shoes and boots, capacious enough to accommodate severe toe deformities or misshapen feet, will protect against abnormal pressure and strain. They are particularly useful in the management of rheumatoid deformities and may avoid the need for operation.*

Elevation of the sole and heel is the easiest way to correct asymmetrical shortening, but patients will rarely tolerate more than a 4 cm raise.

Perhaps the commonest appliance of all is the insole, a thin platform with moulded elevations to support a flat foot or dropped metatarsal heads.

Orthoses (Gr. 'ortho' = straight or correct)

Orthoses are corrective splints, braces or calipers that are designed to stabilize an unstable joint or an incompletely united fracture. Above-knee metal calipers were frequently prescribed to provide stable knee

*Shoe operations are painless: foot operations are not.

extension for patients with paralysed quadriceps muscles, and below-knee calipers for ankle support. They are still used as temporary measures after injury or operation to protect a weak joint while awaiting full recovery, or where other methods are contraindicated or not available. Lightweight orthoses (e.g. polyethylene drop-foot splints or wrist braces) can be worn under normal clothing.

Part 2   Regional Orthopaedics

Examination

Symptoms

Pain from the shoulder or its surrounding tendons is felt anterolaterally and at the insertion of the deltoid; sometimes it radiates down the arm. Pain on top of the shoulder suggests acromioclavicular dysfunction or a cervical spine disorder. The entire shoulder is a common site of referred pain from the cervical spine, heart, mediastinum and diaphragm. Cardiac ischaemia may cause localized pain in either shoulder.

THE PAINFUL SHOULDER

Referred pain
Cervical spondylosis
Mediastinal pathology
Cardiac ischaemia

Joint disorders
Glenohumeral arthritis
Acromioclavicular arthritis

Rotator cuff disorders
Tendinitis
Rupture
Frozen shoulder

Stiffness may be progressive and severe – so much so as to merit the term 'frozen shoulder'.

Deformity may consist of prominence of the acromioclavicular joint or winging of the scapula.

Loss of function is expressed as inability to reach behind the back and difficulty with combing the hair or dressing.

Signs

The patient should always be examined from in front and from behind. Both upper limbs, the neck and the chest must be visible.

● LOOK

Skin Scars or sinuses are noted; don't forget the axilla!

Shape Asymmetry of the shoulders, winging of the scapula, wasting of the deltoid or short rotators and acromioclavicular dislocation are best seen from behind; joint swelling or wasting of the pectoral muscles is more obvious from in front. A joint effusion may 'point' in the axilla.

Position If the arm is held internally rotated, think of posterior dislocation of the shoulder.

● FEEL

Skin Because the joint is well covered, inflammation rarely influences skin temperature.

The *soft tissues* and *bony points* are carefully palpated, following a mental picture of the anatomy. A helpful routine is to start with the sternoclavicular joint, then follow the clavicle laterally to the acromioclavicular joint and so onto the anterior edge of the acromion and around the acromion to the back of the joint. The supraspinatus tendon lies just below the anterior edge of the acromion.

Tenderness and crepitus can often be accurately localized to a particular structure.

● MOVE

Active movements The patient is asked to raise both arms sideways until the fingers point to the ceiling. Abduction may be: (1)

difficult to initiate; (2) diminished in range; (3) altered in rhythm, the scapula moving too early and creating a shrugging effect.

If movement is painful, the arc of pain must be noted; pain in the mid-range of abduction suggests a minor rotator cuff tear or supraspinatus tendinitis; pain at the end of abduction is often due to acromioclavicular arthritis.

Flexion and extension are examined, asking the patient to raise the arms forwards and then backwards. To test adduction he is asked to move the arm across the front of his body. Rotation is tested: first, with the arms close to the body and the elbows flexed to 90 degrees, the hands are separated as widely as possible (external rotation) and brought together again across the body (internal rotation); then the patient is asked to clasp his fingers behind his neck (external rotation in abduction); then to reach up his back with his fingers (internal rotation in adduction).

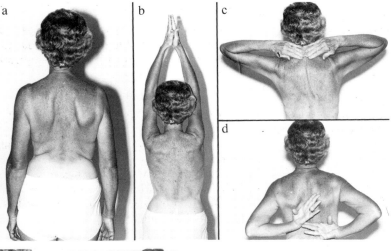

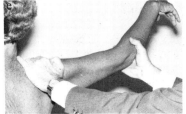

13.1 Examination Small alterations in scapulothoracic and glenohumeral rhythm are best seen from behind. (a) Symmetry of the neck, shoulders and scapulae is assessed. (b) Full abduction (or 'circumduction'), a combination of scapular and glenohumeral movements. (c) Abduction and external rotation. (d) Extension and internal rotation (slightly limited on the right). (e) True glenohumeral movement is gauged by pressing down firmly on the scapula to stop scapulothoracic movement.

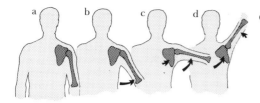

13.2 Scapulohumeral movement (a–c) During the early phase of abduction, most of the movement takes place at the glenohumeral joint. As the arm rises, the scapula begins to rotate on the thorax (c). In the last phase of abduction, movement is almost entirely scapulothoracic (d).

Passive movements These can be deceptive because even with a stiff shoulder the arm can be raised to 90 degrees by scapulothoracic movement. To test true glenohumeral abduction the scapula must first be anchored; this is done by pressing firmly down on the top of the shoulder with one hand while the other hand moves the patient's arm.

Power The deltoid is examined while the patient abducts against resistance. To test serratus anterior (long thoracic nerve, C5, 6, 7) ask the patient to push forcefully against a wall with both hands; if the muscle is weak, the scapula is not stabilized on the thorax and stands out prominently (winged scapula). Pectoralis major is tested by having the patient thrust both hands firmly into the waist.

● IMAGING

At least two x-ray views should be obtained; an AP in the plane of the glenoid, and an axillary projection with the arm in abduction to show the relationship of the humeral head to the glenoid. Look for evidence of subluxation, or dislocation, joint space narrowing, bone erosion and calcification in the soft tissues.

Double contrast arthrography, CT and MRI are useful methods for diagnosing rotator cuff tears or atypical forms of shoulder instability.

● ARTHROSCOPY

Arthroscopy is useful for diagnosing intra-articular lesions, detachment of the glenoid labrum and rotator cuff tears. In some cases the disorder can be dealt with surgically at the same time.

Shoulder deformities

Congenital elevation of the scapula (Sprengel's shoulder)

The scapulae normally complete their descent from the neck by the third month of fetal life; occasionally one remains unduly high. The shoulder on the affected side is elevated; the scapula looks and feels abnormally high, smaller than usual and somewhat prominent. Movements are painless, but abduction may be limited. Associated deformities such as fusion of cervical vertebrae, kyphosis or scoliosis may be present.

Treatment Mild cases are best left untreated. Marked limitation of abduction or severe deformity may necessitate operation to lower the scapula.

Klippel–Feil syndrome

In this rare congenital disorder there is bilateral failure of scapular descent with fusion of several cervical vertebrae. The neck is unusually short and may be webbed; cervical mobility is restricted. The condition is usually left untreated.

Winged scapula

Winging of the scapula causes asymmetry of the shoulders, but may not be obvious until the patient tries to contract the serratus anterior against resistance. Weakness of the serratus anterior may arise from (1) damage to the long thoracic nerve, (2) injury to the

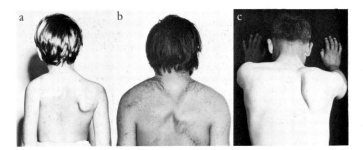

13.3 Scapular disorders
(a) Sprengel shoulder; (b) Klippel–Feil syndrome; (c) winged scapula.

brachial plexus, (3) injury or viral infections of the 5th, 6th and 7th cervical nerve roots, and (4) certain types of muscular dystrophy.

A less obvious type of scapular instability may be caused by weakness of the trapezius following injury of the spinal accessory nerve.

Treatment Disability is usually slight and is best accepted. If function is markedly impaired the scapula can be stabilized by tendon transfer.

Persistent acromioclavicular dislocation

This is a common, though not very troublesome, deformity. An injury (usually on the sports field) causes rupture of the capsule and ligaments around the acromioclavicular joint; the lateral end of the clavicle dislocates and protrudes above the shoulder. If this is not reduced the patient may appear years later with a bony prominence.

Treatment The condition causes little disability and, though operation is feasible, it is seldom indicated (see page 271).

Rotator cuff disorders

The rotator cuff is a sheet of conjoint tendons closely applied over the shoulder capsule and inserting into the greater tuberosity of the humerus. It is made up of subscapularis

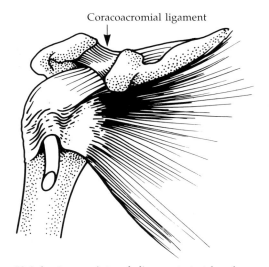

Coracoacromial ligament

13.4 Anatomy A tough ligament stretches from the coracoid to the acromion process; the humeral head moves beneath this arch during abduction and the rotator cuff may be irritated or damaged as it glides in this confined space.

in front, supraspinatus above and infraspinatus and teres minor behind – the 'rotator' muscles, which have an important function in stabilizing the head of the humerus by pulling it firmly into the glenoid whenever the deltoid lifts the arm forwards or sideways.

Arching over the cuff is a fibro-osseous canopy – the coracoacromial arch – formed by the acromion process postero-superiorly, the coracoid process anteriorly and the coracoacromial ligament joining them. Separating the tendons from the arch and

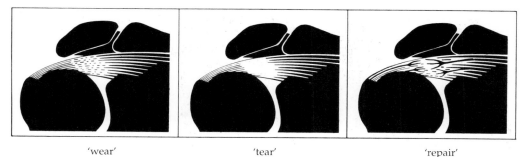

'wear'   'tear'   'repair'

13.5 The pathology of rotator cuff lesions.

allowing them to glide, is the subacromial bursa.

Painful lesions of any of these structures will result in disorganized shoulder movement.

Pathology

The differing clinical pictures stem from three basic pathological processes – degeneration, trauma and vascular reaction.

Degeneration   With advancing age, the cuff degenerates; minute tears develop, and there may be scarring, fibrocartilaginous metaplasia or calcification. The common site is the 'critical zone' of the supraspinatus, the relatively avascular region near its insertion.

Trauma   The supraspinatus tendon is liable to injury if it contracts against firm resistance; this may occur when lifting a weight, or when the patient uses his arm to save himself from falling. This is much more likely if the cuff is already degenerate.

An insidious type of trauma is attrition of the cuff due to impingement against the coracoacromial arch during abduction. The long head of biceps also may be abraded to the point of rupture. Small tears of the cuff or the long head of biceps are found at autopsy in almost everyone aged over 60.

Reaction   In an attempt to repair a torn tendon or to revascularize a degenerate area, new blood vessels grow in and calcium deposits are resorbed. This vascular reaction causes congestion and pain.

WEAR, TEAR AND REPAIR   The three pathological processes may be summed up as 'wear', 'tear' and 'repair'. In the young patient 'repair' is vigorous; consequently, healing is relatively rapid but (because the repair process itself causes pain) it is accompanied by considerable distress. The older patient has more 'wear' but less vigorous 'repair'; healing will be slower but pain less severe. Thus acute tendinitis (which affects younger patients) is intensely painful but rapidly better; chronic tendinitis (a middle group) is only moderately painful but takes many months to recover and may be complicated by partial tears; and a complete tear (which usually occurs in the elderly) becomes painless soon after injury, but never mends.

Acute tendinitis (acute calcification)

Deposits of calcium hydroxyapatite appear in the 'critical zone' of the supraspinatus tendon. Calcification alone is probably not painful; symptoms, when they occur, are due to the florid vascular reaction which produces swelling and tension in the tendon. Resorption of the calcific material is rapid and it may soften or disappear entirely within a few weeks.

Clinical features

An adult, often young, complains of aching, sometimes following overuse. Hourly the pain increases in severity, rising to an

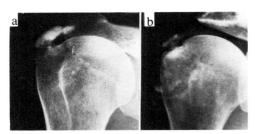

13.6 Acute calcification of supraspinatus The dense mass in the tendon (a) is gradually resorbed or dispersed into the subdeltoid bursa (b).

agonizing climax. After a few days pain subsides and the shoulder gradually returns to normal. During the acute stage the arm is held immobile; the joint is usually too tender to permit palpation or movement.

X-RAY Calcification just above the greater tuberosity is always present. As pain subsides the dense blotch gradually disappears.

Treatment

If symptoms are not very severe the arm is rested in a sling and the patient is given a short course of indomethacin. If pain is more intense a single injection of corticosteroid (methylprednisolone 40 mg) and local anaesthetic (lignocaine 1%) is given into the hypervascular area. If this is not rapidly effective, or if symptoms soon recur, relief can be obtained by an operation at which the calcific material is scooped out.

Chronic tendinitis (the painful arc or impingement syndrome)

Overuse or minor tears of the rotator cuff may initiate a subacute or chronic vascular response in the tendon. Impingement of the rotator cuff against the coracoacromial ligament may play a part in this process.

Clinical features

The patient, usually aged 40–60 years, complains of pain in the shoulder and over the deltoid muscle. It is characteristically worse at night and may be quite severe on attempting certain activities such as putting on a jacket. The shoulder looks normal but is tender just below the anterior edge of the acromion. On abduction, scapulohumeral rhythm is disturbed and pain is aggravated as the arm traverses an arc between 60 and 120 degrees (the 'painful arc'). Repeating the movement with the arm in full external rotation throughout may be much easier and

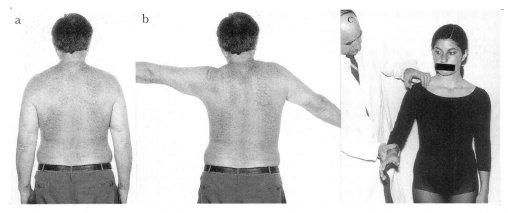

13.7 Supraspinatus tendinitis   (a,b) In abduction, scapulohumeral rhythm is disturbed on the right and the patient has a painful arc starting at about 60 degrees. (c) Supraspinatus tenderness is felt along the anterior edge of the acromion.

relatively painless; this is virtually pathognomonic of supraspinatus tendinitis.

Crepitus or clicking suggests a partial tear of the rotator cuff.

In long-standing cases there is wasting of the muscles and loss of power; movements, especially abduction and external rotation, are restricted.

X-RAYS often show calcification just above the greater tuberosity – a legacy of former events. *MRI* will show changes in the cuff.

Late complications are upward subluxation of the humeral head and osteoarthritis of the shoulder. Sometimes the acromioclavicular joint also is osteoarthritic.

Treatment

Some patients improve with a short course of anti-inflammatory tablets. If this fails,

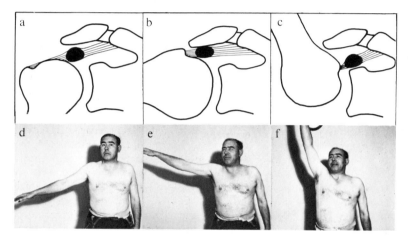

13.8 Painful arc (a–f) The patient registers pain only over a limited arc of abduction, during which the damaged and congested supraspinatus tendon is compressed against the coracoacromial arch (b, e). Before this, and after, the tendon is free in the subacromial space.

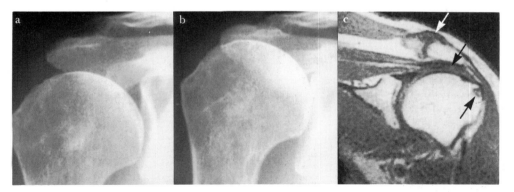

13.9 Chronic tendinitis – imaging (a, b) When the patient attempts to abduct, the head of the humerus rides upwards to abut against the acromion process. Note the marked erosion of the acromioclavicular joint. (c) In another patient, MRI shows thickening of the supraspinatus and an erosion at its insertion. The acromioclavicular joint is also abnormal.

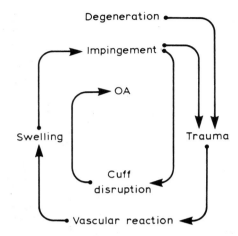

13.10 The vicious spiral of rotator cuff lesions.

local injection of methylprednisolone and lignocaine is tried.

If symptoms keep recurring, operation is advisable. The rotator cuff is 'decompressed' by excising the coracoacromial ligament and part of the acromion. Small tears of the cuff are repaired at the same time.

Rotator cuff disruption

Partial tears of the rotator cuff frequently occur with supraspinatus tendinitis; indeed, it is possible that tendinitis is precipitated by a minor tear.

A complete tear may result from a sudden shoulder strain, or it may appear as a complication of tendinitis or partial rupture. With a partial tear the intact tendon fibres provide continuity and allow vascular ingrowth and repair. With a complete tear there is little or no reaction and no repair; the proximal fibres may retract and become stuck down.

Clinical features

The patient is usually aged 45–75. While lifting a weight or protecting himself from falling he 'sprains' the shoulder. Pain is felt immediately and he is unable to lift the arm sideways.

Often the patient seeks no advice, or is given no effective treatment. If the tear is partial, he may gradually recover, although perhaps with a persistent painful arc of abduction. If the tear is complete the pain soon subsides, but gross weakness of abduction persists.

The appearance is usually normal, but in long-standing cases there is supraspinatus wasting. Tenderness may be diffuse or may be localized to just below the tip of the acromion process. With a recent injury, active abduction is grossly limited and painful. To distinguish between partial and complete tears, pain is abolished by injecting a local anaesthetic; if active abduction is now possible the tear must be only partial.

If some weeks have elapsed since the injury, the two types are easily differentiated. With a complete tear pain has by then subsided and the clinical picture is unmistakable; active abduction is impossible and attempting it produces a characteristic shrug; but passive abduction is full and once the arm has been lifted above a right angle the patient can keep it up by using his deltoid (the 'abduction paradox'); when he lowers it sideways it suddenly drops (the 'drop arm sign'). With a partial tear, abduction slowly recovers.

The diagnosis may be confirmed by ultrasonography, MRI or arthroscopy.

Treatment

In the acute phase treatment is conservative and consists of heat, exercises and one or two injections of local anaesthetic into the tender area.

After 3 weeks it is usually possible to assess the extent of the rupture. *Complete tears* in younger, active individuals, should be repaired; operation is contraindicated in old or sedentary individuals, and in long-standing cases that are painless. *Partial tears* do not require operation unless they cause persistent pain.

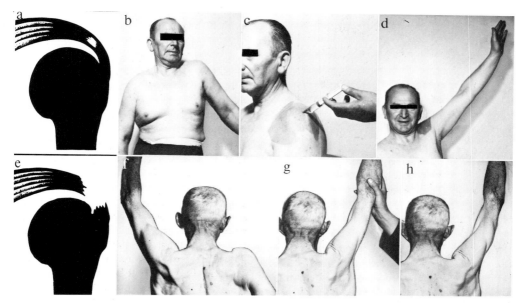

13.11 Torn supraspinatus (a–d) Partial tear of left supraspinatus: the patient can abduct actively once pain has been abolished with local anaesthetic. (e–h) Complete tear of right supraspinatus: active abduction is impossible even when pain subsides (f), or has been abolished by injection; but once the arm is passively abducted (g), the patient can hold it up with his deltoid muscle (h).

Lesions of the biceps tendon

Bicipital tendinitis usually occurs together with rotator cuff impingement; rarely, it presents as an isolated problem in young people after unaccustomed shoulder strain. Tenderness is sharply localized to the bicipital groove.

Rest, local heat and deep transverse frictions usually bring relief; if recovery is delayed, a corticosteroid injection will help.

Tears of the long head of biceps are similar to those of the supraspinatus tendon and are preceded by degeneration and fraying. The patient is usually aged over 50. While lifting, he feels something snap; the shoulder, which previously felt normal, aches for a time and the arm may look bruised. Soon the ache disappears and good function returns, but when the elbow is flexed actively the belly of the muscle contracts into a prominent lump. Function is so little disturbed that treatment is unnecessary.

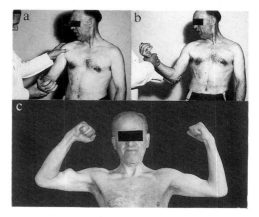

13.12 Biceps tendon Tendinitis: localized tenderness (a), and pain on flexion against resistance (b). (c) Ruptured long head of right biceps: compared with the normal side, the belly of biceps is lower and rounder.

Tears of the distal biceps tendon are rare. They follow an acute flexion strain of the elbow; the tendon is not degenerate but tears cleanly or is avulsed from the radial tuberosity. The diagnosis is often missed: the cardinal features are a suggestive history, pain in the lower forearm, local bruising and loss of power in elbow flexion and supination. If the tendon is not repaired there may be permanent (though not very severe) loss of function.

Adhesive capsulitis (frozen shoulder)

The process probably starts in the same way as a chronic tendinitis but it spreads to involve the entire cuff and joint capsule.

Clinical features

The patient, aged 40–60, may give a history of trauma, often trivial, followed by pain. Gradually it increases in severity and often prevents sleeping on the affected side. After several months it begins to subside, but as it does so stiffness becomes more and more of a problem. Untreated, stiffness persists for another 6–12 months. Gradually movement is regained, but may not return to normal.

Usually there is nothing to see except slight wasting; there may also be some tenderness, but movements are always limited and in a severe case the shoulder is extremely stiff.

X-rays show decreased bone density in the humerus; arthrography shows a contracted joint.

Differential diagnosis

Post-traumatic stiffness After any severe shoulder injury, stiffness may persist for some months. It is maximal at the start and gradually lessens, unlike the pattern of a frozen shoulder.

Disuse stiffness If the arm is nursed overcautiously (e.g. following a forearm

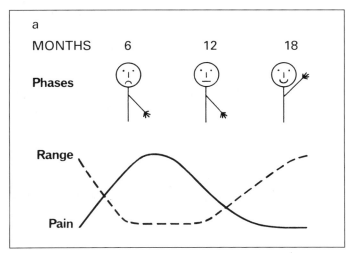

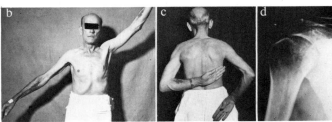

13.13 Frozen shoulder (a) Natural history of frozen shoulder. The face tells the story. (b–d) Patient in phase 2: limited abduction (b); limited internal rotation (c); localized rarefaction (d).

fracture) the shoulder may stiffen. Again, the characteristic pain pattern of a frozen shoulder is absent.

Reflex sympathetic dystrophy Shoulder pain and stiffness may follow myocardial infarction or a stroke. The features are similar to those of a frozen shoulder and it has been suggested that the latter is a form of reflex sympathetic dystrophy.

Treatment

Conservative treatment with analgesics, anti-inflammatory drugs, local heat and exercise aims at relieving pain and preventing further stiffening while recovery is awaited. Injections of corticosteroid and local anaesthetic sometimes help.

Once the acute pain has subsided, manipulation under anaesthesia often hastens recovery. Active exercises should recommence immediately afterwards.

Chronic instability of the shoulder

The shoulder achieves its uniquely wide range of movement at the cost of stability. The shallow glenoid socket is slightly deepened by a fibrocartilaginous labrum and the joint is held secure by the surrounding ligaments and muscles. If these structures give way the shoulder becomes unstable and prone to recurrent dislocation or subluxation.

Anterior dislocation usually follows an acute injury in which the arm is forced into abduction, external rotation and extension. In *recurrent dislocation* the labrum and capsule are often detached from the anterior rim of the glenoid (the classic Bankart lesion).

Anterior subluxation may follow and alternate with episodes of dislocation.

Posterior dislocation is rare; when it occurs it is usually due to a violent jerk in an unusual position, following an epileptic fit or a severe electric shock. Recurrent posterior instability is almost always a *subluxation*, with the humeral head riding back on the posterior lip of the glenoid.

Multidirectional instability is associated with capsular and ligamentous laxity, and sometimes with weakness of the shoulder muscles.

Anterior instability

This is far and away the commonest type of instability, accounting for over 95% of cases.

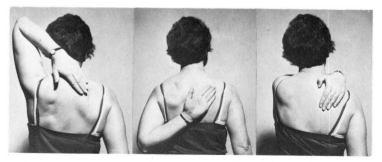

13.14 'Painful shoulder' – the scratch test 'Shoulder' pain may be due to disorders outside the joint (e.g. cervical spondylosis or cardiac ischaemia) or disorders of the shoulder itself (e.g. the rotator cuff syndromes, glenohumeral arthritis, acromioclavicular arthritis or bone disease). If the patient can scratch the opposite scapula in these three ways, the shoulder joint and its tendons are unlikely to be at fault.

Clinical features

The patient is usually a young man who gives a history of his shoulder 'coming out'; he may be able to describe the mechanism precisely: an applied force with the shoulder in abduction, external rotation and extension. This may be the first of many similar episodes: *recurrent dislocation* develops in over 50% of patients under the age of 25 and in about 20% of older patients.

Recurrent subluxation is less obvious. The patient may describe a 'catching' sensation, followed by 'numbness' or 'weakness' – the so-called dead arm syndrome – whenever the shoulder is used in the overhead position (e.g. by throwing a ball, serving at tennis or swimming).

Clinical diagnosis rests on the *apprehension sign*. With the patient seated, the examiner cautiously lifts the arm into abduction, external rotation and then extension; at the crucial moment the patient senses that the humeral head is about to slip out anteriorly and his body tautens in apprehension.

Examination of the other joints may reveal generalized ligamentous laxity.

IMAGING X-rays may show signs of previous dislocation and MRI may reveal a detached glenoid labrum (the Bankart lesion) or deformity of the humeral head.

Treatment

If dislocation recurs at long intervals, the patient may choose to put up with the inconvenience.

The indications for operative treatment are: (1) frequent dislocations, especially if these are painful; and (2) recurrent subluxation or a fear of dislocation sufficient to prevent participation in everyday activities, including sport.

Three types of operation are used: (1) repair or re-attachment of the glenoid labrum (Bankart); (2) shortening and tightening of the anterior capsule (Putti-Platt); and (3) reinforcement of the antero-inferior capsule using adjacent muscles (Bristow).

Posterior instability

Posterior instability usually takes the form of recurrent subluxation rather than full-blown dislocation. The diagnosis is confirmed by x-rays and CT scans.

Treatment is usually conservative – muscle strengthening exercises and voluntary control of the joint. Operative reconstruction is indicated only if disability is marked and there is no gross joint laxity.

(a)   (b)   (c)

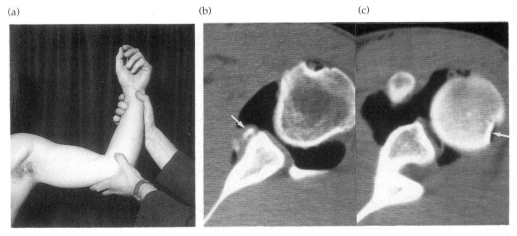

13.15 Anterior instability   (a) Testing for the apprehension sign. MRI may show (b) a Bankart lesion and (c) deformity of the humeral head (the Hill–Sachs lesion).

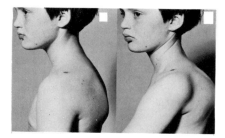

13.16 Habitual subluxation The clue to the diagnosis is the unconcerned expression.

Multidirectional instability

There may be alternating episodes of either anterior or posterior subluxation. Often there is generalized joint laxity and the patient may show a tendency to voluntary or habitual subluxation. Surgical treatment is seldom indicated; muscle strengthening exercises and training in joint control are helpful.

Atraumatic dislocation or subluxation

Displacement of the humeral head can occur even without trauma if there are congenital anatomical abnormalities or ligamentous laxity. The patient can *voluntarily* subluxate or dislocate the shoulder painlessly and can reduce it again; emotionally disturbed patients may find the temptation to do so irresistible. Sometimes displacement occurs so frequently as to justify the term *habitual*. Operative treatment is seldom successful and is best avoided.

Tuberculosis

Tuberculosis of the shoulder is uncommon. It usually starts as an osteitis but is rarely diagnosed until arthritis has supervened. This may proceed to abscess and sinus formation; in some cases fibrous ankylosis

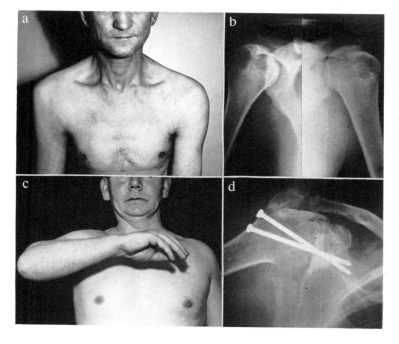

13.17 Tuberculosis (a) Marked wasting of right deltoid. (b) Bone rarefaction and joint damage in arthritis, compared with the normal. After arthrodesis of the glenohumeral joint (c, d) scapulothoracic movement remains, permitting useful abduction.

develops. Patients are usually adults. They complain of a constant ache and stiffness lasting many months. The striking feature is wasting of the muscles around the shoulder. In neglected cases a sinus may be present. There is diffuse warmth and tenderness, and all movements are limited and painful. Axillary lymph nodes may be enlarged.

X-ray Generalized rarefaction is present, usually with erosion of the joint surfaces.

Treatment

In addition to systemic treatment with anti-tuberculous drugs, the shoulder should be rested until acute symptoms have settled. Thereafter movement is encouraged and, provided the articular cartilage is not destroyed, the prognosis for painless function is good. If there are repeated flares, or if the articular surfaces are extensively destroyed, the joint should be arthrodesed.

Rheumatoid arthritis

The acromioclavicular joint, the shoulder joint and the various synovial pouches around the shoulder are frequently involved in rheumatoid disease. Chronic synovitis leads to rupture of the rotator cuff and progressive joint erosion.

Clinical features

The patient, who usually has generalized arthritis, complains of pain in the shoulder and difficulty with tasks such as combing the hair or washing the back.

Active movements are limited, and passive movements are painful and accompanied by marked crepitus. If the supraspinatus is involved the features are similar to those of post-traumatic cuff lesions.

X-RAYS show progressive loss of the cartilage space with periarticular erosions. Often the acromioclavicular joint is involved. Although it may start on one side, the condition usually becomes bilateral.

Treatment

If general measures do not control the synovitis, methylprednisolone may be injected into the joint and the subacromial bursa. If synovitis persists, operative synovectomy is carried out and at the same time cuff tears are repaired. Excision of the

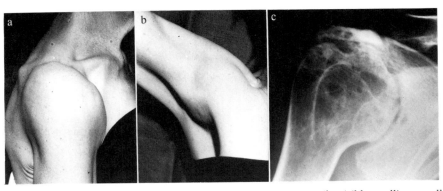

13.18 Rheumatoid arthritis   (a) Large synovial effusions cause easily visible swelling; small ones are likely to be missed – especially if they are present, like this one (b), in the axilla. (c) X-rays show erosion of the joint and of the periarticular bone.

lateral end of the clavicle may relieve acromioclavicular pain.

In advanced cases, pain and stiffness can be very disabling and may call for either arthroplasty or arthrodesis.

Osteoarthritis

Osteoarthritis is usually secondary to congenital dysplasia, local trauma or long-standing rotator cuff lesions. Often chondro-calcinosis is present.

Occasionally with severe cuff tears a rapidly progressive and destructive form of osteoarthritis develops ('Milwaukee shoulder').

Clinical features

The patient is usually aged 50–60 and may give a history of injury or previous painful arc syndrome. There is usually little to see, but shoulder movements are restricted in all directions.

X-rays show distortion of the joint, bone sclerosis and osteophyte formation; the articular 'space' may show calcification.

Treatment

Analgesics and anti-inflammatory drugs relieve pain, and exercises may improve mobility. Most patients manage to live with the restrictions imposed by stiffness, provided pain is not severe.

In advanced cases, if pain becomes intolerable shoulder arthroplasty is justified. It may not improve mobility much, but it does relieve pain. The alternative is arthrodesis.

OSTEOARTHRITIS OF THE ACRO-MIOCLAVICULAR JOINT is common in old people and causes a painful swelling over the top of the shoulder. If analgesics are ineffectual, pain may be relieved by excision of the lateral end of the clavicle.

The elbow

Examination

Symptoms

Pain localized to the medial or lateral condyle is usually due to tendinitis. Pain arising in the joint is more diffuse.

Stiffness, if severe, can be very disabling; the patient may be unable to reach up to the mouth (loss of flexion) or the perineum (loss of extension); limited supination makes it difficult to hold something in the palm or to carry large objects.

Swelling may be due to injury or inflammation; a soft lump on the back of the elbow suggests an olecranon bursitis.

THE PAINFUL ELBOW

Referred pain
Cervical spondylosis

Joint disorders
Rheumatoid arthritis

Periarticular disorders
Olecranon bursitis
Lateral epicondylitis ('tennis elbow')
Medial epicondylitis ('golfer's elbow')

Instability is not uncommon in the late stage of rheumatoid arthritis.

Ulnar nerve symptoms (tingling, numbness and weakness of the hand) may occur in elbow disorders because the nerve is so near the joint.

Signs

Both upper limbs must be completely exposed.

● LOOK

With the arms held alongside the body, varus or valgus deformity is usually obvious. With the arms elevated, palms downwards, wasting or lumps are easily seen.

● FEEL

The back of the joint is palpated for warmth, subcutaneous nodules, synovial thickening and fluid (fluctuation on each side of the olecranon); the back and sides are felt for tenderness and to determine whether the bony points are correctly placed.

The joint line can be located laterally by feeling for the head of the radius (pronating and supinating the forearm makes this easier), but medially it is difficult to find.

The ulnar nerve is fairly superficial behind the medial condyle and here it can be rolled under the fingers to feel if it is thickened or hypersensitive.

● MOVE

Flexion and extension are compared on the two sides. Then, with the elbows tucked into

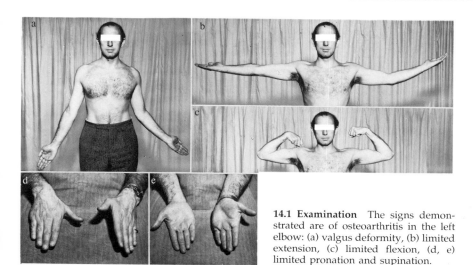

14.1 Examination The signs demonstrated are of osteoarthritis in the left elbow: (a) valgus deformity, (b) limited extension, (c) limited flexion, (d, e) limited pronation and supination.

the sides and flexed to a right angle, the radioulnar joints are tested for pronation and supination.

● X-RAY

The position of each bone is noted, then the joint line and space. Next, the individual bones are inspected for evidence of old injury or bone destruction. Finally, loose bodies are sought.

NOTE   Where appropriate, other parts are examined: the neck (for cervical disc lesions), the shoulder (for cuff lesions) and the hand (for nerve lesions).

Elbow deformities

Cubitus varus

Varus (or 'gun-stock') deformity is most obvious when the elbow is extended and the arms are elevated. The most common cause is malunion of a supracondylar fracture. The deformity can be corrected by a wedge osteotomy of the lower humerus.

Cubitus valgus

The most common cause is non-union of a fractured lateral condyle; this may give

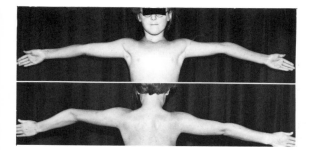

14.2 Cubitus varus This ugly deformity, the sequel to a supracondylar fracture, was later corrected by osteotomy.

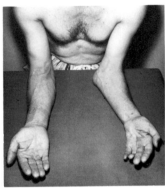

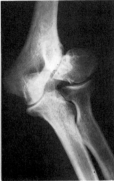

14.3 Cubitus valgus This man's valgus deformity, the sequel to an un-united fracture of the lateral condyle, has resulted in ulnar nerve palsy.

gross deformity and a bony knob on the inner side of the joint. The importance of valgus deformity is the liability for delayed ulnar palsy to develop; years after the causal injury the patient notices weakness of the hand with numbness and tingling of the ulnar fingers. The deformity itself needs no treatment, but for delayed ulnar palsy the nerve should be transposed to the front of the elbow.

Tuberculosis

Although the disease begins as synovitis or osteomyelitis, tuberculosis of the elbow is rarely seen until arthritis supervenes. The onset is insidious with a long history of aching and stiffness. The most striking physical sign is the marked wasting. While the disease is active the joint is held flexed, looks swollen, feels warm and diffusely

tender; movement is considerably limited and accompanied by pain and spasm.

X-rays show generalized rarefaction and often an apparent increase of joint space because of bone erosion.

In addition to antituberculous drugs, the elbow is rested, at first in a splint but later simply by applying a collar and cuff. Surgical debridement is rarely needed.

Rheumatoid arthritis

The elbow is involved in more than 50 per cent of patients with rheumatoid arthritis. There is pain and tenderness, especially around the head of the radius. Eventually the whole elbow may become swollen and stiff. Often both elbows are affected.

X-rays show bone erosion, with gradual destruction of the radial head and widening of the trochlear notch of the ulna.

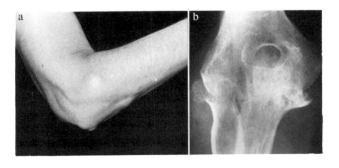

14.4 Rheumatoid arthritis (a) This rheumatoid patient has nodules over the olecranon and a bulge over the radiohumeral joint; (b) his x-rays show deformity of the radial head and marked erosion of the rest of the elbow.

Treatment

In addition to general treatment, the elbow should be splinted during periods of active synovitis. For chronic, painful arthritis of the radiohumeral joint, resection of the radial head and partial synovectomy gives good results. If the joint is diffusely involved, arthroplasty may be necessary; the alternative is long-term splintage, but the limitations of movement may be unacceptable.

Osteoarthritis

Osteoarthritis is usually secondary to intra-articular fractures, loose bodies or crystal deposition disorders.

There may be pain and stiffness but the symptoms are usually not severe. Occasionally ulnar palsy is the presenting feature. The joint may look and feel enlarged and movements are somewhat limited. X-rays show diminution of the joint space with bone sclerosis and osteophytes; one or more loose bodies may be seen.

The osteoarthritis itself rarely requires treatment. Loose bodies, however, if they cause locking, should be removed; if there are signs of ulnar neuritis, the nerve should be transposed.

Loose bodies

The commonest cause of a single loose body in the elbow is osteochondritis dissecans of the capitulum. Multiple loose bodies may occur with osteoarthritis or synovial chondromatosis. If the resulting episodes of sudden locking are troublesome, the loose bodies are excised.

Olecranon bursitis

The olecranon bursa sometimes becomes enlarged as a result of pressure or friction. When it is also painful, the cause is more likely to be infection, gout or rheumatoid arthritis.

Gout is suspected if there is a history of previous attacks, if the condition is bilateral, if there are tophi or if x-ray shows calcification in the bursa. Even then it is not easy to

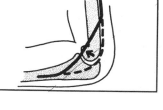

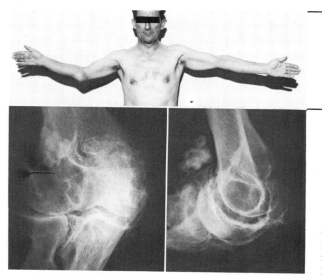

14.5 Osteoarthritis This patient had osteoarthritis and loose bodies in the elbow; the associated ulnar palsy was treated by transposing the nerve (diagram).

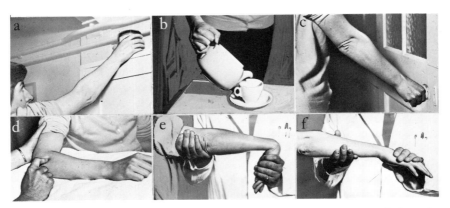

14.6 Tennis elbow Symptoms: (a–c) movements which cause pain – in all three the extensor carpi radialis brevis is in action. Signs: (d) localized tenderness; (e) pain on passive stretching; (f) pain on resisted dorsiflexion.

distinguish from acute infection, unless pus is aspirated.

In rheumatoid arthritis there will be signs of polyarthritis, and subcutaneous nodules may be felt over the olecranon.

The underlying disorder must be treated; septic bursitis may need local drainage. Occasionally a chronically enlarged bursa has to be excised.

Tendinitis of the common extensor origin ('tennis elbow')

The cause of this common disorder is unknown, but it is seldom due to tennis. Most cases probably follow minor trauma to the origin of the wrist extensors and a vascular repair phenomenon similar to that of rotator cuff tendinitis. Often there is a history of unaccustomed activity such as housepainting or carpentry.

Clinical features

Pain is usually localized to the lateral epicondyle, but in severe cases it may radiate widely. It is aggravated by movements such as pouring out tea, turning a stiff door-handle, shaking hands or lifting with the forearm pronated.

The elbow looks normal, and flexion and extension are full and painless. Characteristically there is localized tenderness just below the lateral epicondyle; pain can be reproduced by passively stretching the wrist extensors or actively extending the wrist with the elbow straight.

Treatment

Rest, or avoiding the precipitating activity, may allow the lesion to heal. If pain is severe, the area of maximum tenderness is injected with a mixture of methylprednisolone and lignocaine.

A few cases are sufficiently persistent for operation to be indicated. The origin of the common extensor muscle is detached from the lateral epicondyle.

Golfer's elbow

This condition is comparable to tennis elbow, except that the flexor origin at the medial epicondyle is affected. Treatment is similar.

Examination

Symptoms

Pain may be localized to the radial side (especially in tenovaginitis of the thumb tendons), to the ulnar side (possibly from the radioulnar joint) or to the dorsum (the usual site in disorders of the carpus).

Stiffness is often not noticed until it is severe.

Swelling may signify involvement of either the joint or the tendon sheaths.

Deformity is a late symptom except after trauma.

THE PAINFUL WRIST

Referred pain
Cervical spondylosis

Joint disorders
Infection
RA
OA

Periarticular disorders
de Quervain
Tenosynovitis
Instability

Signs

Examination of the wrist is not complete without also examining the elbow, forearm and hand. Both upper limbs should be completely exposed.

● LOOK

The skin is inspected for scars. Both wrists and forearms are compared to see if there is any deformity. If there is swelling, note whether it is diffuse or localized to one of the tendon sheaths.

● FEEL

Undue warmth is noted. Tender areas must be accurately localized and the bony landmarks compared with those of the normal wrist.

● MOVE

To compare passive dorsiflexion of the wrists the patient places his palms together in a position of prayer, then elevates his elbows. Palmarflexion is estimated in a similar way. Radial and ulnar deviation are measured in the palms-up position. With the elbows at right angles and tucked in to the sides, pronation and supination are assessed. Active movements should be tested against resistance; loss of power may be due to pain, tendon rupture or muscle weakness. Grip strength can be gauged by having the patient squeeze the examiner's hand; mechanical instruments allow more accurate assessment.

● X-RAY

Anteroposterior and lateral views are routinely obtained, and often both wrists must be x-rayed for comparison. Special oblique views are necessary to show up difficult scaphoid fractures. Note the position of the carpal bones and look for evidence of joint space narrowing, especially at the carpometacarpal joint of the thumb.

Wrist deformities

Deformities may be congenital or acquired.

Congenital

Radial club hand   The infant is born with the wrist in marked radial deviation. There is absence of the whole or part of the radius and usually also the thumb. Treatment in the neonate consists of gentle manipulation and splintage. If function deteriorates, centralization of the carpus over the ulna is recommended, preferably before the age of 3 years.

Madelung's deformity   The wrist is deviated forwards, leaving the ulnar head projecting on the back of the wrist. Deformity is seldom marked before the age of 10 years and function is usually excellent. In the worst cases the lower end of the ulna may be excised and the distal radius straightened by osteotomy.

Acquired

Various deformities are seen after *physeal injuries, malunited fractures* or *subluxation of the distal radioulnar joint*. Occasionally osteotomy of the radius or excision of the head of the ulna may be needed.

The typical *rheumatoid deformity* is radial deviation of the wrist, often together with volar subluxation (see below).

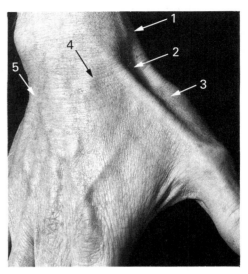

15.1 Tender points at the wrist   The exact site of tenderness may be diagnostic for: (1) de Quervain's disease; (2) scaphoid fracture; (3) carpometacarpal osteoarthritis; (4) tenosynovitis of extensor carpi radialis brevis; (5) tenosynovitis of extensor carpi ulnaris.

Kienböck's disease

After injury or stress, the lunate bone may develop a patchy avascular necrosis. The patient, usually a young adult, complains of ache and stiffness. Tenderness is localized to the centre of the wrist on the dorsum; wrist extension may be limited.

X-rays at first show increased density in the lunate; later the bone looks squashed and irregular.

Treatment   In early cases osteotomy of the radius, to take pressure off the lunate, may prevent bone collapse. In late cases prosthetic replacement, or even wrist arthrodesis, may be necessary.

Tuberculosis

At the wrist, tuberculosis is rarely seen until it has progressed to a true arthritis. Pain and

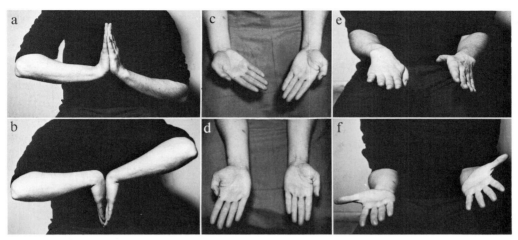

15.2 Movements of the wrist All movements of the left wrist are limited: (a) dorsiflexion, (b) palmarflexion, (c) ulnar deviation, (d) radial deviation, (e) pronation, (f) supination.

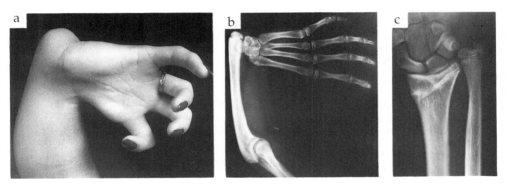

15.3 Deformities (a,b) Radial club hand. (c) X-ray of Madelung's deformity.

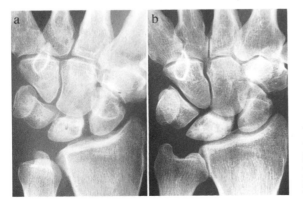

15.4 Kienböck's disease (osteochondritis) (a) Early – the lunate looks mottled and slightly dense. (b) Later – not only is the lunate dense, but also the radiocarpal joint is narrowed. In both these patients the ulna looks slightly short.

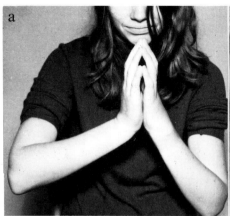
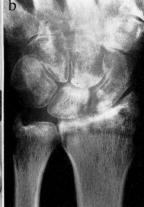

15.5 Tuberculosis (a) This girl presented with chronic ache and swelling of her left wrist; the forearm was wasted and extension absent; (b) her x-ray shows the washed-out appearance of osteoporosis around the wrist.

stiffness come on gradually and the hand feels weak. The forearm looks wasted; the wrist is swollen and feels warm. Involvement of the flexor tendon compartment may give rise to a large fluctuant swelling that crosses the wrist into the palm (compound palmar ganglion). In a neglected case there may be a sinus. Movements are restricted and painful.

X-RAYS show localized osteoporosis and irregularity of the radiocarpal and intercarpal joints, and sometimes bone erosion.

Diagnosis The condition must be differentiated from rheumatoid arthritis. Bilateral arthritis of the wrist is nearly always rheumatoid in origin, but when only one wrist is affected the signs resemble those of tuberculosis. X-rays and serological tests may establish the diagnosis, but often a biopsy is necessary.

Treatment Antituberculous drugs are given and the wrist is splinted. If an abscess forms, it must be drained. If the wrist is destroyed,

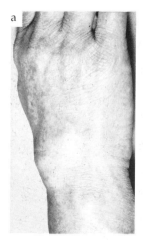
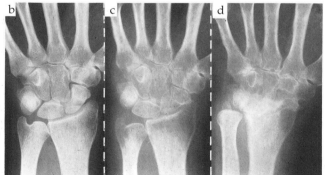

15.6 Rheumatoid arthritis (a) Rheumatoid synovitis of the wrist. (b) At first the x-rays show only soft-tissue swelling; (c) 2 years later, this patient shows early bone changes – periarticular osteoporosis and diminution of the joint spaces; (d) 5 years later still, bony erosions and joint destruction are marked.

systemic treatment should be continued until the disease is quiescent and the wrist is then arthrodesed.

Rheumatoid arthritis

Clinical features

After the metacarpophalangeal joints, the wrist is the most common site of rheumatoid arthritis. Pain, swelling and tenderness may at first be localized to the radioulnar joint, or to one of the tendon sheaths. Sooner or later the whole wrist becomes involved and tenderness is much more ill-defined. In late cases the wrist is deformed and unstable. Extensor tendons may rupture where they cross the dorsum of the wrist, causing one or more of the fingers to drop into flexion.

X-RAYS show osteoporosis and bony erosions. Tell-tale signs are usually obvious in the metacarpophalangeal joints.

Treatment

Management in the early stage consists of splintage and local injection of corticosteroids, combined with systemic treatment.

Persistent synovitis may call for synovectomy and excision of the distal end of the ulna. If deformity has commenced, the wrist should be stabilized by soft-tissue reconstruction. In the late stage joint destruction may require either arthroplasty or arthrodesis.

Chronic carpal instability

This may occur after injury, Kienböck's disease or arthritis. The wrist functions as a system of intercalated segments, stabilized by ligaments and by the scaphoid, which bridges the two rows of carpal bones. Normally the longitudinal axes of the radius, lunate, capitate and third metacarpal form a straight line; if the middle segments collapse this line becomes zig-zag.

Diagnosis

Following an injury (or with a rheumatoid wrist) the patient complains of pain, weakness and sometimes of clicking on movement. There may be localized tenderness, but diagnosis hinges on the x-rays. In scapholunate dissociation, the commonest

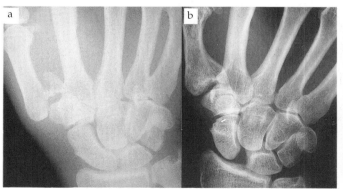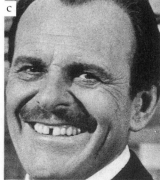

15.7 Carpal instability This patient was first seen after he injured his wrist. (a) The x-ray showed a Bennett's fracture of the base of the first metacarpal and no other injury was apparent. A year later he was still complaining of pain; x-ray at this stage (b) showed a gap between the scaphoid and lunate (the Terry-Thomas sign), (c) The actor, Terry-Thomas (reproduced by permission; © United Artists Inc.).

type of post-traumatic instability, the AP view shows an abnormal gap between the scaphoid and the lunate (the Terry Thomas sign).

The golden rule is never to accept a diagnosis of 'wrist sprain' if, after injury, pain persists for more than a few days.

Treatment

With acute instability the displacement is reduced and held in position in plaster or with K-wires. With chronic instability, treatment is usually conservative: splintage, analgesics and corticosteroid injections. Occasionally operation (arthrodesis) is indicated.

Osteoarthritis

OSTEOARTHRITIS OF THE WRIST is uncommon except as a sequel to injury. Any fracture into the joint may predispose to degeneration, but the most common is a fractured scaphoid, especially with non-union or avascular necrosis. The patient may have forgotten the original injury. Years later he complains of pain and stiffness. The appearance is usually normal and there is no wasting. Movements at the wrist are limited and painful.

X-rays show irregular narrowing at the radiocarpal joint, with bone sclerosis; the proximal portion of the scaphoid or the lunate may be distorted and dense.

Treatment Rest, in a polythene splint, is often sufficient treatment. Excision of the radial styloid process is helpful when osteoarthritis has followed scaphoid injury. Arthrodesis of the wrist is rarely necessary.

OSTEOARTHRITIS OF THE THUMB CARPOMETACARPAL JOINT is quite common in postmenopausal women; it is often acompanied by Heberden's nodes of the finger joints. Pain is more distal than that of de Quervain's disease. There may be swelling or deformity at the base of the thumb metacarpal, and tenderness is sharply localized to the affected joint. Almost invariably the condition is bilateral.

X-rays show narrowing of the space between the trapezium and the thumb metacarpal, often with sclerosis and osteophyte formation.

Treatment If analgesics and local corticosteroid injection do not give relief, operation may be advisable – excision of the trapezium, replacement by a prosthesis or arthrodesis.

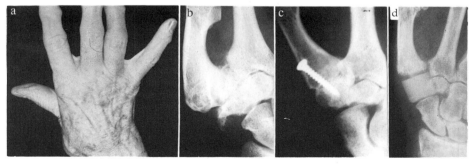

15.8 Osteoarthritis of the carpometacarpal thumb joint (a) Typical deformity in an advanced case, with (b) narrow joint space and osteophytes. (c) Arthrodesis and (d) replacement arthroplasty using a silastic spacer.

Ganglion

The ubiquitous ganglion is seen most commonly on the back of the wrist. It arises from cystic degeneration in the joint capsule or tendon sheath. The distended cyst contains a glairy fluid.

The patient, often a young adult, presents with a painless lump, usually on the back of the wrist. Occasionally there is a slight ache. The lump is well defined, cystic and not tender. It may be attached to one of the tendons.

Treatment may be unnecessary and often the ganglion disappears after some months. If it is troublesome it can be aspirated, and if it recurs, excised.

NOTE: A ganglion should not be confused with rheumatoid tenosynovitis, nor with a 'compound palmar ganglion' in which chronic inflammation distends the flexor tendon sheath above and below the flexor retinaculum.

de Quervain's disease (stenosing tenovaginitis)

The sheath containing the extensor pollicis brevis and abductor pollicis longus becomes inflamed and thickened. Usually this is due to excessive or unaccustomed activity such as pruning roses or wringing out clothes.

Clinical features

The condition is most common in women aged 30–50, who complain of pain on the

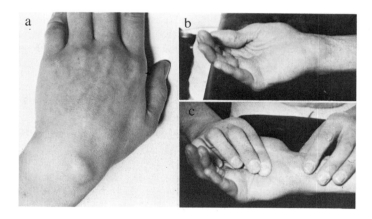

15.9 Wrist swellings (a) Simple ganglion; (b, c) compound palmar ganglion with cross-fluctuation.

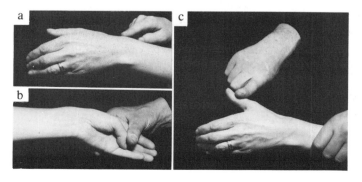

15.10 de Quervain's disease (a) The patient can point to the painful area; (b) forced adduction is painful; (c) pain on active extension against resistance.

radial side of the wrist. There may be swelling along the course of the thumb tendons. The tendon sheath is often thick and hard. Tenderness is most acute at the very tip of the radial styloid. Abduction of the thumb against resistance and passive adduction of the thumb across the palm (Finkelstein's test) are both painful.

Treatment

The early case can be relieved by a corticosteroid injection into the tendon sheath, sometimes combined with plaster splintage of the wrist. Resistant cases need an operation, which consists of slitting the thickened tendon sheath.

Carpal tunnel syndrome

In the normal carpal tunnel there is barely room for all the tendons and the median nerve; consequently any swelling is likely to result in compression and ischaemia of the nerve. Usually the cause eludes detection; the syndrome is, however, common in menopausal women, in rheumatoid arthritis and in pregnancy.

Clinical features

Pain and paraesthesia occur in the distribution of the median nerve in the hand. Night

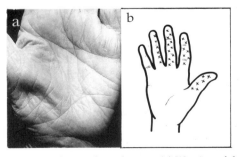

15.11 Carpal tunnel syndrome   (a) Wasting of the thenar muscles; (b) area of sensory abnormality.

after night the patient is woken in the early hours with burning pain, tingling and numbness. Hanging the arm over the side of the bed, or shaking the arm, may relieve the symptoms. During the day little pain is felt except with such activities as knitting or holding a newspaper, where the arms are kept immobile. In advanced cases there may be clumsiness and weakness.

The condition is eight times more common in women than men. The usual age group is 40–50 years; in younger patients it is not uncommon to find related factors such as pregnancy or rheumatoid disease.

Both hands, or only the dominant hand, may be involved. Abnormal physical signs are usually absent; ideally the condition should be diagnosed before signs are obvious. The pattern of sensory change can sometimes be reproduced by holding the wrist fully palmarflexed for 1 minute, or by compressing the arm with a sphygmomanometer cuff. In late cases there is wasting of the thenar muscles and weakness of thumb abduction. Electrical studies show slowing of nerve conduction across the wrist.

Diagnosis

The symptoms of carpal tunnel syndrome are easily mistaken for those of cervical spondylosis involving C6 and C7. X-ray signs of cervical disc degeneration are common in older people and this adds to the confusion. The classic complaint of pain and paraesthesia at night, together with nerve conduction changes, help to establish the diagnosis.

Treatment

In the vast majority of cases, operative division of the anterior carpal ligament offers a quick and simple cure; this can be done open or arthroscopically. Conservative treatment may be preferable during pregnancy; the wrist is splinted at night to prevent it folding into flexion.

The hand

Examination

The hand is (in more senses than one) the medium of introduction to the outside world. Deformity and loss of function are quickly noticed – and often bitterly resented.

Symptoms

Pain is usually felt in the palm or in the finger joints. A poorly defined ache may be referred from the neck, shoulder or mediastinum.

Deformity may appear suddenly (due to tendon rupture) or slowly (suggesting bone or joint pathology).

Swelling may be localized, or may occur in many joints simultaneously. Characteristically, rheumatoid arthritis causes swelling of the proximal joints and osteoarthritis the distal joints.

Loss of function is particularly troublesome in the hand. The patient may have difficulty handling eating utensils, holding a cup or glass, grasping a doorknob (or a crutch), dressing or (most trying of all) attending to personal hygiene.

THE PAINFUL HAND

Referred from
Neck
Shoulder
Mediastinum

Joint disorders
RA
OA

Periarticular disorders
Carpal tunnel
Tenosynovitis
Infection

Signs

Both upper limbs should be bared for comparison. Examination of the hand needs patience and meticulous attention to detail.

● LOOK

The skin may be scarred, altered in colour, dry or moist, and hairy or smooth. Wasting and deformity, and the presence of any lumps, should be noted. The resting posture is an important clue to nerve or tendon damage. Swelling may be in the subcutaneous tissue, in a tendon sheath or in a joint.

● FEEL

The temperature and texture of the skin are noted. If a nodule is felt, the underlying tendon should be moved to discover if it is attached. Swelling or thickening may be in the subcutaneous tissue, a tendon sheath, a joint or one of the bones. Tenderness should be accurately localized to one of these structures.

● MOVE

Active movements With palms facing upwards the patient is asked to curl the fingers into full flexion; a 'lagging finger' is

immediately obvious. Individual movements are then examined, first at the metacarpophalangeal joints and then at each interphalangeal joint in turn.

Passive movements are examined in a similar manner, recording the range of movement at each joint.

● GRIP STRENGTH

Grip strength is assessed by asking the patient to squeeze the examiner's fingers; it may be diminished because of muscle weakness, finger stiffness or wrist instability. Strength can be measured more accurately by having the patient squeeze a partially inflated sphygmomanometer cuff (normally a pressure of 150 mmHg can be achieved easily) or a mechanical dynamometer.

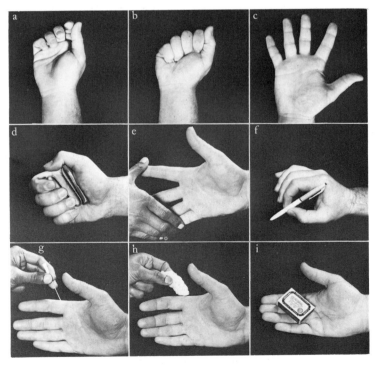

Positions: (a) resting, (b) full flexion, (c) full extension.

Strength: (d) power grip, (e) finger abduction, (f) pinch grip.

Sensation: (g) pin prick, (h) light touch, (i) stereognosis.

16.1 Examination

● NEUROLOGICAL ASSESSMENT

If symptoms such as numbness, tingling or weakness exist – and in all cases of trauma – a full neurological examination of the upper limbs should be carried out, testing power, reflexes and sensation. Further refinement is achieved by testing two-point discrimination, sensibility to heat and cold, and stereognosis.

Congenital deformities

The hand and foot are much the most common sites of congenital deformities of the locomotor system; the incidence is no less than 1 in 2500 live births. Early recognition is important, and definitive treatment should be timed to fit in with the functional demands of the child. There are five types of malformation.

FAILURE OF DEVELOPMENT Total or partial absence of parts may be transverse ('congenital amputations') or axial (missing rays).

FAILURE OF DIFFERENTIATION Fingers may be partly or wholly joined together (syndactyly). This may be corrected by separating the fingers and repairing the defects with skin grafts.

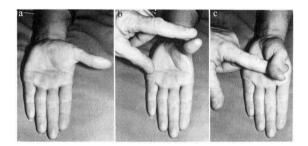

16.2 Movements of the thumb With the hand held flat on the table and palm upwards, the patient is asked (a) to stretch the thumb away from the hand (extension), (b) to lift it towards the ceiling (abduction) and (c) to squeeze down onto the examiner's finger (adduction).

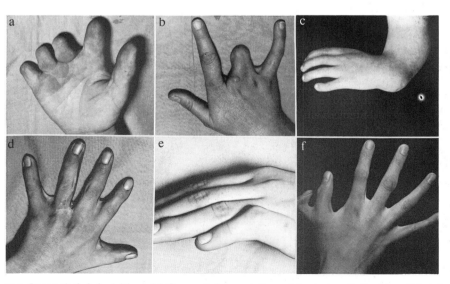

16.3 Congenital deformities (a) Congenital amputations; (b) missing digits; (c) radial club hand; (d) syndactyly; (e) camptodactyly; (f) extra digits.

FOCAL DEFECTS Polydactyly (extra digits) is the most common hand malformation. The extra finger should be amputated, if only for cosmetic reasons.

OVERGROWTH A giant finger is unsightly, but attempts at operative reduction are fraught with complications.

GENERALIZED MALFORMATIONS The hand may be involved in generalized disorders such as Marfan's syndrome ('spider hands') or achondroplasia ('trident hand').

Acquired deformities

Deformity of the hand may be due to disorders of the skin, subcutaneous tissues, muscles, tendons, joints, bones or neuromuscular function.

Skin contracture

Cuts and burns of the palmar skin are liable to heal with contracture; this may cause puckering of the palm or fixed flexion of the fingers. Surgical incisions should never cross flexor creases. Established contractures may require excision of the scar and Z-plasty of the overlying skin.

Dupuytren's contracture

This is a nodular hypertrophy and contracture of the palmar aponeurosis. The condition is familial, but there is a higher than usual incidence in diabetics, in patients with AIDS and in epileptics receiving phenytoin therapy. Occasionally the plantar aponeurosis also is affected.

Clinical features

The patient – usually a middle-aged man – complains of a nodular thickening in the palm. Gradually this extends distally to involve the ring or little finger. Pain may occur but it is seldom a marked feature. Often both hands are involved, one more than the other. The palm is puckered,

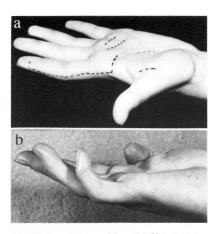

16.4 Deformities – skin   (a) Skin incisions should never cross the creases on the flexor surface; those shown are safe. (b) Postoperative contracture of a badly placed scar.

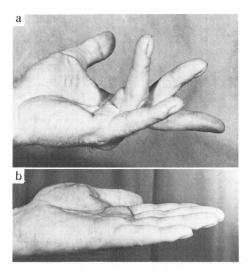

16.5 Dupuytren's contracture   (a, b) Moderately severe contracture before and after fasciotomy.

nodular and thick. If the subcutaneous cords extend into the fingers they may produce flexion deformities at the metacarpophalangeal and proximal interphalangeal joints. Sometimes the dorsal knuckle pads are thickened.

Similar nodules may be seen on the soles of the feet. There is a rare, curious association with fibrosis of the corpus cavernosum (Peyronie's disease).

Diagnosis

Dupuytren's contracture must be distinguished from skin contracture (where the previous laceration is usually obvious) and tendon contracture (where the 'cord' moves on passive flexion of the finger).

Treatment

Operation is indicated if the deformity is progressive. By careful dissection the thickened part of the aponeurosis is excised. A Z-plasty may be needed to lengthen the wound and permit adequate skin closure. Postoperative splintage and physiotherapy are rewarded by the restoration of painless hand function.

Muscle contracture

Ischaemic contracture of the forearm muscles may follow circulatory insufficiency due to injuries at or below the elbow (Volkmann's ischaemic contracture: page 257). There is

shortening of the long flexors; the fingers are held in flexion and can be straightened only when the wrist is flexed. Sometimes the picture is complicated by associated damage to the ulnar or median nerve (or both). If disability is marked, some improvement may be obtained by releasing the shortened muscles at their origin above the elbow, or else by excising the dead muscles and restoring finger movement with tendon transfers.

Shortening of the intrinsic muscles of the hand produces a characteristic deformity: flexion at the metacarpophalangeal joints with extension of the interphalangeal joints and adduction of the thumb. The main causes of intrinsic contracture are spasticity (e.g. in cerebral palsy) and scarring (after trauma or infection). Moderate contracture can be treated by releasing the intrinsic muscles where they cross the metacarpophalangeal joints.

Tendon lesions

'Mallet' finger ('baseball' finger) This results from injury to the extensor tendon of the terminal phalanx. The patient cannot actively straighten the terminal joint, but passive movement is normal. The finger should be splinted for 6 weeks with the distal joint extended and the middle joint flexed, to allow the tendon to reattach.

Ruptured extensor pollicis longus The long thumb extensor may rupture after fraying where it crosses the wrist (e.g. after a Colles' fracture, or in rheumatoid arthritis). Direct

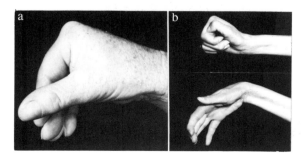

16.6 Deformities – muscle (a) Flexion deformity due to ischaemic contracture of the intrinsic hand muscles (the 'intrinsic-plus' hand). (b) Ischaemic contracture of the long flexors in the forearm; with the wrist in extension, the fingers involuntarily curl into flexion; when the wrist flexes, the pull on the finger flexors is released.

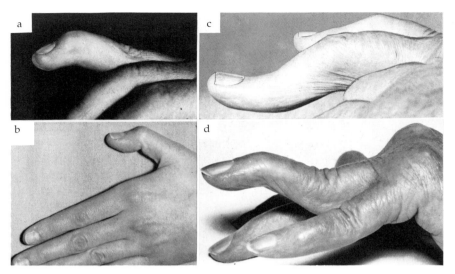

16.7 Deformities – tendons   (a) Mallet finger. (b) Ruptured extensor pollicis longus. (c) Boutonnière. (d) Swan-neck deformity.

repair is unsatisfactory and a tendon transfer, using the extensor indicis, is needed.

Dropped finger   Sudden loss of finger extension at the metacarpophalangeal joint is usually due to tendon rupture at the wrist (e.g. in rheumatoid arthritis). If direct repair is not possible, the distal portion can be attached to an adjacent finger extensor.

Boutonnière   This is a flexion deformity of the proximal interphalangeal joint, due to interruption of the central slip of the extensor tendon. The lateral slips separate and the head of the proximal phalanx pops through the gap like a finger through a buttonhole. It is seen after trauma or in rheumatoid disease. Post-traumatic rupture can sometimes be repaired; the chronic deformity in rheumatoid disease usually defies correction.

Swan-neck deformity   This is the reverse of boutonnière; the proximal interphalangeal joint is hyperextended and the distal interphalangeal joint flexed. It is due to imbalance of extensor versus flexor action in the finger, and is often seen in rheumatoid arthritis. If the joints are mobile, the deformity may be corrected by tendon rebalanc-

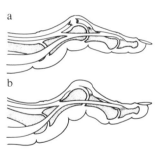

16.8 Deformities – boutonniére   (a) When the middle slip of the extensor tendon first ruptures there is no more than an inability to extend the proximal interphalangeal joint. If it is not repaired, (b) the lateral slips slide towards the volar surface, the knuckle 'buttonholes' the extensor hood, and the distal joint is drawn into hyperextension.

ing and joint stabilization. If the deformity is fixed, surgical treatment is futile.

Bone lesions

Malunited fractures may cause metacarpal or phalangeal deformity. Occasionally this needs correction by osteotomy and internal fixation.

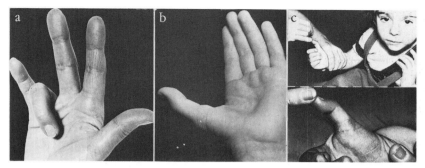

16.9 Stenosing tenovaginitis   (a) Trigger finger; (b) trigger thumb – the only variety which occurs in children, in whom (c) the thumb may be stuck bent.

Stenosing tenovaginitis (trigger finger)

A flexor tendon may become trapped at the entrance to its sheath; on forced extension it passes the constriction with a snap ('triggering'). The usual cause is thickening of the fibrous tendon sheath (often following local trauma or unaccustomed activity), but a similar hold-up may occur in rheumatoid tenosynovitis.

Clinical features

Any digit may be affected, but the ring and middle fingers most commonly. The patient notices that the finger clicks as he bends it; when the hand is unclenched, the affected finger remains bent but with further effort it suddenly straightens with a snap. A tender nodule can be felt in front of the affected sheath.

Treatment

Early cases may be cured by an injection of methylprednisolone carefully placed at the entrance of the tendon sheath. Refractory cases need operation: the fibrous sheath is incised, allowing the tendon to move freely.

Rheumatoid arthritis

The hand, more than any other part of the body, is where rheumatoid arthritis carves its story. Early on there is *synovitis* of the proximal joints and tendon sheaths; later, joint and tendon *erosions* prepare the ground for mechanical derangement; in the final stage joint instability and tendon rupture cause progressive *deformity* and loss of function.

Clinical features (see also page 21)

Pain and stiffness of the fingers are early symptoms; often the wrist also is affected. Examination may show swelling of the metacarpophalangeal and proximal interphalangeal joints; both hands are affected, more or less symmetrically. Joint mobility and grip strength are diminished.

As the disease progresses, deformities begin to appear (and are increasingly difficult to correct). In the late stage one sees the characteristic ulnar deviation of the fingers and subluxation of the metacarpophalangeal joints, often associated with swan-neck or boutonnière deformities. When these abnormalities become fixed, functional loss may be so severe that the patient needs help with washing, dressing and feeding.

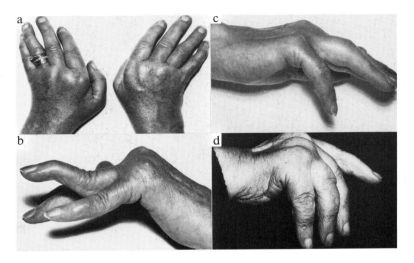

16.10 Rheumatoid arthritis – typical deformities   (a) Ulnar drift; (b) swan-neck deformity; (c) dropped finger; (d) three dropped fingers.

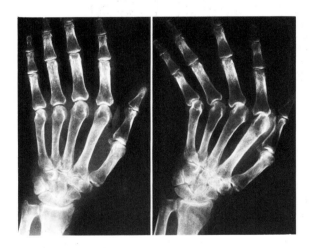

16.11 Rheumatoid arthritis – ulnar drift These x-rays were taken 2 years apart; they show how the progressive finger deformity is accompanied by (perhaps preceded by) an equal and opposite wrist deformity, in which the entire carpus moves ulnarwards and rotates radialwards.

X-RAYS   During the initial stages x-rays show only soft-tissue swelling and osteoporosis around the joints. Later there is narrowing of the joint spaces and small periarticular erosions appear. In the last stage articular destruction may be marked, with joint deformity and dislocation.

Treatment

In early cases treatment is directed at controlling the systemic disease and the local synovitis. In addition to general measures (page 24), splints may reduce pain and swelling and improve mobility. Persistent

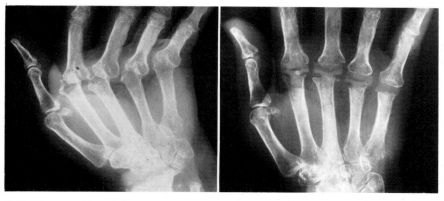

16.12 Rheumatoid arthritis – treatment In advanced rheumatoid arthritis the metacarpophalangeal joints may be completely dislocated, as they were in this patient; joint replacement with flexible Silastic spacers corrected her deformity and restored stability.

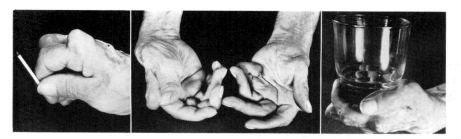

16.13 Rheumatoid arthritis – does it need treatment?   Not always. Why interfere if deformities have been present for years and the hand still works? Despite gross deformity this patient can manipulate tiny objects and large ones.

synovitis may benefit from local injections of methylprednisolone, but sometimes surgical synovectomy is needed.

As the disease progresses it becomes increasingly important to prevent deformity. Uncontrolled synovitis requires synovectomy followed by physiotherapy. Isolated tendon ruptures are repaired or bypassed by appropriate tendon transfers. Joint instability may require stabilization or arthroplasty.

In late cases with established deformities, reconstructive surgery may be needed, but treatment should be directed at restoring function rather than correcting deformity.

Osteoarthritis

Osteoarthritis of the distal interphalangeal joints is very common in postmenopausal women. It often starts with pain in one or two fingers; the distal joints become swollen and tender, the condition usually spreading to all the fingers of both hands. On examination there is bony thickening around the distal interphalangeal joints (Heberden's nodes) and some restriction of movement. Not infrequently some of the proximal interphalangeal joints are involved (Bouchard's nodes) and the carpometacarpal joint of the thumb may show similar changes. *X-rays* show narrowing of the joint spaces and osteophyte formation. *Treatment* is symptomatic; pain and tenderness gradually subside and the patient is left with painless, knobbly fingers.

Acute infections of the hand

Infection of the hand is frequently limited to one of several well-defined compartments: under the nailfold (paronychia); the pulp space (whitlow); subcutaneous tissues elsewhere; the tendon sheaths; and the deep fascial spaces. Almost invariably the cause is a staphylococcus which has been implanted by trivial or unobserved injury.

Clinical features

Usually there is a history of trauma, but it may have been so trivial as to pass unnoticed. A few hours or days later the finger (or hand) becomes painful and swollen. The patient is ill and pyrexial. There is obvious redness and tension in the tissues, and exquisite tenderness over the site of infection. Finger movements may be markedly restricted.

Treatment

The principles of treatment are as follows:

Antibiotics As soon as the diagnosis is made, antibiotic treatment is started – usually with flucloxacillin and, in severe cases, with fusidic acid as well, or, for bite wounds, metronidazole. This may later be changed when bacterial sensitivity is known.

Rest and elevation In a mild case the hand is rested in a sling. In a severe case the arm is elevated in a roller towel while the patient is kept under observation.

Drainage If there are signs of an abscess – throbbing pain, marked tenderness and toxaemia – the pus should be drained. A

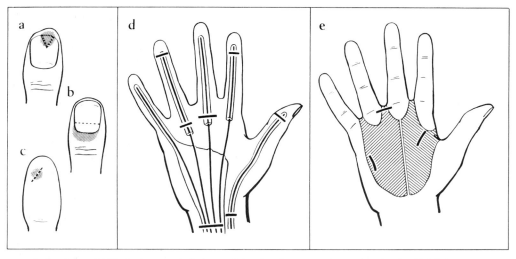

16.14 Infections (a) To drain an apical abscess it is often best to excise a triangle of nail. (b) Acute parony-chia is most efficiently drained by excising the proximal part of the nail. (c) A pulp abscess should be drained over the point of maximal tenderness. (d) Synovial sheath infections can be drained by incisions near their proximal and distal ends. (e) Incisions for web abscess and for the rare infections of the mid-palmar and thenar spaces (partly redrawn from The Infected Hand by D.A. Bailey, published by H.K. Lewis, London).

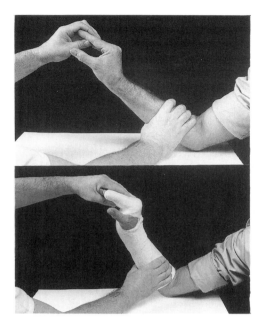

16.15 The 'position of safety' The knuckle joints are 90 degrees fixed, the finger joints extended and the thumb abducted. This is the position in which the ligaments are at their longest and splintage is least likely to result in stiffness.

tourniquet and either general or regional block anaesthesia are essential. The incision should be made at the site of maximal tenderness, but never across a skin crease.

Splintage After draining tendon sheath or fascial space infections, a removable splint should be applied, with the joints in the 'position of safety'.

Individual lesions

PARONYCHIA   Infection under the nail-fold is common. The area is swollen, red and tender. If pus is present it can often be released simply by lifting the nailfold from the nail; otherwise it must be incised. Occasionally a portion of the nail needs to be removed.

WHITLOW   Pulp space infection causes throbbing pain. The fingertip is swollen, red and acutely tender. Early drainage is essential. Under antibiotic cover a small incision over the site of maximal tenderness is usually sufficient.

OTHER   SUBCUTANEOUS   INFEC-TIONS   Anywhere in the hand a blister or superficial cut may become infected, causing redness, swelling and tenderness. A local collection of pus should be drained through a small incision over the site of maximal tenderness. It is important to exclude a deeper pocket of pus in a nearby tendon sheath or in one of the deep fascial spaces.

TENDON   SHEATH   INFECTION Suppurative tenosynovitis is uncommon but dangerous. Unless treatment is swift and effective, the patient may end up with a useless finger. The affected digit is painful and swollen; it is held bent, is very tender and the patient will not move it or permit it to be moved. Pus must be drained through two incisions – one at the proximal end of the sheath and one at the distal end; using a fine catheter the sheath is then irrigated with an antibiotic solution. Delayed healing may be caused by necrosis of the tendon.

Tendon-sheath infection in the thumb or little finger may spread proximally to the synovial bursa. This has to be drained through a further incision just above the wrist.

FASCIAL   SPACES   Infection from a web space or from an infected tendon sheath may spread to either of the deep fascial spaces of the palm. The palm is ballooned, so its normal concavity is lost. There is extensive tenderness and the whole hand is held still. For drainage an incision is made directly over the abscess, and sinus forceps inserted; if the web space also is infected it, too, should be incised.

The neck   17

Examination

Symptoms

The common symptoms of neck disorder are pain and stiffness.

Pain is felt in the neck itself, but it may also be referred to the shoulders or arms.

Stiffness may be either intermittent or continuous. Sometimes it is so severe that the patient can scarcely move the head.

Deformity usually appears as a wry neck; occasionally the neck is fixed in flexion.

Numbness, tingling and weakness in the upper limbs may be due to pressure on a nerve root; weakness in the lower limbs may result from cord compression in the neck.

Headache sometimes emanates from the neck, but if this is the only symptom other causes should be suspected.

Signs

No examination of the neck is complete without examination of both upper limbs. Two arms = one neck; if both arms are affected suspect the neck.

● LOOK

Any deformity is noted. From the back, skin blemishes, scapular abnormalities or muscular asymmetry can be seen. One shoulder may be higher and there may be muscle wasting in the arm or hand.

● FEEL

The neck is examined for tender areas or lumps. Muscle spasm may be felt. The anterior structures (trachea, thyroid, oesophagus) should be carefully palpated.

● MOVE

Forward flexion, extension, lateral flexion and rotation are tested, and then shoulder movements

● NEUROLOGICAL EXAMINATION

Neurological examination of the upper limbs is mandatory in all cases; in some the lower limbs also should be examined. Muscle power, reflexes and sensation should be carefully tested; even small degrees of abnormality may be significant.

● PULSES

The radial pulse is felt with the arm at rest and on traction; it may weaken or disappear if the thoracic outlet is abnormally tight.

● X-RAY

The anteroposterior view should show the regular, undulating outline of the lateral

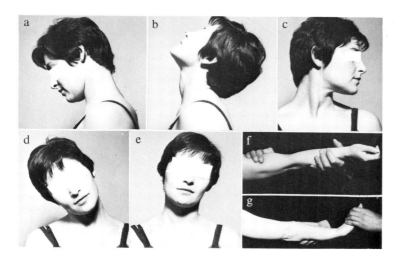

17.1 Examination (a) Flexion; (b) extension; (c) rotation; (d, e) sideways tilt; (f, g) testing power in the elbow and wrist extensors. In this patient with signs of a prolapsed disc, flexion and tilting to the left are limited.

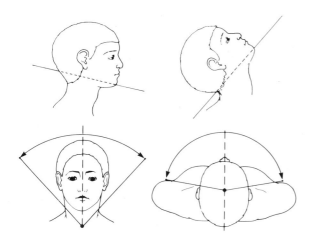

17.2 Normal range of movement In full flexion the chin normally touches the chest; in full extension the imaginary line joining the chin to the posterior occipital protuberance (the occipitomental line) forms an angle of at least 45 degrees with the horizontal, and usually over 60 degrees in young people. Lateral flexion and rotation are equal in both directions.

masses; their symmetry may be disturbed by destructive lesions or fractures. A projection through the mouth is required to show the upper two vertebrae. In the lateral view the disc spaces are inspected; narrowing indicates disc degeneration. Osteophytes are sought; in oblique views their relationship to the intervertebral foramina can be seen. Flexion and extension views are required to demonstrate instability.

Deformities of the neck

Torticollis ('wry neck')

In torticollis the chin is twisted upwards and towards one side. It may be either congenital or secondary to other local disorders.

INFANTILE (CONGENITAL) TORTICOLLIS The sternomastoid muscle on

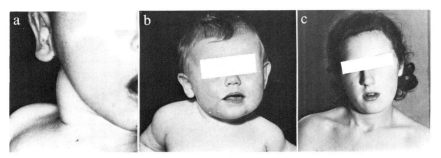

17.3 Torticollis   (a) Sternomastoid tumour in a young baby; (b) early wry neck; (c) deformity with facial hemiatrophy in the adolescent.

one side is fibrous and fails to elongate as the child grows. Sometimes a well-defined lump is felt in the muscle during the first few weeks of life, but deformity may not become apparent until the child is 2 or 3 years old. As the neck grows, the contracted sternomastoid tethers the skull on one side, thus twisting the chin towards the opposite side. Secondary facial deformities may occur.

Treatment   If a child has a sternomastoid 'tumour' subsequent deformity may be prevented by gentle, daily manipulation of the neck. In the established case the sternomastoid can be divided or elongated.

SECONDARY TORTICOLLIS   Wry neck may develop as a result of acute disc prolapse (the most common cause in adults), inflamed neck glands, vertebral infection, injuries of the cervical spine or ocular disorders.

Prolapsed cervical disc

Cervical disc prolapse may be precipitated by local strain or injury, especially sudden unguarded flexion and rotation. In many cases (perhaps in all) there is a predisposing abnormality of the disc with increased nuclear tension.

Prolapsed material may press on: (1) the posterior longitudinal ligament, causing neck pain and stiffness; and (2) the nerve roots, causing pain and paraesthesia in one

or both arms. Prolapse usually occurs immediately above or below the sixth cervical vertebra, so the nerve roots affected are C6 or C7.

Clinical features

The original attack may occasionally be related to a definite and severe strain. Subsequent attacks may be sudden or gradual in onset, and with trivial cause. The patient may complain of: (1) pain and stiffness of the neck, the pain often radiating to the scapular region and sometimes to the occiput; (2) pain and paraesthesia in one upper limb (rarely both), often radiating to the outer elbow, back of the wrist and to the index and middle fingers. Weakness is rare. Between attacks the patient feels well, although the neck may feel a bit stiff.

The neck may be tilted forwards and sideways. The muscles are tender and movements are restricted. The arms should be examined for neurological deficit.

IMAGING   X-rays may show slight narrowing of the disc space. The disc itself is best displayed by MRI.

Differential diagnosis

Acute cervical disc prolapse should be differentiated from the following.

Neuralgic amyotrophy   Pain is sudden and severe, and situated over the shoulder rather

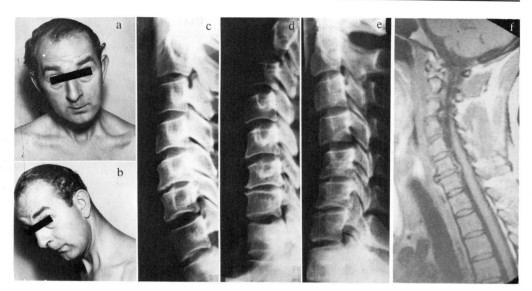

17.4 Cervical disc lesions   (a, b) Acute wry neck due to prolapsed disc. (c) A reduced disc-space at C5/6 is not necessarily significant; in (d) the disc space is reduced and the lordosis is obliterated, while in (e) the lordosis is reversed – both suggest a prolapsed disc. (f) MRI showing a prolapsed disc at C5/6.

than in the neck itself. Multiple neurological levels are affected.

Cervical spine infections   Pain is unrelenting and local spasm severe. X-rays show erosion of the vertebral end-plates.

Cervical tumours   Neurological signs are progressive and x-rays show bone destruction.

Treatment

Heat and analgesics are soothing but, as with lumbar disc prolapse, there are only three satisfactory ways of treating the prolapse itself.

Rest   A collar will prevent unguarded movement; it may be made of felt, sponge-rubber or polythene.

Reduce   Traction may enlarge the disc space, permitting the prolapse to subside. The head of the couch is raised and weights (up to 8 kg) are tied to a harness fitting under the chin and occiput. Traction is applied intermittently for no more than 30 minutes at a time.

Remove   If symptoms are refractory and severe enough, the disc may be removed through an anterior approach; bone grafts are inserted to fuse the affected area and to restore the normal intervertebral height.

Cervical spondylosis

Spondylosis is the most common disorder of the cervical spine. The intervertebral discs degenerate and flatten. Bony spurs appear at the anterior and posterior margins of the vertebral bodies; those that develop posteriorly may encroach upon the intervertebral foramina, causing pressure on the nerve roots.

Clinical features

The patient, usually aged over 40, complains of neck pain and stiffness. The symptoms come on gradually and are often worse on first getting up. The pain may radiate widely: to the occiput, the scapular muscles

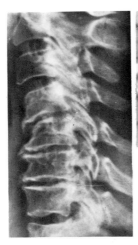

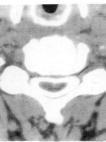

17.5 Cervical spondylosis (a) Typical x-ray showing multiple disc degeneration and osteophytes, (b) MRI showing encroachment upon the intervertebral foramina.

and down one or both arms. Paraesthesia, weakness and clumsiness are occasional symptoms. Typically there are exacerbations of more acute discomfort, and long periods of relative quiescence.

The appearance is normal. Tenderness occurs in the posterior neck muscles and scapular region; all movements are limited and painful.

In one or both upper limbs numbness or weakness may be found and one of the reflexes may be depressed.

X-RAY Several disc spaces are narrowed and the corners of the vertebrae show bony outgrowths or spurs (often referred to, somewhat inaccurately, as osteophytes). Oblique views may show encroachment of the intervertebral foramina.

Differential diagnosis

Other disorders associated with neck or arm pain and sensory symptoms must be excluded. Cervical spine lipping is very common in people over 40 and this can be misleading in patients with other disorders.

Thoracic outlet syndrome   Pain is felt usually in the ulnar forearm and hand; this is sometimes associated with paraesthesia. A lump may be palpable in the neck and x-ray may show a cervical rib.

Carpal tunnel syndrome   Pain and paraesthesia are worse at night. Nerve conduction is slowed across the wrist.

Rotator cuff lesions   Pain may resemble that of a prolapsed cervical disc, but shoulder movements are abnormal and there are no neurological signs.

Cervical tumours   With tumours of the spinal cord, nerve roots or lymph nodes, the symptoms are not intermittent; and the x-ray may be abnormal.

Treatment

Heat and massage are often soothing, but restricting neck movements in a collar is the most effective treatment during painful attacks. Physiotherapy is the mainstay of treatment, patients usually being maintained in relative comfort by various measures including exercises, gentle passive manipulation and intermittent traction.

Operation is seldom indicated, but if severe symptoms are relieved only by a rigid and irksome support, anterior fusion is appropriate.

Infections

Pyogenic infection (usually staphylococcal) is uncommon and tuberculous infection rare. In both, destructive changes usually involve the intervertebral disc spaces and the neighbouring vertebrae. Later, pus may spread to form a retropharyngeal abscess, or into the spinal canal where it may compress the cord. Rest and appropriate antibiotics are essential. Abscesses may need drainage and the spinal cord may need to be decompressed – this may be combined with fusion, though with pyogenic infection spontaneous fusion is usual.

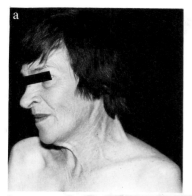

17.6 Rheumatoid arthritis (a) Movement is severely restricted; attempted rotation causes pain and muscle spasm. (b) Atlantoaxial subluxation is common; erosion of the joints and the transverse ligament has allowed the atlas to slip forward about 2 cm; (c) reduction and posterior fusion with wire fixation. (d) This patient has subluxation not only at the atlantoaxial joint but also at two levels in the mid-cervical region.

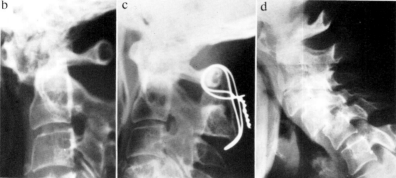

Rheumatoid arthritis

The cervical spine is severely affected in 30 per cent of patients with rheumatoid arthritis. Three types of lesion are common: (1) erosion of the atlantoaxial joints and the transverse ligament, with resulting instability; (2) erosion of the atlanto-occipital articulations, allowing the odontoid peg to ride up into the foramen magnum; and (3) erosion of the facet joints in the mid-cervical region, sometimes ending in fusion but more often leading to subluxation.

The patient is usually a woman with advanced rheumatoid arthritis. She has neck pain and movements are markedly restricted. Symptoms and signs of root compression may be present in the upper limbs; less often there is lower limb weakness and upper motor neuron signs due to cord compression.

X-rays show an erosive arthritis, usually at several levels. Flexion and extension views may reveal subluxation at the atlanto-axial joint or in the mid-cervical region.

Treatment Despite the startling x-ray appearances, serious complications are uncommon. Pain can usually be relieved by wearing a collar. Only if it is persistent and severe, or associated with increasing neurological deficit, is posterior spinal fusion advised.

Neuralgic amyotrophy (acute brachial neuritis)

This unusual cause of severe shoulder pain and weakness is believed to be a viral infection of the cervical nerve roots; there is often a history of an antecedent viral infection and sometimes a small epidemic occurs among inmates of an institution.

Pain in the shoulder and arm is intense and sudden in onset. It may extend into the neck and down as far as the hand; usually it lasts a few days but may continue for weeks. Other symptoms are paraesthesia in the arm or hand, and weakness of the muscles of the shoulder, forearm and hand.

Wasting of the deltoid or the small muscles of the hand may be obvious after only a few days, and winging of the scapula is common. Shoulder movement is limited by pain but this is always transient. Sensory loss in one or more of the cervical dermatomes is not uncommon.

There is no specific treatment; pain is controlled with analgesics. The prognosis is usually good, but full neurological recovery may take months or years.

The back   18

Examination

Symptoms

The usual symptoms of back disorders are pain, stiffness and deformity in the back, and pain, paraesthesia or weakness in the legs. The mode of onset is very important: did it start suddenly (perhaps after lifting) or gradually? Are the symptoms constant, or are there periods of remission? Are they related to any particular posture?

Pain may be felt in the back, usually low down and on either side of the midline, or extending into the buttock and down the limb. Pain felt in the thigh and calf, though called *sciatica*, is rarely due to sciatic nerve disorder. It is *referred pain*, either from the dural sleeve of a lumbar or sacral nerve root or from an abnormal vertebral joint; pain referred from the root dura is characteristically more intense and often accompanied by numbness or paraesthesia, whilst pain referred from a joint or ligament is more inconstant and is not accompanied by neurological symptoms – but both are distributed more or less along the path of the sciatic nerve.

Stiffness may be sudden and almost complete (after a disc prolapse) or continuous and predictably worse in the mornings (suggesting arthritis or ankylosing spondylitis).

Deformity is usually noticed by others, but the patient may become aware of shoulder asymmetry or of clothes not fitting well.

Numbness or paraesthesia is felt anywhere in the lower limb, but can usually be mapped fairly accurately over one of the dermatomes. It is important to ask if it is aggravated by standing or walking and relieved by sitting down – the classic symptom of spinal stenosis.

Other symptoms important in back disorders are *urethral discharge, diarrhoea* and *sore eyes* – the features of Reiter's disease.

Signs with the patient standing

Adequate exposure is essential; patients must strip to pants and bra.

● LOOK

Skin Scars, pigmentation, abnormal hair or unusual skin creases may be seen.

Shape and posture Asymmetry of the chest, trunk or pelvis may be obvious, or may appear only when the patient bends forwards. Lateral deviation of the spine is described as a list; lateral curvature is scoliosis.

Seen from the side the thoracic spine may seem unduly bent (kyphosis); if it is sharply angulated the prominence is called a kyphos. The lumbar spine may be unusually flat or excessively lordosed.

● FEEL

The spinous processes and the interspinous ligaments are palpated, noting any prominence or a 'step'.

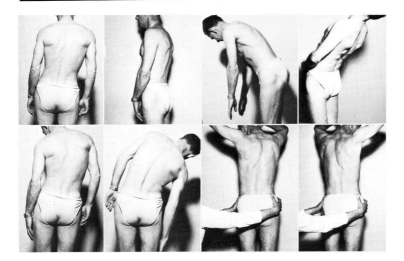

18.1 Examination (1) This patient has a prolapsed lumbar disc. He stands with a tilt. Forward flexion and tilting to the left are limited – other movements are full.

● MOVE

Flexion: ask the patient to try to touch his toes. Even with a stiff back he may be able to do this by flexing the hips; so watch the lumbar spine to see if it really moves, or better still, measure the spinal excursion. The mode of flexion is also important; hesitant movements, especially on regaining the upright position, may signify localized instability. *Extension:* ask the patient to lean backwards; with a stiff spine he may cheat by bending the knees. The 'wall test' will unmask a disguised loss of extension: standing with the back flush against a wall, the heels, buttocks, shoulders and occiput should all make contact with the surface. *Lateral flexion:* ask the patient to bend sideways, sliding his hand down the outer side of his leg; the two sides are compared. *Rotation:* ask the patient to twist the trunk to each side in turn while the pelvis is anchored by the examiner's hands; this is essentially a thoracic movement and is not limited in lumbosacral disease. Rib excursion is assessed

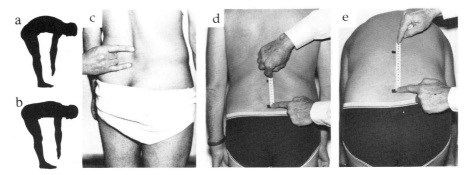

18.2 Examination (2) In both diagrams the hands nearly reach the toes; to distinguish spine flexion (a) from hip flexion (b), watch the lumbar lordosis undoing as the patient bends. Alternatively (c) note the separation of fingers placed on the spinous processes. Better still (d, e) *measure* the lumbar excursion; with the patient upright, two bony points 10 cm apart are selected – in full flexion they should separate by at least a further 5 cm.

by measuring the *chest circumference* in full expiration and then full inspiration; the normal excursion is about 7 cm.

Muscle power in the feet and ankles is conveniently tested with the patient standing. Ask him to stand up on his toes (plantarflexion) and then to rock back on his heels (dorsiflexion); small differences between the two sides are easily spotted.

Signs with the patient prone

Bony outlines and small lumps can be felt more easily with the patient lying face down. Deep *tenderness* is easy to localize, but difficult to ascribe to a particular structure.

The popliteal and posterior tibial *pulses* are felt, hamstring *power* is tested and *sensation* on the back of the limbs assessed. The *femoral stretch test* (for lumbar root tension) is carried out by flexing the patient's knee and lifting the hip into extension; pain may be felt in the front of the thigh and the back.

Signs with the patient supine

The patient is observed as he turns – is there pain or stiffness? Hip and knee mobility are examined before testing for cord or root involvement.

The straight leg raising test discloses lumbosacral root tension. With the knee held absolutely straight, the leg is lifted from the couch until the patient experiences pain – not merely in the thigh (which is common and not significant) but in the buttock and back; the angle at which this occurs is noted. At this point passive dorsiflexion of the foot may cause an additional stab of pain. If the knee is slightly flexed, buttock pain is suddenly relieved; pain may then be reinduced without extending the knee by simply pressing on the common peroneal nerve, to tighten it like a bowstring. Sometimes straight leg raising on the unaffected side produces pain on the affected side. This 'crossed sciatic tension' is indicative of severe root irritation, usually due to a prolapsed disc.

Muscle bulk and tone, power, reflexes and *sensation* are then assessed. The pedal and femoral *pulses* are felt.

While the patient is lying undressed, rapid appraisal helps to exclude disease or tumour of the breasts, abdomen or genitalia.

Imaging

In the AP x-ray the spine should look perfectly straight. Individual vertebrae may

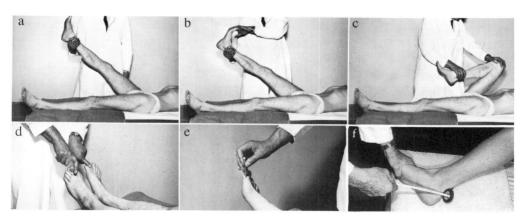

18.3 Examination (3) The legs are examined for nerve root involvement. (a) Straight leg raising is limited, and (b) the sciatic stretch is positive; but (c) flexion of the hip with the knee bent is painless, demonstrating that the hip is not at fault. (d) Muscle power, (e) skin sensation and (f) the tendon reflexes are tested.

show alterations in structure and the intervertebral spaces may be edged by bony spurs. The sacroiliac joints may show erosion or ankylosis.

In the lateral view the normal thoracic kyphosis and lumbar lordosis should be regular and uninterrupted. There may be anterior shift of an upper segment upon a lower (spondylolisthesis). Individual vertebrae, which should be rectangular, may be wedged or biconcave.

Special techniques such as contrast myelography, CT and MRI are useful for outlining the discs and the spinal canal.

Scoliosis

Seen from behind, the normal back is straight; in scoliosis it is curved to the side, and sometimes twisted. The deformity may be *postural* and correctible, or *structural* and fixed.

Postural scoliosis

In postural scoliosis the deformity is secondary or compensatory to some condition outside the spine, such as a short leg or pelvic tilt due to contracture of the hip; when the patient sits (thereby cancelling leg asymmetry) the curve disappears. Local muscle spasm associated with a prolapsed lumbar disc may cause a skew back: although sometimes called 'sciatic scoliosis' this, too, is a spurious deformity.

Structural scoliosis

Structural scoliosis is always accompanied by bony abnormality or vertebral rotation. The deformity is fixed and does not disappear with changes in posture. Secondary curves nearly always develop to counterbalance the primary deformity; they, too, may later become fixed. Once established, the deformity is liable to increase throughout the growth period.

Several types of structural scoliosis are recognized.

Adolescent idiopathic scoliosis is far and away the most common, and this will be described in detail.

Infantile idiopathic scoliosis is seen in young children; some cases resolve spontaneously but others progress to severe deformity.

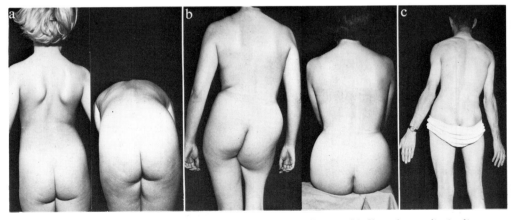

18.4 Postural scoliosis (a) Postural scoliosis disappears on flexion. (b) Short leg scoliosis disappears when the patient sits. (c) Sciatic scoliosis disappears when the underlying cause (a prolapsed disc) has been treated.

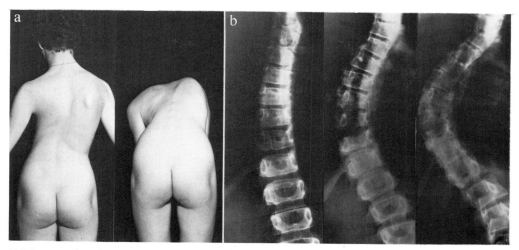

18.5 Structural scoliosis   (a) A fixed (structural) curve is more obvious on flexion. (b) Over a period of 4 years this curve has increased – most rapidly in the last 12 months, during the prepubertal spurt of growth.

Osteopathic scoliosis is due to congenital vertebral anomalies. Although rare, curves may be severe and dangerously progressive.

Neuropathic scoliosis is due to asymmetrical muscle weakness (e.g. in poliomyelitis or cerebral palsy).

Myopathic scoliosis is sometimes seen in the rare muscular dystrophies.

Neurofibromatosis may be associated with a short, and often severe, deformity; why this occurs is not known.

Adolescent idiopathic scoliosis

Idiopathic scoliosis usually presents before puberty and progresses until skeletal growth ceases; thereafter further deterioration is slight. The cause is unknown but any *extension deformity* of the normally kyphotic dorsal spine inevitably forces the spine to swivel round, thus producing the appearance of a lateral curvature.

Pathology

The curvature may occur anywhere in the thoracic or lumbar spine. The vertebrae that make up the curve are always rotated around the vertical axis, so the bodies point to the convexity and the spinous processes to the concavity of the curve. The ribs on the convex side are also carried around posteriorly and stand out as a prominent hump.

Clinical features

Patients usually present between the ages of 10 and 15. Deformity is the only symptom and the severity depends largely on which part of the spine is involved: high curves are noticed early while lumbar curves may pass virtually unnoticed. Whatever the deformity when the patient stands upright, it always looks worse on flexion; this is in sharp contrast to a postural curve, which disappears on flexion. The shoulder is elevated on the side of the convexity and the hip sticks out on the side of the concavity. With thoracic scoliosis the breasts are asymmetrical and the rib angles protrude.

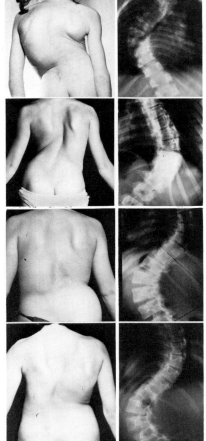

Infantile thoracic

60% male
90% convex to left
Associated with ipsilateral plagio-cephaly. May be resolving or progressive
Progressive variety becomes severe

Adolescent thoracic

90% female
90% convex to right
Rib rotation exaggerates the deformity
50% develop curves of greater than 70 degrees

Lumbar

More common in females
80% convex to left
One hip prominent but no ribs to accentuate deformity
Therefore not noticed early, but backache in adult life

Combined

Two primary curves, one in each direction
Even when radiologically severe, clinical deformity is relatively slight because it is always well balanced

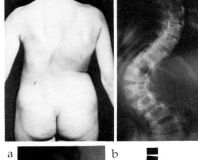

a   b

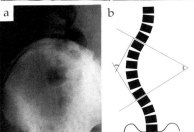

(a) *Risser's sign* (a) The iliac apoplysis is fully ossified but not yet completely fused. (b) *Cobb's angle* Measuring the angle of curvature.

18.6 Structural scoliosis – idiopathic curve patterns

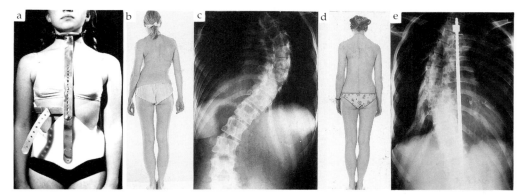

18.7 Structural scoliosis – treatment   (a) A Milwaukee brace may delay progress of the curve. (b,c,d,e) before and after operative correction and fusion.

X-RAY This should include full length views of the spine. The angle of curvature (Cobb's angle) is measured. X-ray of the pelvis shows when the iliac apophysis has ossified and fused (Risser's sign), a sign of skeletal maturity after which progression of the curve is minimal.

Treatment

Prognosis is the key to treatment: the aim is to prevent the curve becoming severe. Generally speaking, the younger the child and the higher the curve the worse the prognosis. A period of preliminary observation may be needed before deciding between conservative and operative treatment. At 4-monthly intervals the patient is examined, photographed and x-rayed so that the curves can be measured and checked for progression. School screening should permit early diagnosis and regular assessment of the need for active treatment.

Exercises alone have no effect on the curve, but they are useful to maintain suppleness.

Supports are used: (1) for all progressive curves over 20 degrees but less than 40 degrees; (2) for well-balanced double curves; (3) with younger children needing operation, to hold the curve stationary until aged 10, when fusion is more likely to succeed; and (4) to prevent recurrence after spinal fusion in young children.

Operation is indicated for curves of more than 40 degrees. The vertebrae are exposed and the curve is corrected, as far as possible, by special instrumentation. Bone grafts are then added in order to achieve spinal fusion. A rigid external splint may be needed for a few months.

Kyphosis

Rather confusingly, the term 'kyphosis' is used to describe both the normal (the gentle rounding of the dorsal spine) and the abnormal (excessive dorsal curvature). In the latter sense it signifies a well-recognized deformity which may be progressive.

Postural kyphosis is common ('round back' or 'drooping shoulders') and may be associated with other postural defects such as flat feet.

Structural kyphosis is fixed and associated with changes in the shape of the vertebrae. It may occur in osteoporosis of the spine (the common round back of elderly people), in ankylosing spondylitis and in Scheuermann's disease (adolescent kyphosis).

Kyphos (gibbus) is a sharp posterior angulation due to localized collapse or wedging of one or more vertebrae. This may be the result of a congenital defect, a fracture (sometimes pathological) or spinal tuberculosis.

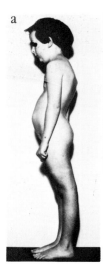
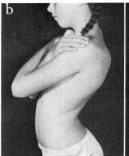
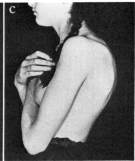
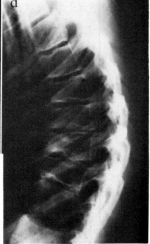

18.8 Kyphosis (a) Postural kyphosis and (b) kyphosis compensatory to a lumbar 'sway-back'. Unlike these two varieties, the deformity in Scheuermann's disease (c, d) is fixed.

Scheuermann's disease (adolescent kyphosis)

This is a growth disorder of the spine in which the vertebrae become slightly wedge shaped. If this happens in the thoracic spine – and especially if several vertebrae are involved – the normal kyphosis is exaggerated. The condition is thought to result from damage to the vertebral growth plates in children who outgrow their bone strength during the pubertal growth spurt; there may also be vertebral osteoporosis and the discs herniate into the fragile bone.

Clinical features

The condition starts at puberty and is twice as common in girls as boys. The parents notice that the child, an otherwise fit teenager, is becomingly increasingly round-shouldered. She may complain of backache and fatigue.

A smooth thoracic kyphosis is seen; it may produce a distinct hump. The deformity cannot be corrected by changes in posture.

X-RAY   Early on there is some irregularity of the vertebral end-plates and notching of the anterior corners of the vertebral bodies. In the lumbar spine this produces no visible deformity; in the thoracic spine (usually T6–10) the vertebral bodies may become wedged (i.e. narrower in front).

Treatment

Mild curves require only back-strengthening exercises and postural training. More severe curvature in a child who still has some years of growth ahead responds well to a period of 12–24 months in a brace.

The older adolescent or young adult with a rigid curve of more than 60 degrees may need operative correction and fusion.

Tuberculosis

The spine is the most common site of skeletal tuberculosis, and the most dangerous.

Pathology

Blood-borne infection settles in a vertebral body adjacent to the intervertebral disc. Bone destruction and caseation follow, with infection spreading to the disc space and to the

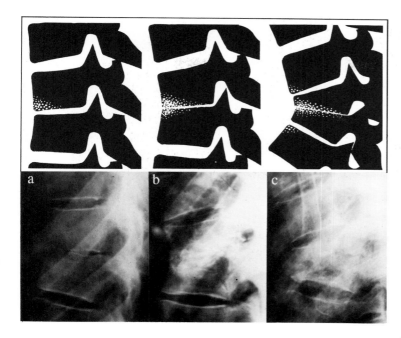

18.9   Tuberculosis – pathology (a–c) Progressively increasing destruction of the front of the vertebral bodies leads to forward collapse.

next vertebra. As the vertebral bodies collapse into each other, a sharp angulation (or kyphos) develops. Caseation and cold abscess formation may extend to neighbouring vertebrae or escape into the paravertebral soft tissues. There is a major risk of cord damage due to pressure by the abscess or displaced bone.

Clinical features

There is usually a long history of ill-health and backache. In some cases deformity is the dominant feature. Occasionally the patient presents with a cold abscess pointing in the groin, or with paraesthesia and weakness of the legs.

On examination the characteristic finding in the thoracic spine is an angular kyphos; in the lumbar spine this is scarcely visible. There is local tenderness and muscle spasm. All movements are restricted.

The groins and lumbar regions should be examined for abscess formation, and the lower limbs must be examined for neurological changes.

X-RAYS Early on there may be no more than disc space narrowing. With bone destruction there is collapse of adjacent vertebrae and obliteration of the disc space. A paravertebral abscess may be present. In long-standing cases there may be marked deformity involving a considerable length of the spine.

Investigations

The Mantoux test is positive and the erythrocyte sedimentation rate may be raised. If there is an abscess, pus should be sent for bacteriological examination and culture.

Diagnosis

It is often difficult to distinguish tuberculosis from other types of infection or (in older patients) from metastatic disease. If there is doubt, a needle biopsy may provide the answer.

Treatment

Except for the more advanced cases with progressive bone destruction, conservative

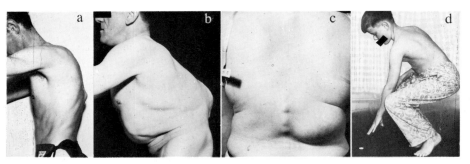

18.10 Tuberculosis – clinical features   (a) This kyphos is slight but diagnostic. If collapse continues (b), kyphos becomes severe. (c) Large lumbar abscess. (d) The coin test – he bends his hips and knees rather than bending his back.

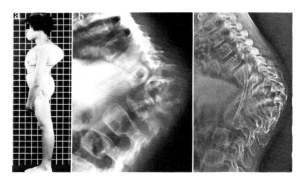

18.11 Tuberculosis – operative treatment A severe kyphos (a) may benefit from operation. This curve (b) has been partially corrected and held (c) by both anterior strut grafts and posterior fusion (this film is a xerographic tomograph.

treatment is usually sufficient and curative. Antituberculous chemotherapy should be rigidly supervised and continued for 6–12 months. If pain and spasm are marked, a period in hospital (sometimes on a frame) may be advisable; otherwise a well-fitting brace is all that is needed.

The indications for operation are: (1) abscess formation (this must be drained); (2) marked bone destruction and progressive deformity (this requires spinal fusion); (3) threatened paraplegia that does not respond to conservative treatment.

Pott's paraplegia

The spinal cord may be compressed by soft inflammatory material (an abscess, a caseous mass or granulation tissue) or by hard solid material (a bony sequestrum, a sequestrated disc or the ridge of bone at the kyphos). Occasionally fibrous tissue is the compressing agent.

Clinically the patient presents with signs of paraplegia added to those of spine tuberculosis. Clumsiness and weakness are early symptoms; later, muscle tone is increased and the tendon reflexes are brisk; clonus and extensor plantar responses may be found. Paraesthesia, or numbness, and disturbance of bladder control are common.

Early-onset paresis is due to pressure by an abscess or bony sequestrum. It usually produces a block on myelography. It is treated by early anterior decompression and debridement followed by spinal fusion. About 80 per cent recover, usually within a few weeks.

Late-onset paresis is due to increasing deformity, or reactivation of disease, or vascular insufficiency of the cord. Investigations should be carried out to establish the precise diagnosis. If the myelogram shows a block, operative debridement is still worth while even in late cases. If there is no block, operation is unlikely to be of use.

Pyogenic infection

Pyogenic organisms – usually staphylococci – may infect the vertebral body (pyogenic spondylitis) or the intervertebral disc (discitis).

Clinical features

Pain is the chief complaint. It may be associated with acute muscle spasm; spinal movements are markedly restricted.

X-RAYS reveal narrowing of the disc space and destruction of the adjacent bone. Even before these signs appear, *radioscintigraphy* will almost always show increased activity. In late cases, new bone formation is common – a point of distinction from tuberculous spondylitis. With healing, there may be fusion of adjacent vertebrae.

INVESTIGATIONS   The ESR is usually raised. A positive blood culture is unusual. Antistaphylococcal antibodies may be present in high titres. Agglutination tests for salmonella and brucella should always be performed. A needle biopsy may be required to discover the offending organism.

Treatment

Treatment consists of bed rest and intravenous antibiotics for 4–6 weeks; with a positive blood culture or biopsy sample, the most suitable drug can be selected. Once the acute infection has subsided, the patient is allowed up in a spinal brace, which is worn until x-rays and blood tests show that healing has occurred.

Intervertebral disc lesions

Lumbar backache is one of the most common causes of chronic disability in Western societies, and in the majority of cases the backache is associated with some abnormality of the intervertebral discs at the lowest two levels of the spine (L4/5 and L5/S1).

Prolapsed intervertebral disc

In acute disc herniation the gelatinous nucleus pulposus squeezes through the fibres of the annulus fibrosus and bulges posteriorly or posterolaterally beneath the posterior longitudinal ligament. Local oedema may add to the swelling, causing pressure on one of the nerve roots. With a complete rupture part of the nucleus may sequestrate and lie free in the spinal canal.

Symptoms depend on the structure involved and the degree of compression. Pressure on the ligament probably accounts

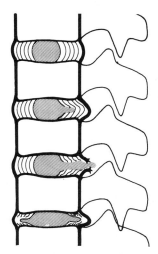

18.12   Disc   pathology   (1) From   above, downwards: an abnormal increase in pressure within the nucleus causes splitting and bulging of the annulus; the posterior ligament may rupture, allowing disc material to extrude into the spinal canal; with chronic degeneration (lowest level) the disc space narrows and the posterior facet joints are displaced, giving rise to osteoarthritis.

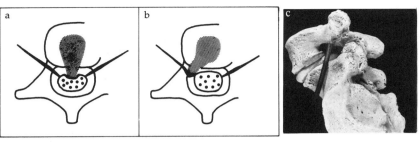

18.13 Disc pathology (2) (a, b) The bulging disc may press on the dura or on a nerve root. (c) The nerve is particularly vulnerable near the entrance to the intervertebral foramen.

for backache; pressure on the dural envelope of the nerve root causes severe pain referred to the lower limb (sciatica); and compression of the nerve itself causes numbness, paraesthesia and muscle weakness.

Clinical features

The patient is usually a fit young adult, though children and old people can be affected. Typically, while lifting or stooping (or perhaps merely coughing) the patient is seized with back pain and is unable to straighten up. Either then or a day or two later pain is felt in the buttock and lower limb (sciatica). Both backache and sciatica are made worse by coughing or straining. Later there may be paraesthesia or numbness in the leg or foot, and occasionally muscle weakness. Cauda equina compression is rare but may cause urinary retention.

The patient usually stands with a slight list to one side ('sciatic scoliosis'). All back movements are severely limited, and during forward flexion the list may increase.

There is often tenderness in the midline of the low back, and paravertebral muscle spasm. Straight leg raising is limited and painful on the affected side; dorsiflexion of the foot and bowstringing of the lateral popliteal nerve may accentuate the pain. Sometimes raising the unaffected leg causes acute sciatic tension on the painful side ('crossed sciatic tension'). With a prolapse at L3/4 the femoral stretch test may be positive.

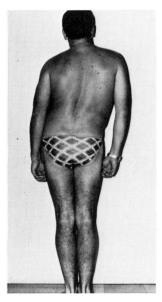

18.14 Lumbar disc – signs The patient has a sideways list or tilt. If the disc protrudes medial to the nerve root the tilt is towards the painful side (to relieve pressure on the root); with a far lateral prolapse the tilt is away from the painful side.

NEUROLOGICAL EXAMINATION may show muscle weakness (and, later, wasting), diminished reflexes and sensory loss corresponding to the affected level. L5 impairment causes weakness of big toe extension and knee flexion, with sensory loss

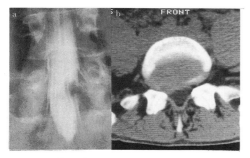

18.15 Lumbar disc – imaging (a) Radiculogram in which absence of the contrast medium shows where a disc has protruded. (b) CT scan showing how disc protrusion can obstruct the intervertebral foramen.

on the outer side of the leg and the dorsum of the foot. S1 impairment causes weak plantarflexion and eversion of the foot, a depressed ankle jerk and sensory loss along the lateral border of the foot. Cauda equina compression causes urinary retention and sensory loss over the sacrum.

X-RAYS are essential, not to show an abnormal disc space but to exclude bone disease. After several attacks the disc space may be narrowed. A myelogram or radiculogram outlines the disc well, but side-effects are unpleasant. CT and MRI are the best ways of identifying the disc and localizing the lesion.

Differential diagnosis

The full-blown syndrome is unlikely to be misdiagnosed, but with repeated attacks and with lumbar spondylosis gradually supervening the features often become atypical. Three groups of disorders must be excluded.

1. Inflammatory conditions, such as ankylosing spondylitis or tuberculosis, cause severe stiffness and a raised ESR.
2. Vertebral tumours cause constant pain; x-rays show bone destruction or a pathological fracture.
3. Nerve tumours may cause sciatica but pain is continuous; CT or MRI may delineate the lesions.

Treatment

Heat and analgesics soothe, and exercises strengthen muscles; but there are only three ways of treating the prolapse itself – *rest*, *reduction* and *removal*; equally important is the *rehabilitation* afterwards.

REST With an acute attack the patient should be kept in bed, with hips and knees slightly flexed and 10 kg traction to the pelvis. An anti-inflammatory drug such as indomethacin is useful. For mild attacks a spinal corset and reduced activity may suffice.

REDUCTION Continuous bed rest and traction for 2 weeks will reduce the herniation in over 90 per cent of cases. If the symptoms and signs have not improved significantly by then, an *epidural injection* of corticosteroid and local anaesthetic may help. Percutaneous *intradiscal injection of chymopapain* may 'dissolve' the nucleus (chemonucleolysis); however, this is potentially dangerous and operation is more certain.

REMOVAL The indications for operative removal of a disc are: (1) a cauda equina compression syndrome which does not clear up within 6 hours of starting bed rest and traction – this is an emergency; (2) persistent pain and severely limited straight leg raising after 2 weeks of conservative treatment; (3) neurological deterioration while under conservative treatment; and (4) frequently recurring attacks. Through a posterior approach between adjacent vertebral laminae, the dural sac is retracted to one side and the bulging disc is exposed. The friable, partially shredded material is removed. This can be done by open operation or by endoscopic surgery (microdiscectomy).

REHABILITATION After recovery from an acute disc rupture, or disc removal, the patient is taught isometric exercises and how to lie, sit, bend and lift with the least strain. Light work is resumed after a month and heavy work after 3 months. At that stage, if recovery is anything but total, the patient should be advised to avoid heavy lifting tasks altogether.

Lumbar instability and spondylosis

With disc degeneration, and especially after recurrent disc prolapse, there may be gradual flattening of the disc and displacement of the posterior facet joints. The disturbed movement in flexion and extension constitutes a type of instability; symptoms are due to mechanical derangement and secondary osteoarthritis of the facet joints.

Clinical features

The patient often gives a history of acute disc rupture and recurrent attacks of pain over several years. Backache may be intermittent and related to spells of hard work, standing or walking a lot, or sitting in one position during a long journey; it is relieved by lying down. Pain is often referred to the buttock and sometimes it extends down the leg like sciatica. There may be acute incidents of pain, 'locking' or 'giving way'.

The patient is usually over 40 and otherwise fit. Often, tender areas are felt in the back and buttocks. Lumbar movements are limited and may be painful at their extremes; there may be a typical 'heave' or 'jerk' as the patient straightens up after bending forward. Neurological examination may show residual signs of an old disc prolapse (e.g. an absent ankle jerk).

X-RAYS show narrowing of the disc space and marginal bony spurs ('osteophytes').

Treatment

Because the disability is seldom severe, and may even decrease with time (as the spine stabilizes itself), conservative measures are encouraged for as long as possible. These consist of instruction in modified activities, isometric exercises, manipulation during acute episodes, the wearing of a lumbar corset and small doses of anti-inflammatory drugs. If these measures, conscientiously applied, cannot control pain, spinal fusion is indicated.

Chronic back pain can be psychologically debilitating; counselling and support are often welcomed by the patient.

Spinal stenosis

One of the long-term consequences of disc degeneration and osteoarthritis is narrowing of the spinal canal due to hypertrophy at the posterior disc margin and the facet joints. This is more likely if the canal was always small, or if a spondylolisthesis decreases its anteroposterior diameter.

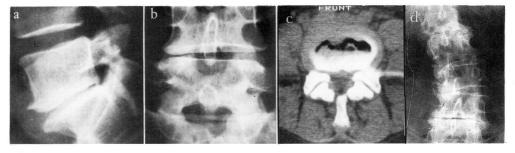

18.16 Spondylosis   (a, b) with chronic disc degeneration the space at L5/S1 has become narrow and the anterior edges have developed 'traction spurs'. Secondary osteoarthritis of the posterior facet joints is almost inevitable. (c) CT showing hypertrophic osteoarthritis of the facet joints. (d) In advanced cases several levels are involved, with deformity of the spine.

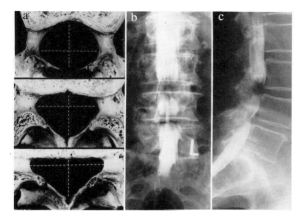

18.17 Spinal stenosis (a) The shape of the lumbar spinal canal varies from oval (with a large capacity) to trefoil (with narrow lateral recesses); further encroachment on an already narrow canal can cause an ischaemic neuropathy and 'spinal claudication'. (b, c) Myelogram showing marked narrowing of the radio-opaque column at the level of stenosis.

Clinical features

Typically, the patient complains of aching, numbness and paraesthesia in the thighs and legs; it comes on only after standing upright or walking for 5–10 minutes, and is consistently relieved by sitting, squatting or leaning against a wall to flex the spine (hence the confusing term 'spinal claudication'). Symptoms are often unilateral, suggesting an asymmetrical stenosis ('root canal stenosis').

Examination, especially after getting the patient to reproduce the symptoms by walking, may show neurological deficit in the lower limbs.

X-RAYS Lateral views may show degenerative spondylolisthesis or advanced disc degeneration and osteoarthritis. Measurement of the spinal canal may be carried out on plain films, but more reliable information is obtained from CT. If operation is planned, myelography or MRI is useful to show the extent of spinal canal narrowing.

Treatment

Conservative measures, including instruction in spinal posture, may suffice. If they fail, operative decompression is almost always successful.

Spondylolisthesis

'Spondylolisthesis' means forward shift of the spine. The shift is nearly always between L4 and L5, or between L5 and the sacrum. Normal laminae and facets constitute a locking mechanism which prevents each vertebra from moving forwards on the one below. Forward shift (or slip) occurs only when this mechanism has failed. This usually happens for one of the following reasons:

1. Dysplasia of the lumbosacral facet joints.
2. Separation or stress fracture through the neural arch, allowing the anterior part of the vertebra to slip forward (the commonest variety).

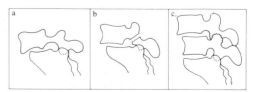

18.18 Spondylolisthesis – varieties (a) The pars interarticularis may be long and attenuated, with forward shift of the upper vertebra on the lower; (b) there may be a break in the pars interarticularis – a type of stress fracture or (c) degeneration of the facet joints (usually at L4/5) may allow slipping of the upper vertebra.

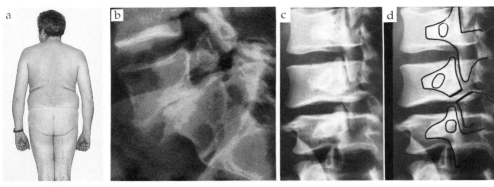

18.19 Spondylolisthesis – clinical and x-ray   (a) The transverse loin creases, short lumbar spine and long sacrum are characteristic. In the lateral x-ray (b) the slip may be obvious, but the defect in the pars interarticularis is better seen in the oblique view (c, d) where it is likened to a 'collar' around the 'neck' of an illusory 'dog'.

3. Osteoarthritic degeneration of the facet joints (usually at L4/5).

Clinical features

In children the condition is painless but the mother may notice the unduly protruding abdomen. In adolescents and adults backache is the usual presenting symptom; it is often intermittent, coming on after exercise or strain.

Degenerative spondylolisthesis usually occurs in women over 40 years; the other varieties may be seen at any age.

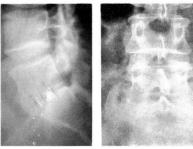

18.20 Spondylolisthesis – treatment Stability may be restored by (a) an anterior inter-body fusion with bone grafts or (b) posterolateral grafting and fusion.

On examination the buttocks look curiously flat, the sacrum appears to extend to the waist and transverse loin creases are seen. Sometimes there is a scoliosis.

A 'step' can often be felt when the fingers are run down the spine. Movements are usually normal in younger patients; in the degenerative group the spine is often stiff.

X-RAYS show the forward shift of the upper part of the spinal column on the stable vertebra below; elongation of the arch or defective facets may be seen. The gap in the pars interarticularis is best seen in the oblique views.

Treatment

Conservative treatment is indicated (1) if the patient is no longer young and symptoms are not disabling, or (2) if there is doubt whether the symptoms arise from the slip or from an associated disc prolapse. It consists of bed rest during an acute attack and a supporting corset between attacks.

Operative treatment is indicated (1) at any age if the symptoms are disabling, or (2) in the young adult with even moderate symptoms, and (3) if neurological compression is marked. Spinal fusion is carried out to fix the unstable segment.

The backache problem

Backache is such a frequent cause of disability that it has become almost a disease in itself. Careful history taking and examination will uncover one of five patterns.

Transient backache following muscular activity This suggests a simple back strain, which will respond to a short period of rest followed by gradually increasing exercise.

Sudden, acute pain and sciatica In young people (those under 20) it is important to exclude infection and spondylolisthesis. Patients aged 20–40 years are more likely to have an acute disc prolapse. Elderly patients may have osteoporotic compression fractures.

Chronic low back pain, with or without sciatica If the patient is over 40 and has had recurrent episodes of pain, the most likely diagnosis is facet joint dysfunction, segmental instability or osteoarthritis. However, disorders such as ankylosing spondylitis, chronic infection or other bone disease must be excluded by appropriate imaging and blood investigations. Treatment is almost always conservative.

Back pain plus pseudoclaudication These patients are usually aged over 50 and give a history of long-standing back trouble. The diagnosis of spinal stenosis should be confirmed by suitable imaging studies.

Severe and constant pain This suggests local bone pathology such as a fracture, Paget's disease, a tumour or infection.

'Chronic pain syndrome'

Patients with chronic backache may despair of finding a cure and they often develop psychosomatic ailments. When this occurs they are unlikely to respond to surgery and may require prolonged support and management in a special Pain Clinic – but only after every effort has been made to exclude organic pathology.

The hip

19

Examination

Symptoms

Pain arising in the hip joint is felt in the groin, down the front of the thigh and, sometimes, in the knee; occasionally knee pain is the only symptom! Pain at the back of the hip is seldom from the joint; it usually derives from the lumbar spine.

Stiffness may cause difficulty with putting on socks or sitting in a low chair.

Limp is common, and sometimes the patient complains that the leg is 'getting shorter'.

Walking distance may be curtailed; or, reluctantly, the patient starts using a walking stick.

THE PAINFUL HIP

Referred pain
Discogenic disease

Joint disorders
Infection
Perthes' disease
Slipped epiphysis
RA
OA
Osteonecrosis

Periarticular disorders
Hernia
Tendinitis
Bursitis

Signs with the patient upright

The gait is noted, and also whether the patient uses any form of support. If there is a *limp* it may be due to pain (the antalgic gait), to shortening (the short-leg limp) or to abductor weakness (the Trendelenburg lurch).

The Trendelenburg test is used to assess stability. The patient is asked to stand, unassisted, on each leg in turn; he lifts the other leg by bending the knee (but not the hip). Normally the weight-bearing hip is held stable by the abductors and the pelvis rises on the unsupported side; if the hip is unstable, or very painful, the pelvis drops on the unsupported side. A positive Trendelenburg test is found in: (1) dislocation or subluxation of the hip; (2) weakness of the abductors; (3) shortening of the femoral neck; or (4) any painful disorder of the hip.

Signs with the patient lying supine

● LOOK

Skin   Scars or sinuses may be seen (or they may be at the back of the hip). In babies, asymmetry of skin creases may be important.

Shape   Swelling or wasting is noted.

Position   The limb may lie in an abnormal position; excessive rotation is easy to detect but other deformities are often obscured by tilting of the pelvis.

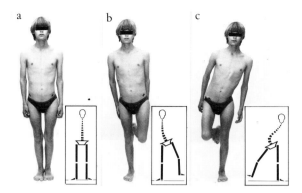

19.1 Trendelenburg's sign   (a) Standing normally on two legs. (b) Standing on the right leg which has a normal hip whose abductor muscles ensure correct weight transference. (c) Standing on the left leg whose hip is faulty, so that abduction cannot be achieved; the pelvis drops on the unsupported side and the shoulder swings over to the left.

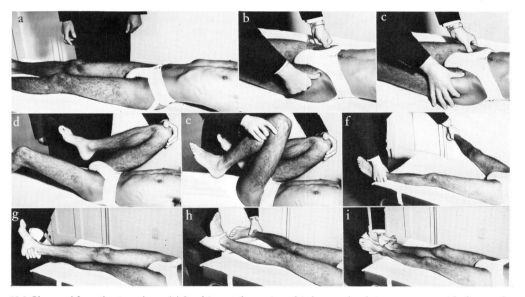

19.2 Signs with patient supine   (a) Looking at the patient: his legs and pelvis are square with the couch; the lordosis indicates fixed flexion of the hip. (b) Feeling the anterior superior iliac spines. (c) Locating the top of the greater trochanter (d) Flexing the right hip causes the left to lift off the couch (fixed flexion). The left hip also has limitation of (e) flexion, (f) abduction, (g) adduction, (h) internal rotation, and (i) external rotation.

Limb length can be gauged by looking at the ankles or heels; but first it is necessary to position the pelvis so that the anterior superior iliac spines are at the same level. Provided the pelvis is truly at right angles to the trunk and lower limbs, any visible discrepancy in limb length is real. This can be checked by placing the two lower limbs in comparable positions in relation to the pelvis and then measuring the distance from the anterior superior iliac spine to the medial malleolus on each side.

If shortening is present it is usually possible to establish where the fault lies. With the

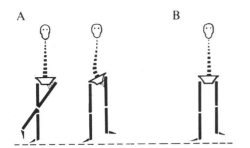

19.3 Shortening (1) – real or apparent? A leg may look short without actually being short. Thus A, with fixed adduction of his left hip, has to hitch up his pelvis in order to uncross his legs; this makes the leg *appear* short.
B has no hip deformity; unlike A he is able to stand (or lie) with his legs at right angles to his pelvis. His leg really *is* short.

knees flexed and the heels together, it can be seen whether the discrepancy is below or above the knee. If it is above, the next question is whether the abnormality lies above the greater trochanter. The thumbs are pressed firmly against the anterior superior iliac spines and the middle fingers grope for the tops of the greater trochanters; any elevation of the trochanter on one side is readily felt.

Measurement may show that the discrepancy in limb length is only *apparent* and not real. This occurs when the pelvis is tilted and one limb is hitched upwards. Almost invariably this is due to an uncorrectable deformity in the hip: with fixed adduction on one

side, the limbs would tend to be crossed; when the legs are placed side by side the pelvis has to tilt upwards on the affected side, giving the impression of a shortened limb. The exact opposite occurs when there is fixed abduction, and the limb seems to be longer on the affected side.

● FEEL

Skin temperature and *soft tissue* contours can be felt, but are unhelpful unless the patient is very thin.

Bone contours are felt when levelling the pelvis and judging the height of the greater trochanters. Tenderness may be elicited in and around the joint.

● MOVE

The assessment of hip movements is difficult because any limitation can easily be obscured by movement of the pelvis. Thus, even a gross limitation of extension, causing a *fixed flexion deformity*, can be completely masked simply by arching the back into excessive lordosis. Fortunately it can be just as easily unmasked by performing *Thomas' test*: both hips are flexed simultaneously to their limit, thus completely obliterating the lumbar lordosis; holding the 'sound' hip firmly in this position (and thus keeping the pelvis still), the other limb is lowered gently; with any flexion deformity the knee will not

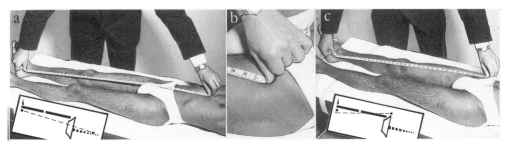

19.4 Shortening (2) – measurements Apparent length (a) is measured from a fixed point in the midline (e.g. the xiphisternum) to the bottom of the medial malleolus. Real length is measured from the anterior superior iliac spine; note how the thumb is pressed hard up against it (b) – also to the medial malleolus (c).

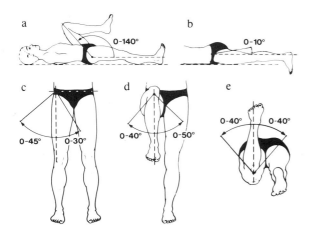

19.5 Normal range of movements (a) The hip should flex until the thigh meets the abdomen, but (b) only extends a few degrees. (c) Abduction is usually greater than adduction. The relative amounts of internal and external rotation vary according to whether the hip is in (d) flexion or (e) extension; in flexion the unwary may confuse internal with external rotation, but a hand on the thigh resolves the difficulty.

rest on the couch. Meanwhile the full range of *flexion* will also have been noted; the normal range is about 130 degrees.

Similarly, when testing *abduction* the pelvis must be prevented from tilting sideways. This is achieved by placing the 'sound' hip (the hip opposite to the one being examined) in full abduction and keeping it there, thus fixing the pelvis in the coronal plane. A hand is placed on one iliac crest to detect the slightest movement of the pelvis. Then after checking that the anterior superior iliac spines are level, the affected joint is moved gently into abduction. The normal range is about 45 degrees. *Adduction* is tested by crossing the one limb over the other; the pelvis must be watched and felt to determine the point at which it starts to tilt. The normal range of adduction is about 30 degrees.

To test *rotation* both legs, lifted by the ankles, are rotated first internally then externally; the patellae are watched to estimate the amount of rotation. Rotation in flexion is tested with the hip and knee each flexed 90 degrees.

Abnormal movement Telescoping may be elicited by alternately pulling and pushing the limb in its long axis; this is a sign of marked instability.

Signs with the patient lying prone

Scars, sinuses or wasting are noted. Extension of the two hips is most accurately compared with the patient lying prone. Rotation also can be assessed by flexing both knees and then moving the legs (like two handles) first away from each other and then crossing each other.

X-rays

The minimum required is an anteroposterior view of the pelvis showing both hips and a lateral view of each hip separately. The two sides can be compared: any difference in the size, shape or position of the femoral heads is important. With a normal hip Shenton's line, which continues from the inferior border of the femoral neck to the inferior border of the pubic ramus, looks continuous; any interruption in the line suggests an abnormal position of the femoral head. Narrowing of the joint 'space' is a sign of arthritis.

The diagnostic calendar

Hip disorders are characteristically seen in certain well-defined age groups. Whilst there are exceptions to this rule, it is sufficiently true to allow the age of onset to serve as a guide to the probable diagnosis.

Age of onset (years)	Probable diagnosis
0 (birth)	Congenital dislocation
0–5	Infections
5–10	Perthes' disease
10–20	Slipped epiphysis
Adults	Osteoarthritis
	Avascular necrosis
	Rheumatoid arthritis

Congenital dislocation of the hip

Normally at birth the hips are completely stable and held partially flexed. Occasionally, however, the joint is 'unstable' in the sense that it is either dislocated or is dislocatable – that is, though usually in place, it can easily be made to dislocate by gentle manipulation. Most dislocatable hips become stable within 3 weeks. The incidence of persistent dislocation is about 2 per 1000 births. The condition is much more common in girls than in boys. The left hip is more often affected than the right; in nearly a third of all cases both hips are affected. There is a familial tendency which may be related to an underlying acetabular dysplasia or to joint laxity.

Intrauterine malposition has been blamed for the condition; these babies have a higher than usual incidence of breech presentation. Postnatal posture is also important: dislocation is commonest of all in North American Indians who swaddle their babies tightly with hips fully extended, and least common in African Negroes who carry their babies across their backs with hips widely abducted.

Pathology

The acetabulum is unusually shallow (shaped like a saucer instead of a cup) and its roof slopes too steeply; the femoral head slides out posteriorly and then rides upwards. The joint capsule, though stretched, remains intact and, by folding inwards, may impede reduction. The fibro-cartilaginous labrum is often turned into the acetabulum and this acts as a further obstacle to reduction. Maturation of the acetabulum and femoral epiphysis is retarded and the femoral neck is unduly anteverted.

Clinical features

The ideal, still unrealized, is to diagnose every case at birth. For this reason, every newborn child should be examined for signs of hip instability. Where there is a family history of congenital dislocation, and with breech presentations, extra care is taken and the infant may have to be examined more than once.

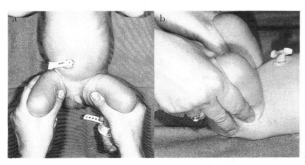
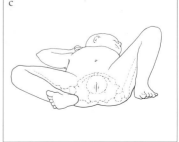

19.6 Congenital dislocation – early signs   (a, b) Position of the hands for performing Ortolani's test. (c) Showing why abduction is limited.

IN THE NEONATE there are several ways of testing for instability. In *Ortolani's test*, the baby's thighs are held with the thumbs medially and the fingers resting on the greater trochanters; the hips are flexed to 90 degrees and gently abducted. Normally there is smooth abduction to almost 90 degrees. In congenital dislocation the movement is usually impeded, but if pressure is applied to the greater trochanter there is a soft 'clunk' as the dislocation reduces, and then the hip abducts fully (the 'jerk of entry'). If abduction stops half-way and there is no jerk of entry, there may be an irreducible dislocation.

Barlow's test is performed in a similar manner, but here the examiner's thumb is placed in the groin and, by grasping the upper thigh, an attempt is made to lever the femoral head in and out of the acetabulum during abduction and adduction. If the femoral head is normally in the reduced position, but can be made to slip out of the socket and back in again, the hip is classed as 'dislocatable' (i.e. unstable).

Every hip with signs of instability – however slight – is examined by *ultrasonography*. This shows the shape of the cartilaginous socket and the position of the femoral head.

LATE FEATURES   With unilateral dislocation the skin creases are asymmetrical, the hip does not abduct fully and the leg is slightly short and rotated externally. The Trendelenburg test is positive.

Bilateral dislocation is more difficult to detect because there is no asymmetry and the characteristic waddling gait may be mistaken for normal toddling. However, the perineal gap is abnormally wide and abduction is limited.

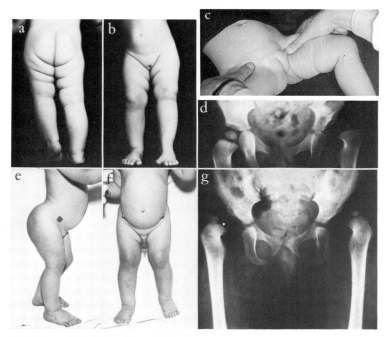

Unilateral dislocation of the left hip. (a, b, c) Asymmetrical creases and absence of the femoral head in the left groin. (d) X-ray shows the dislocated hip.

Bilateral dislocation. (e, f) Lordosis and a wide perineal gap. (g) X-ray shows that both hips are dislocated.

19.7 Congenital dislocation – late signs

X-RAY   In the established case the bony part of the acetabular roof slopes upwards abnormally and the socket is unusually shallow. The ossific centre of the femoral head is underdeveloped, and from its position it may be apparent that the head is displaced upwards and outwards.

Prognosis

Untreated, congenital dislocation leads to progressive deformity and disability, although with bilateral involvement, because the changes are symmetrical, disability is, for some years, less marked.

Where treatment is started after the age of 6, the outlook is still not good; however, for unilateral cases with asymmetrical deformity, reduction is worth while if only to provide a more favourable anatomy for later reconstructive surgery.

Treatment between 6 months and 6 years often gives good results, although this may require prolonged conservative treatment and operation.

The best way to attain a normal outcome is to start treatment within a week or two of birth; even then careful follow-up is necessary to be certain that redislocation has not occurred and that the acetabulum is developing normally.

Management

THE FIRST 3–6 MONTHS   The simplest and safest policy is to regard all infants with a positive Ortolani or Barlow test, as probably unstable and to nurse them in double napkins or an abduction pillow for the first 6 weeks. At that stage they are re-examined: those with stable hips are left free but kept under observation for at least 6 months; those with persistent instability are treated by more formal abduction splintage (see below) until the hip is stable and x-ray shows that the acetabular roof is developing satisfactorily (usually 3–6 months).

Where facilities for ultrasound scanning are available, newborn infants with a high-risk background (a family history or extended breech delivery) or a suggestion of hip instability are examined by ultrasonography. If this shows that the hip is reduced and has a normal cartilaginous outline, no treatment is required but the child is kept under observation for 3–6 months. If the anatomy is less than perfect, the hip is splinted in abduction and at 6 weeks ultrasound scanning is repeated. Some hips will now appear normal and these need no further treatment, apart from routine observation for 3–6 months. A few will show persistent abnormality and for these splintage is continued until a further scan at 3

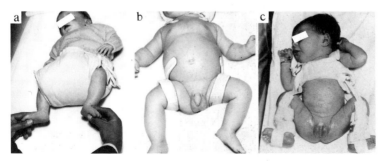

19.8 Congenital dislocation – treatment before weight-bearing   Reduction is usually easy and can be held by (a) an abduction pillow, (b) Von Rosen's malleable splint, or – best of all – by (c) the Pavlik harness. The hips should not be more than about 60 degrees abducted, though flexion sometimes needs to be well beyond a right angle.

months or an x-ray at 6 months shows a well-formed acetabular roof.

Splintage It is crucial to ensure that the hip is properly reduced before it is splinted; this can be checked by ultrasound. The object is to hold the hips about 100 degrees flexed and somewhat abducted. Extreme positions are avoided and the joints should be allowed some movement in the splint. For the newborn, double napkins or a soft abduction pillow may suffice. For larger infants, Von Rosen's splint or the Pavlik harness is better.

PERSISTENT   DISLOCATION: 6 MONTHS TO 6 YEARS   If, after early treatment, the hip is still incompletely reduced, or if the child presents late with a 'missed' dislocation, the hip must be reduced and held reduced until acetabular development is satisfactory.

Closed reduction Manipulation under anaesthesia carries a high risk of femoral head necrosis. To minimize this risk reduction must be gradual; traction is applied to both legs, preferably on a vertical frame, and abduction is gradually increased until, by 3 weeks, the legs are widely separated. This manoeuvre alone (aided if necessary by adductor tenotomy) may achieve stable,

concentric reduction. Arthrography at this stage will show whether the femoral head is fully seated in the acetabulum.

Splintage If concentrically reduced, the hips (both) are held in a plaster spica at 60 degrees of flexion, 40 degrees of abduction and 20 degrees of internal rotation. After 6 weeks the plaster is replaced by a splint that prevents adduction but allows movement. Within a few months x-rays may show a concentric femoral head with a normal acetabular roof; if so, splintage is gradually discarded.

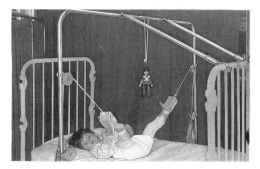

19.9 Congenital dislocation – treatment after weight-bearing Vertical traction with gradually increasing abduction.

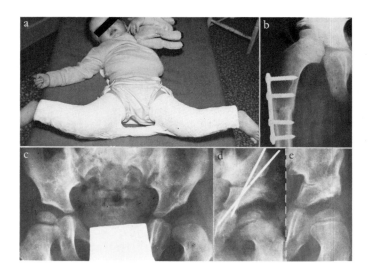

19.10 Congenital dislocation – operative   treatment (a) Reduced open, but stable only in medial rotation; 6 weeks later (b) derotation osteotomy. (c) Reduced open, but head poorly covered; (d, e) innominate osteotomy.

Operation   If, at any stage, concentric reduction has not been achieved, then open operation is needed. Any obstruction is dealt with and the hip is reduced and held in a spica for 3 months. If reduction can be achieved only by markedly internally rotating the hip, a corrective osteotomy of the femur is carried out either at the time of open reduction or 6 weeks later. If the head, though reduced, is poorly covered, it should be provided with a bony roof – usually by repositioning the innominate bone and acetabulum (innominate osteotomy).

AFTER THE AGE OF 6   For unilateral dislocation, operative reduction is still feasible, at least up to the age of 10; as in the former group, it may be necessary to combine this with corrective osteotomy of the femur or innominate osteotomy of the pelvis. In older children, the force needed for reduction may damage the hip and cause avascular necrosis, so it may be better to leave well alone and wait until pain and abnormal function call for further reconstructive surgery.

With bilateral dislocation the deformity is symmetrical and therefore less noticeable; the risk of operative intervention is also greater because failure on one or other side results in asymmetrical deformity. Therefore, most surgeons avoid operation unless pain or deformity is unusually severe. The untreated patient waddles through life and may be surprisingly uncomplaining. However, if disability becomes severe, hip replacement may be justified.

Subluxation of the hip

In subluxation the femoral head is not fully seated in the acetabulum. It may follow unsuccessful treatment of congenital dislocation or it may be an incomplete form of dislocation. The acetabulum is unusually shallow and the roof is sloping (acetabular dysplasia); the femoral head is liable to drift upwards and outwards. The faulty load transmission leads to secondary osteoarthritis.

Clinical features

In babies the signs are less obvious than those of congenital dislocation, but abduction may be limited and this should arouse suspicion. Ultrasonography may show a deficient acetabulum. In older children there may be a limp and a positive Trendelenburg sign. X-ray examination at this stage shows a sloping acetabular roof and uncovering of the femoral head.

In the infant *treatment* is similar to that for dislocation; the hip is splinted in abduction until the acetabular roof looks normal. In

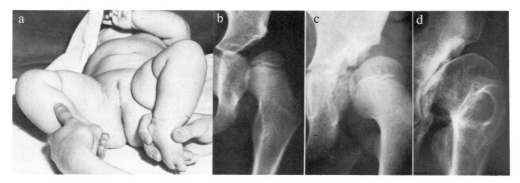

19.11 Congenital subluxation   (a) The cardinal physical sign; (b) x-ray in childhood; (c) in adolescence; (d) degeneration in early adult life.

children aged more than a year operation may be needed to restore joint congruity; either a varus osteotomy of the femur or an osteotomy of the pelvis to reposition the acetabular roof.

Acquired dislocation of the hip

Dislocation occurring after the first year of life is due to one of three causes: pyogenic arthritis, muscle imbalance or trauma.

Dislocation following sepsis

Pyogenic arthritis in infants may lead to destruction of the cartilaginous femoral head and a pathological dislocation. There may be a tell-tale scar or sinus and marked shortening of the limb. On x-ray the femoral head appears to be completely absent; however, some part of it often survives, although it is too osteoporotic to be seen.

The dislocation should be treated by traction, followed, if necessary, by open reduction. In the absence of a femoral head, the greater trochanter can be placed in the acetabulum; varus osteotomy of the upper femur helps to achieve stability.

Dislocation due to muscle imbalance

Unbalanced paralysis in childhood may result in the hip abductors being weaker than the adductors. The greater trochanter fails to develop properly, the femoral neck becomes valgus and the hip may subluxate or dislocate. Treatment is similar to that of congenital dislocation, but in addition a muscle rebalancing operation is essential.

Traumatic dislocation

Occasionally dislocation of the hip is missed while attention is focused on some more distal (and more obvious) injury. Reduction is essential, if necessary by open operation; even if avascular necrosis or hip stiffness supervenes, a hip in the anatomical position presents an easier prospect for reconstructive surgery than one that remains persistently dislocated.

Femoral anteversion (intoe gait)

The commonest cause of intoe gait is excessive anteversion of the femoral neck, so that

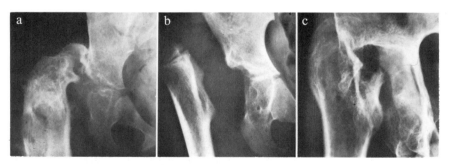

19.12 Acquired dislocation (non-traumatic) (a) Acute suppurative arthritis following osteomyelitis of the femoral neck in a child. (b) Acute suppurative arthritis in infancy has resulted in complete disappearance of the femoral head and neck. (c) Pathological dislocation in tuberculosis.

internal rotation of the hip is increased and external rotation diminished. The gait may look clumsy, but is no bar to athletic prowess and usually improves with growth. These children often sit on the floor in the 'television position' (with the knees facing each other) but should be encouraged to adopt the 'Buddha position'. Correction by osteotomy is feasible, but seldom indicated, and certainly not before the age of 8.

Protrusio acetabuli (Otto pelvis)

In this condition the socket is too deep and bulges into the cavity of the pelvis. The 'primary' form shows a slight familial tendency. It affects females much more often than males and develops soon after puberty; at this stage there are usually no symptoms although movements are limited. X-rays show the sunken acetabulum, with the inner wall bulging beyond the iliopectineal line. Secondary osteoarthritis may develop in later life, but until then the condition does not require treatment.

Protrusio may occur in later life secondary to bone 'softening' disorders, such as osteomalacia or Paget's disease, and in longstanding cases of rheumatoid arthritis. If pain is severe, or movements are markedly restricted, joint replacement is indicated.

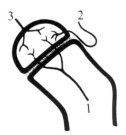

19.13 Perthes' disease – the background 1, Metaphyseal (nutrient) vessels; 2, lateral epiphyseal (capsular) vessels; 3, vessels in the ligamentum teres.

Perthes' disease (coxa plana)

Perthes' disease is a disorder of childhood characterized by necrosis of the femoral head. Although the incidence is only 1 in 10 000, it should always be considered in the differential diagnosis of hip pain in young children. Patients are usually 4–8 years old and often show delayed skeletal maturity; boys are affected 4 times as often as girls.

Pathogenesis

Up to the age of 4 months, the femoral head is supplied by: (1) metaphyseal vessels which penetrate the growth disc; (2) lateral epiphyseal vessels running in the retinacula; and (3) scanty vessels in the ligamentum teres. The metaphyseal supply gradually declines until, by the age of 4 years, it has virtually disappeared; by the age of 7, however, the vessels in the ligamentum teres have developed. Between 4 and 7 years of age the femoral head may depend for its blood suppy almost entirely on the lateral epiphyseal vessels whose situation in the retinacula makes them susceptible to stretching and to pressure from an effusion. The precipitating cause is probably an effusion into the hip joint following either trauma, of which there is a history in over half the cases, or a non-specific synovitis.

Pathology

The pathological process takes 2–4 years to complete, passing through three stages.

Stage 1: *bone death* Following one or more episodes of ischaemia, part of the bony femoral head dies; it still looks normal on plain x-ray but it stops enlarging.

Stage 2: *revascularization and repair* New blood vessels enter the necrotic area and new bone is laid down on the dead trabeculae, producing the appearances of increased density on the x-ray. If only part of the epiphysis is involved and the repair process is rapid, the bony architecture may be completely restored.

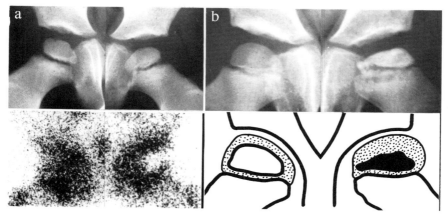

19.14 Perthes' disease – early features (a) This boy had an irritable left hip, his x-ray is virtually normal, but a scan on the same day shows a void in the lateral portion of the femoral head. (b) Later the head becomes radiologically dense; it stops growing but the cartilage does not – the diagram shows how this results in an increased 'joint space'.

Stage 3: *distortion and remodelling* If a large part of the bony epiphysis is damaged, or the repair process is slow, the epiphysis may collapse and subsequent growth at the head and neck will be distorted. Sometimes the epiphysis ends up flattened ('coxa plana') but enlarged ('coxa magna') and the femoral head is incompletely covered by the acetabulum.

Clinical features

The patient – usually a boy of 4–8 years – complains of pain and starts to limp. The hip looks deceptively normal, although there may be a little wasting. Early on, the joint is irritable, so all movements are diminished and their extremes painful. Often the child is not seen till later, when most movements are full; but abduction is nearly always limited and usually internal rotation also.

X-RAY Even before x-ray changes appear, the ischaemic area can sometimes be demonstrated as a 'void' on radioisotope scanning. The earliest changes are increased density of the bony epiphysis and apparent widening of the joint space. Flattening, fragmentation and lateral displacement of the epiphysis follow, with rarefaction and broadening of the metaphysis. The picture varies with the age of the child, the stage of the disease and the amount of head which has been ischaemic.

A prognostic grading has been devised by Catterall, in which increasing amounts of femoral head involvement are related to a worsening outcome.

Differential diagnosis

The commonest cause of hip pain in children is a non-specific *transient synovitis* – the so-called irritable hip. Ultrasound may show a joint effusion, but the x-rays are always normal. Symptoms last for a week or two and clear up completely. The child should be kept in bed until pain disappears and the effusion resolves.

Treatment

As long as the hip is irritable the child should be in bed with skin traction applied to the affected leg. Once irritability has subsided, which usually takes about 3 weeks, further treatment is dictated by an assessment of prognosis in each case.

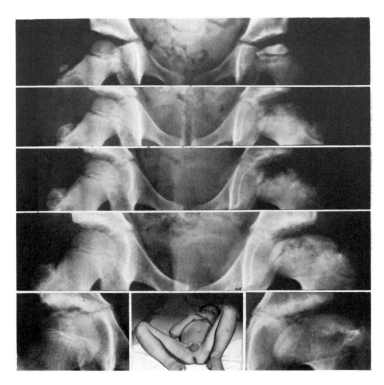

19.15 Perthes' disease
Serial x-rays over a period of 5 years. Despite radiological severity the clinical signs are usually slight, but abduction in flexion is nearly always limited (*inset*).

Favourable prognostic signs are: (1) onset under the age of 6; (2) only partial involvement of the femoral head; (3) absence of metaphyseal rarefaction; and (4) normal femoral head shape. Children in this category need no active treatment, though they should be followed up; 'supervised neglect' is an apt description.

Unfavourable signs are: (1) onset over the age of 6; (2) involvement of the whole femoral head; (3) severe metaphyseal rarefaction; and (4) lateral displacement of the femoral head. Children in this category need treatment by containment of the femoral head.

'Containment' The aim is to counteract lateral displacement and to contain the femoral head within the acetabulum; seated in its socket it is more likely to retain its normal shape. Containment is achieved either by holding the hips widely abducted, in plaster or in a removable splint (ambulation,

though awkward, is just possible, but the position must be maintained for at least a year), or by operation – a varus osteotomy of the femur or an innominate osteotomy of the pelvis. Surgery is not devoid of risk but has the great merit of achieving containment rapidly, so that the child's social development is less affected.

In those with the very worst x-ray changes the outcome is dubious whatever the treatment, so some surgeons prefer not to subject these children to unrewarding splintage or operation.

Slipped upper femoral epiphysis

Displacement of the proximal femoral epiphysis – also known as epiphysiolysis – is uncommon and virtually confined to

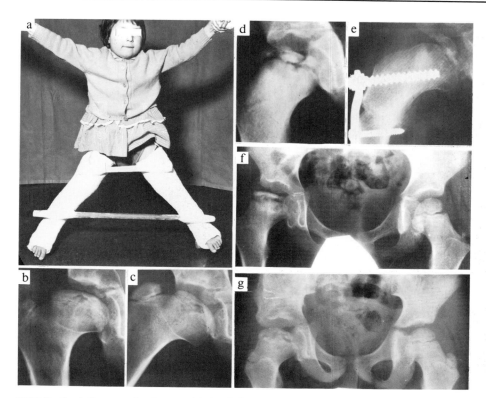

19.16 Perthes' disease – treatment   (a) An abduction splint (the so-called 'broomstick' plaster) can provide containment of the femoral head, as shown by x-rays taken in the neutral (b) and abducted (c) positions. The same effect can be achieved more rapidly (and with less inconvenience) by femoral osteotomy (d, e) or by innominate osteotomy (f, g).

children going through the pubertal growth spurt. Boys are affected more often than girls.

Cause and pathology

A slipped epiphysis is, to all intents and purposes, an insufficiency fracture through the hypertrophic zone of the cartilaginous growth plate. Trauma may be the precipitating cause, but often an underlying abnormality predisposes to slipping. The disorder occurs around puberty, and often in very tall children or very fat children with delayed gonadal development. Perhaps this means that these children have an imbalance between pituitary growth hormone (which

stimulates bone growth) and gonadal hormone (which promotes physeal fusion). Thus, during the pubertal growth spurt the relatively immature physis might be too weak to resist the stress imposed by the increased body weight.

Clinical features

The patient – usually a boy of 14 or 15 years – presents with pain in the groin, the anterior part of the thigh or the knee (referred pain); he may also limp. The onset may be sudden and in 30 percent there is a history of trauma ('acute slip'). However in the majority symptoms are protracted ('chronic slip'), or else a long period of pain may culminate in

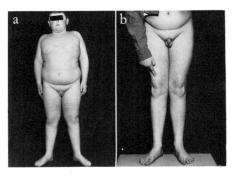

19.17 Slipped epiphysis – clinical features (a) The build is unmistakable; (b) this boy complained of pain only in the knee.

a sudden climax following minor trauma ('acute-on-chronic slip'). Two-thirds of the patients are fat and sexually underdeveloped, or unusually tall and thin.

On examination the leg is externally rotated and is 1 or 2 cm short. Characteristically there is limitation of abduction and medial (internal) rotation. Following an acute slip, the hip is irritable and all movements are accompanied by pain.

X-RAY   Even when slipping is trivial, changes can be seen. In the anteroposterior view the epiphyseal plate seems to be too wide and too 'woolly'. A line drawn along the superior surface of the neck remains superior to the head instead of passing through it (Trethowan's sign). In the lateral view the femoral epiphysis is tilted backwards.

Complications

Avascular necrosis is the most serious complication. It is seen only after a slip has been reduced or pinned, and is presumably due to the remaining leash of vessels being damaged.

Coxa vara may result if the displacement is not reduced and the epiphysis fuses in its deformed position. The patient limps but the condition is usually painless. Osteotomy may be needed to correct the deformity and in the hope of preventing secondary osteoarthritis.

Slipping at the opposite hip occurs in a third of cases – sometimes while the patient is in bed.

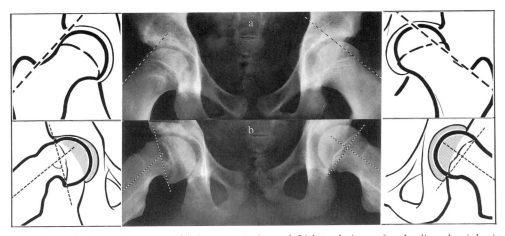

19.18 Slipped epiphysis – x-rays   (a) Anteroposterior and (b) lateral views of early slipped epiphysis of the right hip. The upper diagrams show Trethowan's line passing just above the head on the affected side, but cutting through it on the normal side. The lateral view is diagnostically more reliable; even minor degrees of slip can be shown by drawing lines through the base of the epiphysis and up the middle of the femoral neck – if the angle indicated is less than 90 degrees, the epiphysis has slipped posteriorly.

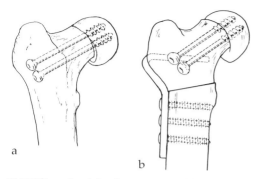

19.19 Slipped epiphysis treatment   (a) A mild or moderate slip (less than half the epiphyseal width) can be treated by pinning alone. (b) A severe slip also can be pinned without reduction, but then a compensatory osteotomy must be performed lower down.

Forewarned is forearmed: at the least suspicion of symptoms the epiphysis should be pinned.

Secondary osteoarthritis is a likely sequel if displacement has not been reduced, and inevitable if there has been avascular necrosis.

Treatment

Manipulation is dangerous and should be avoided.

Minor displacement (less than one-third the width of the epiphysis) is treated by accepting the position and fixing the epiphysis with two thin threaded pins. This is always done under x-ray control.

Moderate displacement (one-third to one-half the epiphyseal width) can often be treated by pinning alone. With further growth the proximal femur may be remodelled to an acceptable degree; if this does not happen the residual deformity can be corrected later by an osteotomy lower down.

Severe displacement (more than half the epiphyseal width) demands surgical correction. In skilled hands this can be achieved by exposing the slip, removing a small piece of the femoral neck in order to permit replacement

of the epiphysis, and pinning. A safer method is to fix the epiphysis in the displaced position and follow this with a compensatory osteotomy lower down.

Pyogenic arthritis

Pyogenic arthritis of the hip is usually seen in children under 2 years. The organism (usually a staphylococcus) reaches the joint either directly from a distant focus or by local spread from osteomyelitis of the femur. Unless the infection is rapidly aborted the femoral head, which is largely cartilaginous at this age, is liable to be destroyed by the proteolytic enzymes of bacteria and pus.

Clinical features

The child is ill and in pain, but it is often difficult to tell exactly where the pain is! The affected limb may be held absolutely still and all attempts at moving the hip are resisted. With care and patience it may be possible to localize a point of maximum tenderness over the hip; the diagnosis is confirmed by aspirating pus from the joint.

In the acute stage x-rays are of little value but ultrasound scans may show an effusion.

Treatment

Antibiotics should be given as soon as the diagnosis is reasonably certain. The joint is aspirated under general anaesthesia and, if pus is withdrawn, arthrotomy is advisable; antibiotics are instilled locally and the wound is closed without drainage. The hip is kept on traction or splinted in abduction until all evidence of disease activity has disappeared.

Tuberculosis

The disease may start as a synovitis, or as an osteomyelitis in one of the adjacent bones.

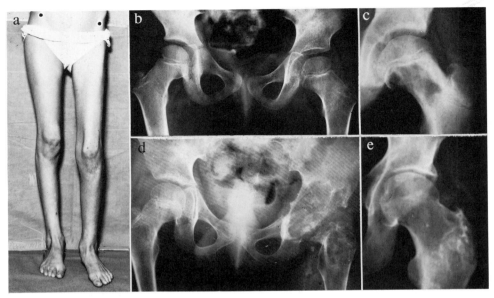

19.20 Tuberculosis – active   (a) Apparent lengthening in early disease of the left hip. (b) Synovitis of left hip. (c) Osteomyelitis of the femoral neck. (d) Florid arthritis. (e) Trochanteric infection – this rarely extends to the joint.

Once arthritis develops, destruction is rapid and may result in pathological dislocation. Healing usually leaves a fibrous ankylosis with considerable limb shortening and deformity.

Clinical features

The patient, usually a child, limps and complains of pain in the groin or thigh. Muscle wasting is characteristic. Occasionally a cold abscess may point in the thigh or buttock. All movements are limited and painful.

The first x-ray change is general rarefaction; the femoral epiphysis may be enlarged or a bone abscess visible; later there is destruction of the articular surfaces.

Early disease may heal leaving a normal or almost normal hip; but if there has been arthritis the usual result is an unsound fibrous ankylosis. The leg is scarred and thin, and shortening is often severe.

Treatment

Antituberculous drugs are essential. Skin traction is applied and, for a child, an abduction frame may be used. An abscess in the femoral neck is best evacuated; if the arthritis does not settle, joint 'debridement' is performed. As the disease subsides, traction is discontinued and the patient is got up.

If the joint has been destroyed, arthrodesis may be necessary once all signs of activity have disappeared, but usually not before the age of 14. In adults joint replacement is feasible.

Rheumatoid arthritis

The hip joint is frequently affected in rheumatoid arthritis. The hallmark of the disease is progressive bone destruction on both sides of the joint without any reactive osteophyte formation.

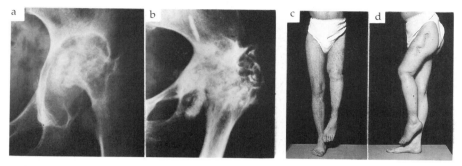

19.21 Tuberculosis – healing and aftermath   (a) Healing arthritis with enlargement of the acetabulum. (b, c, d) Joint destruction with calcification, fibrous ankylosis and gross deformity.

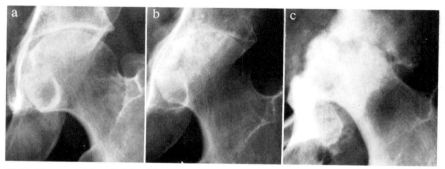

19.22 Rheumatoid arthritis   Three stages in the development of rheumatoid arthritis: (a) loss of joint space; (b) erosion of bone after cartilage has disappeared; (c) perforation of the acetabular floor – such marked destruction is more likely to occur if the patient is having corticosteroids.

Clinical features

Usually the patient already has rheumatoid disease affecting many joints. Pain in the groin comes on insidiously; limp, though common, may be ascribed to pre-existing arthritis of the foot or knee. With advancing disease the patient has difficulty getting into or out of a chair, and even movement in bed may be painful.

Wasting of the buttock and thigh is often marked, and the limb is usually held in external rotation and fixed flexion. All movements are restricted and painful.

X-RAYS   During the early stages there is osteoporosis and diminution of the joint space; later, the acetabulum and femoral head are eroded. In the worst cases (and especially in patients on corticosteroids) there is gross bone destruction and the floor of the acetabulum may be perforated.

Treatment

If the disease can be arrested by general treatment, hip deterioration may be slowed down. But once cartilage and bone are eroded, no treatment will influence the progression to joint destruction. Total joint replacement is then the best answer. It relieves pain and restores a useful range of movement. It is advocated even in younger patients, because the polyarthritis so limits activity that the implants are not unduly stressed.

Osteoarthritis

Osteoarthritis may develop in a relatively young adult as the sequel to congenital subluxation, Perthes' disease, coxa vara, acetabular deformities or injury. In the older patient it may also be secondary to rheumatoid arthritis, avascular necrosis or Paget's disease. When no underlying cause is discovered it is referred to as primary osteoarthritis.

Pathology

The articular cartilage becomes soft and fibrillated whilst the underlying bone shows cyst formation and sclerosis. These changes are most marked in the area of maximal loading (chiefly the top of the joint); at the margins of the joint there are the characteristic osteophytes. Synovial hypertrophy and capsular fibrosis may account for joint stiffness.

Clinical features

Pain is felt in the groin but may radiate to the knee. Typically it occurs after periods of activity but later it is more constant and sometimes disturbs sleep. Stiffness at first is noticed chiefly after rest; later it increases progressively until putting on socks and shoes becomes difficult. Limp is often noticed early and, if the hip is adducted, the patient may think the leg is getting shorter.

The patient is usually fit and over 50, but secondary osteoarthritis can occur at 30 or even 20. There may be an obvious limp and, except in early cases, a positive Trendelenburg sign. The affected leg usually lies in external rotation and adduction, so it appears short; there is nearly always some fixed flexion, although this may only be revealed by Thomas' test. Muscle wasting is detectable but rarely severe. Deep pressure may elicit tenderness, and the greater trochanter is somewhat high and posterior. Movements, though often painless within a limited range, are restricted.

X-RAY   The earliest sign is a decreased joint space, usually maximal in the superior weight-bearing region but sometimes affecting the entire joint. Later signs are subarticular sclerosis, cyst formation and osteophytes.

Treatment

Analgesics and anti-inflammatory drugs may be helpful, and warmth is soothing. The

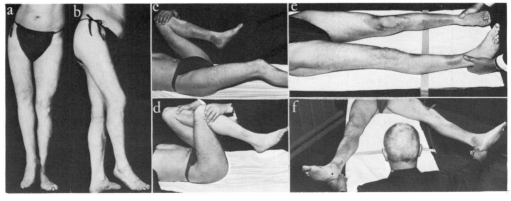

19.23 Osteoarthritis – signs   The right hip is osteoarthritic and shows: (a, b) apparent shortening, with adduction and flexion deformity; (c) demonstrating fixed flexion; (d, e, f) limitation of flexion, internal rotation and abduction.

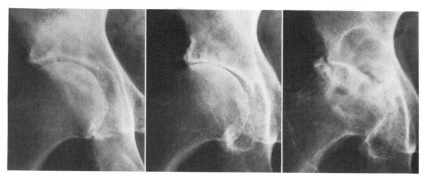

19.24 Osteoarthritis – x-rays   Over a period of 4 years this patient developed progressive diminution of the joint space, subarticular sclerosis, cysts and peripheral osteophytes.

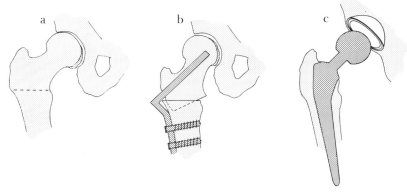

19.25 Osteoarthritis – treatment   (a) When only part of the joint is damaged, a realignment osteotomy may allow redistribution of stress to a less damaged part of the articular surface (b). In older patients, and when articular destruction is marked, joint replacement (c) is indicated.

patient is encouraged to use a walking-stick and to try to preserve movement and stability by non-weight-bearing exercises. In early cases physiotherapy, including manipulation, may relieve pain for long periods. If conservative methods fail, operation is indicated.

There are three main operations: osteotomy, arthrodesis and arthroplasty.

Osteotomy, if performed early, often relieves pain and can arrest the degenerative process. Arthrodesis is now rarely performed; the tide of opinion is against it, despite its advantages in the young. Arthroplasty (joint replacement) is much the most popular operation for patients over 55.

The knee

20

Examination

Symptoms

Pain is the most common knee symptom. With inflammatory or degenerative disorders it is usually diffuse, but with mechanical disorders and especially after injury it is often localized – the patient can, and should, point to the painful spot.

Stiffness also is common and, like pain, may result in a limp.

Swelling may be localized or diffuse. If there was an injury, it is important to ask whether the swelling appeared immediately (suggesting a haemarthrosis) or only after some hours (typical of a torn meniscus).

Locking is an ambiguous term: patients often use it to describe stiffness; with true locking the knee suddenly becomes unable to extend fully, though flexion is unaffected. This happens when a torn meniscus is caught between the articular surfaces. By wiggling the knee around, the patient may be able to 'unlock' it.

Giving way also suggests a mechanical disorder (such as a torn ligament) although it can result from muscle weakness; when it occurs particularly on stairs, the patellofemoral joint is suspect. Instability sufficient for the patient to fall suggests patellar dislocation.

3 CAUSES OF:	
Giving way	Torn meniscus
	Torn ligaments
	Unstable patella
Acute swelling	Synovitis
	Haemarthrosis
	Septic arthritis
Chronic swelling	Rheumatoid arthritis
	Osteoarthritis
	Tuberculosis

Signs with the patient upright

Valgus or varus deformity is best seen with the patient standing. He should also be observed walking, noting any instability or limp.

Signs with the patient supine

● LOOK

Skin The colour of the skin and any sinuses or scars are noted.

Shape Wasting of the quadriceps is usually obvious. The visual impression can be checked by measuring the girth of the thigh at the same level (usually a hand's breadth above the patella) in each limb. *Swelling* of the knee and lumps around the joint are observed.

Position The knee may lie in valgus or varus, partially flexed or hyperextended.

● FEEL

Skin Increased warmth is detected by comparing the two knees.

Fluid There are three tests for fluid. (1) Cross-fluctuation: the left hand compresses and empties the suprapatellar pouch while the right hand straddles the front of the joint below the patella; by squeezing with each hand alternately, a fluid impulse is transmitted across the joint. (2) The patellar tap: again the suprapatellar pouch is compressed with the left hand, while the index finger of the right pushes the patella sharply backwards; with a positive test the patella can be felt striking the femur and bouncing off again. (3) The bulge test: this is useful when only very little fluid is present. The medial compartment is emptied by pressing on that side of the joint; the hand is then lifted away and the lateral side is sharply compressed; a distinct ripple is seen on the flattened, medial surface.

The soft tissues and bony outlines are then palpated systematically, feeling for thickening and localized tenderness. This is easier if the knee is bent. The medial joint line can be felt quite easily, the lateral with a little more difficulty. The *patellofemoral joint* is accessible if the patella is pushed first to one side and then to the other. Rubbing the patella against the femur may elicit tenderness – the patellar friction test.

● MOVE

Flexion and extension Normally the knee flexes until the calf meets the ham and extends completely with a snap; even slight loss of extension, or 'springiness' on attempt-

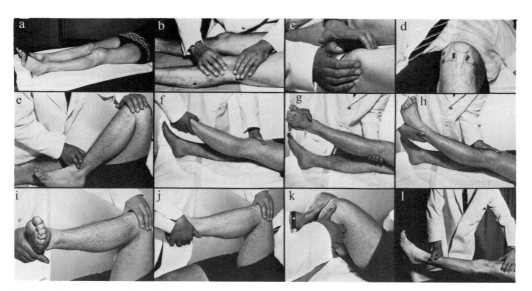

20.1 Examination – supine (a) Looking at both knees – the left is swollen and the thigh wasted; (b) testing for fluid by cross-fluctuation; (c) feeling for synovial thickening; (d) the points which should be palpated for tenderness.
Testing movements: (e) flexion, (f) extension, (g) abduction, (h) adduction. Lateral rotation (i), medial rotation (j) and anteroposterior glide (k) are tested with the knee bent; (l) testing quadriceps power.

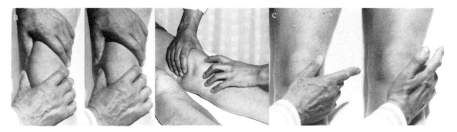

20.2 Tests for fluid   (a) Cross-fluctuation, the easiest test for large quantities of fluid; (b) the patellar tap, most likely to be positive with a moderate amount of fluid; and (c) the bulge test, with which small quantities can be detected.

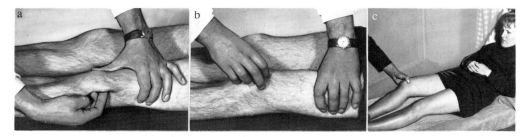

20.3 Examination of patella   (a) Feeling for tenderness behind the patella; (b) the patellar friction test; (c) the apprehension test.

ing it, is important. While moving feel for crepitus – a sign of patellofemoral degeneration.

Rotation   Flex the knee as far as it will go. Place your left hand so that your middle finger is on one side of the joint line and your thumb is on the other. Now with your right hand rotate the leg internally and externally; then repeat these rotations at different angles of flexion, feeling and listening for a catch or click in the joint. *McMurray's test* is similar but, in addition, the leg is externally rotated and stressed into valgus while being slowly extended; the manoeuvre is repeated with the leg internally rotated and stressed into varus. In this way a torn meniscal tag can sometimes be trapped between the articular surfaces and then induced to snap free with a palpable and audible click.

The patellar apprehension test   This is a test for recurrent subluxation or dislocation. As flexion commences, press the patella laterally with the thumb: if the patella is unstable, the patient will go rigid in anticipation of impending dislocation.

● TESTS FOR LIGAMENTOUS STABILITY

The medial and lateral liagments are tested by stressing the knee into valgus and varus. If the leg is very heavy, this is best done by tucking the patient's foot under your arm and holding the extended knee firmly with one hand on each side of the joint; the leg is then angulated alternately towards abduction and adduction. The test is performed at full extension and again at 30 degrees of flexion. There is normally some mediolateral movement at 30 degrees, but if this is excessive (compared to the normal side) it suggests a torn or stretched collateral ligament.

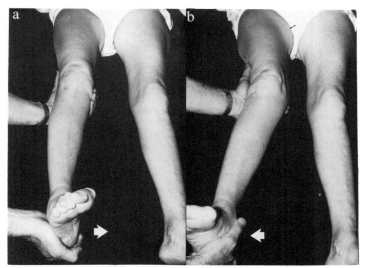

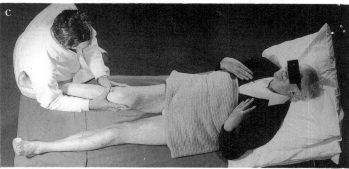

20.4 Testing for instability (1) The collateral ligaments can be tested by stressing first the lateral and then the medial side (a,b).

If the leg is tucked under the examiner's arm (c), the knee can be 'steered' medially and laterally with greater control.

The cruciate ligaments are tested by examining for abnormal gliding movements in the antero-posterior plane. With both knees flexed 90 degrees and the feet resting on the couch, the upper tibia is inspected from the side; if its upper end has dropped back, or can be gently pushed back, this indicates a tear of the posterior cruciate ligament (the 'sag sign'). With the knee in the same position, the foot is anchored by the examiner sitting on it (provided this is not painful); then, using both hands, the upper end of the tibia is grasped firmly and rocked backwards and forwards to see if there is any anteroposterior glide (the *'drawer test'*). Excessive anterior movement denotes anterior cruciate laxity; excessive posterior movement signifies posterior cruciate laxity. More sensitive is the *Lachman test*. The patient's knee is flexed 20 degrees; with one hand grasping the lower thigh and the other the upper part of the leg, the joint surfaces are shifted backwards and forwards upon each other. If the knee is stable, there should be no gliding.

Signs with the patient lying prone

Scars or lumps in the popliteal fossa are noted. If there is a swelling, is it in the midline (most likely a bulging capsule) or to one side (possibly a bursa)? A semimembranous bursa is usually just above the joint line, a Baker's cyst below it.

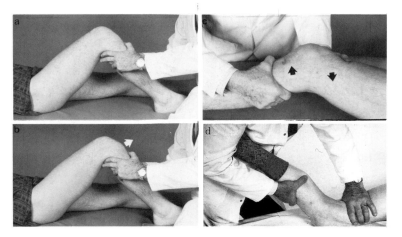

20.5 Testing for instability (2) Cruciate laxity can be revealed by performing the 'drawer test' (a,b). More reliable is the Lachman test (c): with the knee at 30°, the leg and thigh are moved firmly in opposite directions; this is sometimes easier with the patient prone (d).

The popliteal fossa is carefully palpated. If there is a lump, where does it originate? Does it pulsate? Can it be emptied into the joint?

Apley's test   The knee is flexed to 90 degrees and rotated while a compression force is applied; this, the grinding test, reproduces symptoms if a meniscus is torn. Rotation is then repeated while the leg is pulled upwards with the surgeon's knee holding the thigh down; this, the distraction test, produces increased pain only if there is ligament damage.

● IMAGING

Anteroposterior and lateral x-rays usually suffice, but special views may be needed to show up the patellofemoral joint and the intercondylar area.

Arthrography and MRI are useful in doubtful meniscal or ligament injuries.

● ARTHROSCOPY

Arthroscopy is useful: (1) to establish or refine the accuracy of diagnosis; (2) to help in deciding whether to operate, or to plan the operative approach with more precision; (3) to record the progress of a knee disorder; and (4) to perform certain operative procedures. Arthroscopy is not a substitute for clinical examination; a detailed history and

meticulous assessment of the physical signs are indispensable preliminaries and remain the sheet anchor of diagnosis.

Deformities of the knee

Bow leg (genu varum) and knock knee (genu valgum)

Bow leg in babies and knock knee in 4 year olds are so common that they are thought of as normal stages of development. They almost invariably correct spontaneously after a few years. If deformity is still marked by the age of 10, it can be corrected by staples, to slow epiphyseal growth, or osteotomy.

SECONDARY   DEFORMITY   Genu varum or genu valgum may be seen in a number of disorders that distort the bone ends or the joint itself. *Metaphyseal deformity* is common in rickets, in certain bone dysplasias (e.g. dyschondroplasia), in Paget's disease and following fractures. *Joint deformity* occurs in rheumatoid arthritis (usually valgus) or osteoarthritis (usually varus).

Treatment involves the management of the underlying condition. However, the deformity, once established, is permanent and this may require osteotomy.

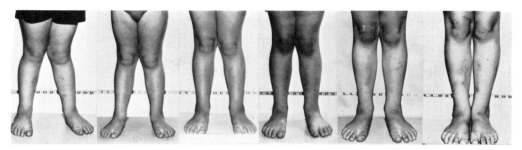

20.6 Genu valum (1)   Idiopathic knock knee – natural history without treatment. Age: 3 years, 3-1/2, 4, 5, 6 and 7.

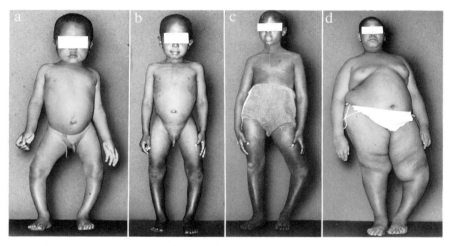

20.7 Bow legs   (a) Blount's disease, in which there is defective growth of the medial part of the tibial physis; (b) healed rickets; (c) trauma has damaged the upper tibial epiphysis; (d) this patient has an endocrine disorder and her upper tibial epiphysis has slipped.

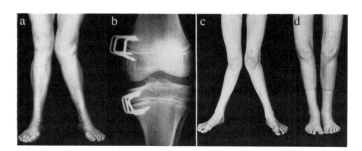

20.8 Genu valgum (2)   Only rarely does knock knee persist: (a, b) an adolescent treated by stapling the growth-plate on the medial side; (c, d) before and after bilateral osteotomy for severe deformity.

Lesions of the menisci

Meniscal tears

Tears of the menisci are common in young adults; they usually result from a twisting injury during sport. The meniscus splits in its length. If the separated fragment remains attached front and back, the lesion is called a *bucket-handle tear*. The torn portion sometimes displaces and becomes jammed between femur and tibia, causing a block to extension ('locking'). Sometimes there is only an *anterior horn tear* or a *posterior horn tear*. The meniscus is avascular and spontaneous repair does not occur unless the tear is peripheral. The loose tag acts as a mechanical irritant, giving rise to recurrent synovial effusion and/or articular cartilage damage.

Even in the absence of injury, there is gradual degeneration and stiffening of the menisci, so splits and tears are quite common in later life.

Clinical features

The patient usually sustains a twisting injury of the knee . Pain may be severe and further activity is avoided; occasionally the knee is 'locked' in partial flexion. Almost invariably swelling appears some hours later, or perhaps the following day.

With rest the initial symptoms subside, only to recur periodically after trivial twists or strains. Sometimes the knee gives way spontaneously and this is again followed by pain and swelling.

With medial meniscus tears (much the more common) pain is localized to the joint line; when the lateral meniscus is involved, pain is more ill-defined.

'Locking' – that is, the sudden inability to extend the knee fully – suggests a bucket-handle tear. The patient sometimes learns to 'unlock' the knee by bending it fully or by twisting it from side to side.

On examination the joint may be held slightly flexed and there is often an effusion. In long-standing cases the quadriceps will be wasted. Tenderness along the medial joint line is typical of a medial meniscus tear; tenderness on the lateral side is less well localized. Flexion is usually full but extension is often slightly limited.

Between attacks of pain and effusion there is a disconcerting paucity of signs. The history is helpful, and McMurray's test may be positive. Apley's grinding test may also be positive.

IMAGING   *Plain x-rays* are normal but *arthrography* may reveal the tear. *MRI* is even more reliable.

ARTHROSCOPY   has the advantage that if a lesion is identified, it can be treated at the same time.

Treatment

The displaced portion can be excised arthroscopically, but if difficulty is encountered an open operation is preferable. For a peripheral tear, operative repair is feasible and often successful. Postoperative physiotherapy is an important part of the treatment.

Meniscal cysts

A meniscal cyst is similar to a ganglion, arising from the outer part of the meniscus and forming a tense swelling at the joint line.

The patient presents with a small lump, usually on the lateral side of the joint. Often there is a history of injury to the joint. The cyst is sometimes so tense that it feels bony hard, and it is tender on pressure.

If the symptoms warrant operation, the cyst can be decompressed or removed arthroscopically; any meniscal lesion can be dealt with at the same operation.

Chronic ligamentous instability

The knee depends on its ligaments for stability. Ligament injuries are common in sportsmen, athletes and dancers. Whatever the

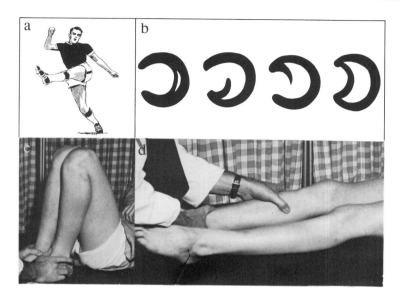

20.9 Torn medial meniscus (a) The meniscus is torn by a twisting force with the knee bent and taking weight; (b) the initial split may result in an anterior or posterior tag or may extend to become a 'bucket-handle' tear; (c) a locked knee flexes fully but (d) lacks full extension.

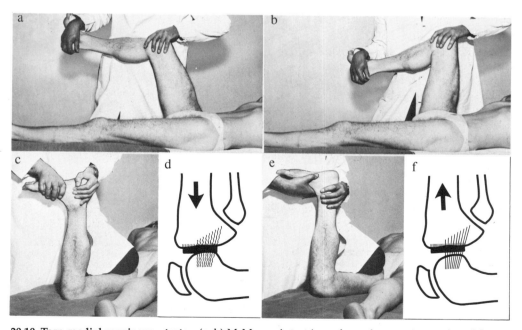

20.10 Torn medial meniscus – tests (a, b) McMurray's test is performed at varying angles of flexion. (c, d) Apley's grinding test relaxes the ligaments but compresses the meniscus – it causes pain with meniscus lesions. (e, f) The distraction test releases the meniscus but stretches the ligaments and causes pain if these are injured.

nature of the acute injury, the victim may be left with chronic instability of the knee – a sense of the joint wanting to give way, or actually giving way, during unguarded activity. Sometimes this is accompanied by pain and recurrent episodes of swelling.

Examination should include special tests for ligamentous instability (see page 196) as well as radiological investigation, MRI and arthroscopy. It is important not only to establish the nature of the lesion but also to measure the level of functional impairment against the needs and demands of the individual patient before advocating treatment.

Treatment

Stability is desirable but operation often does not succeed and may not last; so conservative treatment is important. Vigorous quadriceps and hamstring exercises are employed; they are an indispensable preliminary to operation and may allow the patient to lead a normal life even without operation. With the addition of an external brace, games may be possible.

If symptoms are unacceptable or a higher athletic standard is demanded, stabilization must be considered. Stabilization (or reconstruction) involves one or more of the three Rs – Reattachment, Reinforcement and Replacement. Reattachment implies tightening loose ligaments or capsule by securing one or both ends. Reinforcement diverts healthy muscles or tendons to strengthen weak structures. Replacement may involve rerouting living structures, or inserting synthetic material (such as Dacron) to take the place of the ligament and to act as a scaffold along which new fibrous tissue may grow.

Osgood–Schlatter's disease

This condition is common. Although often called apophysitis or osteochondritis, it is nothing more than a traction injury of the

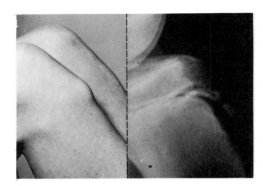

20.11 Osgood–Schlatter's disease This boy complained of a painful bump below the knee. The x-ray shows the traction injury of the tibial apophysis.

apophysis into which part of the patellar ligament is inserted.

A young adolescent complains of pain after activity, and of a lump. The lump is tender and its situation over the tibial tuberosity is diagnostic. Sometimes active extension of the knee against resistance is painful. *X-rays* show fragmentation or displacement of the tibial apophysis.

Spontaneous recovery is usual, but takes time, and it is wise to restrict such activities as cycling and football.

Osteochondritis dissecans

A small osteocartilaginous fragment sometimes separates from the medial femoral condyle and appears as a loose body in the joint. The most likely cause is trauma, and the lesion is probably an osteochondral fracture. Deprived of its blood supply, the bony part of the fragment undergoes necrosis. A small crater remains on the medial femoral condyle.

Clinical features

The patient, usually aged 15–20 years, presents with intermittent ache or swelling. Later, there are attacks of giving way, and locking may occur.

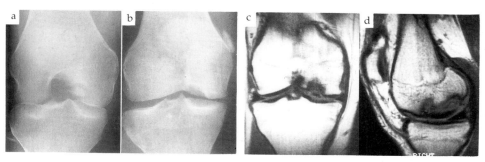

20.12 Osteochondritis dissecans   At first the affected area separates ('dissects') but still remains in position. (a) The 'tunnel' view may be the most helpful. (b) The anteroposterior view shows the loose fragment and the crater on the medial femoral condyle from which it came. (c,d) MRI shows that the surrounding bone, too, is abnormal.

On examination there is little to be found apart from a small effusion. If the fragment has separated, a loose body may be present.

X-RAY shows the fragment, often still in place but separated from the femoral condyle by a clear zone. Later it may be seen lying free in the joint. MRI gives a better idea of the surrounding bone changes.

Treatment

Small osteochondral fragments are probably best removed. Large ones may be fixed back in position, especially if they have not separated completely from the condyle; at the same time the bed is drilled to promote union. After operation the knee is held in a cast for 6 weeks; thereafter movement is encouraged but weightbearing is deferred until x-rays show signs of healing.

Recurrent dislocation of the patella

When the patella dislocates, it always does so towards the lateral side. A single dislocation occasionally results from an unusual injury; in recurrent dislocation there are other predisposing factors, such as: (1)

generalized ligamentous laxity; (2) anatomical abnormalities of the patella or the lateral femoral condyle; or (3) valgus deformity of the knee.

Clinical features

Girls are more commonly affected than boys and the condition is often bilateral. Dislocation occurs unexpectedly when the quadriceps muscle is contracted with the knee in flexion. There is acute pain and the patient cannot straighten the knee; sometimes the knee collapses and the patient falls to the ground.

If the knee is seen while the patella is dislocated, the diagnosis is obvious.

Between attacks the patella may be too high (patella alta) or too small, and the knee may hyperextend. The *apprehension test* is nearly always positive.

Treatment

Only rarely is the patient seen during the first attack, when the ideal treatment would be operative repair of the torn medial structures. Usually the patella has been reduced and a back slab applied. Treatment then should concentrate on strengthening the quadriceps (especially vastus medialis). As the child grows older the extensor mechanism often becomes more stable.

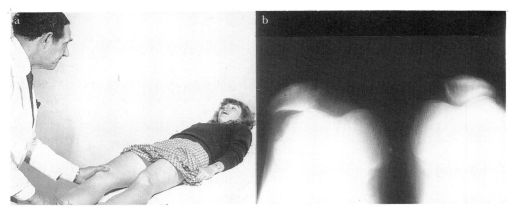

20.13 Patellar instability   (a) The apprehension test – the patient's facial expression shows that she is apprehensive that the patella may dislocate. (b) Subluxation of the patella.

If conservative measures fail to prevent repeated dislocation, operation is advised. The principle is to medialize the line of pull in the extensor apparatus. This may be achieved either by soft-tissue re-alignment to augment the pull on the medial side or by transposing the patellar ligament more medially.

Chondromalacia patellae

Softening of the articular cartilage of the patella is a common finding at arthroscopy. The cause is unknown, the condition is not necessarily symptomatic, and there is no consistent relationship to later development of osteoarthritis. Its significance lies in the fact that it is often associated with *anterior knee pain* in teenage girls.

ANTERIOR KNEE PAIN

1. Referred from hip
2. Chondromalacia patellae
3. Osteochondritis dissecans
4. Meniscal disorders
5. Tendinitis
6. Bursitis
7. Osgood–Schlatter's disease
8. Patellofemoral OA

Pathogenesis

The most likely cause is chronic or recurrent overload of the patellar articular surface, due to malcongruence of the patellofemoral surfaces or to abnormal tracking of the patella during flexion and extension.

Clinical features

The patient, often a teenage girl, complains of diffuse pain in front of the knee, chiefly on going up or down stairs. The knee looks normal but sometimes fluid is detectable. If the patella is pushed sideways, its posterior surface can be felt and is usually tender. Pressing the patella against the femur and then moving it (the friction test) causes pain. The tibiofemoral joint has full movement, although occasionally there is painful grating.

X-RAYS should include skyline views of the patella. The most accurate way of showing and measuring patellofemoral malposition is by CT.

ARTHROSCOPY may reveal cartilage softening. Other possible causes of knee pain should be looked for.

Treatment

The patient is given analgesics and advised to avoid undue activity. Physiotherapy, concentrating on exercises to strengthen the vastus medialis, is useful. Often the pain disappears after a year or two, but if it persists operation may be considered. A variety of procedures has been tried: shaving of the softened articular cartilage, arthroscopic lavage, realignment of the patella and even (in desperation) patellectomy.

Tuberculosis

Tuberculosis of the knee may appear at any age, but it is more common in children than in adults.

Clinical features

Pain and limp are early symptoms; or the child may present with a swollen joint. The thigh muscles are wasted, thus accentuating the joint swelling. The knee feels warm and there is synovial thickening. Movements are restricted and often painful. The Mantoux test is positive and the ESR may be increased.

X-RAY shows marked osteoporosis and (in children) enlargement of the bony epiphysis. In late cases the joint surfaces are eroded.

DIAGNOSIS Monarticular rheumatoid synovitis, or juvenile chronic arthritis, may closely resemble tuberculosis. A synovial biopsy may be necessary to establish the diagnosis.

Treatment

Antituberculous chemotherapy should be given for 3–6 months, while the knee is rested in a splint. At that stage, if the swelling has disappeared and x-rays show that the joint surfaces are intact, the knee is mobilized and the patient is allowed to start walking. However, if the joint surfaces are destroyed and the knee is stiff, arthrodesis is recommended; in adults this can be done as soon as the disease is inactive, but in children the operation is deferred until growth ceases.

Rheumatoid arthritis

Occasionally, rheumatoid arthritis starts in the knee as a chronic monarticular synovitis. Sooner or later, however, other joints become involved.

Clinical features

During stage 1 (synovitis) the patient complains of pain and chronic swelling. There may be a large effusion and the thickened synovium is easily palpable.

In stage 2 (articular erosion) there is increasing instability of the joint and some loss of flexion and extension. X-rays show loss of joint space and marginal erosions; the condition is easily distinguishable from osteoarthritis by the complete absence of osteophytes.

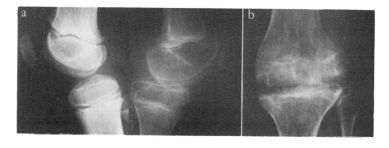

20.14 Tuberculosis – clinical and x-ray In synovitis (a) the bones are porotic and the epiphyses enlarged compared with the normal side; (b) arthritis.

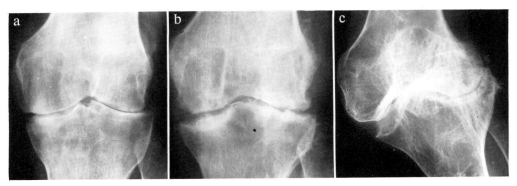

20.15 Rheumatoid arthritis (a) Early changes are cartilage erosion (giving a narrow joint space) and osteoporosis. (b) Later, joint destruction becomes more obvious, and (c) in severe cases gross deformity may result.

In stage 3 (deformity) pain and disability are usually severe. In some patients the joint has only a jog of painful movement; in others, it becomes increasingly unstable and deformed. X-rays show the bone destruction characteristic of advanced disease.

Treatment

In addition to general treatment, local splintage and injection of methylprednisolone usually reduce the synovitis promptly; a more prolonged effect may be obtained by injecting radiocolloids such as yttrium-90. The majority of patients can be managed by conservative methods and synovectomy is rarely indicated.

If deformity is marked, a femoral or tibial osteotomy may improve function and relieve pain. However, once bone destruction is present and the joint is unstable, total replacement is advised.

Osteoarthritis

The knee is one of the commonest sites for osteoarthritis. Often there is a predisposing factor: injury to the articular surface, a torn meniscus, ligamentous instability or pre-existing deformity of the knee. However, in many cases no obvious cause can be found; sometimes the condition is part of a generalized osteoarthritis.

Cartilage breakdown usually starts in an area of excessive loading. Thus, with long-standing varus the changes are most marked in the medial compartment. The characteristic features of cartilage fibrillation, sclerosis of the subchondral bone and peripheral osteophyte formation are usually present; in advanced cases the articular surface may be denuded of cartilage and underlying bone may eventually crumble.

Clinical features

Patients are usually over 50 years old; they tend to be overweight and may have long-standing bow-leg deformity.

Pain is the leading symptom, worse after use, or (if the patellofemoral joint is affected) on stairs. After rest, the joint feels stiff and it hurts to 'get going' after sitting for any length of time. Swelling is common, and giving way or locking may occur.

On examination there may be an obvious deformity or the scar of a previous operation. The quadriceps muscle is usually wasted.

Except during an exacerbation, there is little fluid and no warmth; nor is the synovial membrane thickened. Movement is

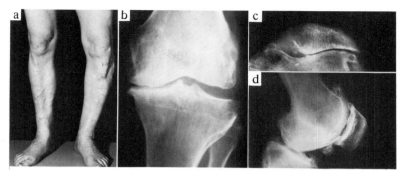

20.16 Osteoarthritis of the knee   (a, b) Varus deformity and degeneration on the medial side. (c, d) Sometimes it is the patellofemoral joint that is mainly affected.

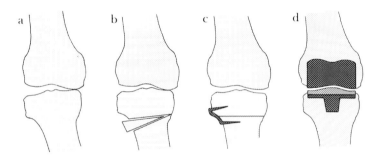

20.17 Osteoarthritis – treatment (a) Medial compartment damage can be treated by wedge osteotomy of the tibia (b, c), which produces a redistribution of stress on the articular surfaces. In more advanced cases, joint replacement (d) may be more appropriate.

somewhat limited and is often accompanied by patellofemoral crepitus. Pressure on the patella may elicit pain.

X-RAY   A weight-bearing view is essential. The tibiofemoral joint space is diminished (often only in one compartment) and there is subchondral sclerosis. Osteophytes are usually present and occasionally there is soft-tissue calcification in the suprapatellar region or in the joint itself (chondrocalcinosis).

Treatment

If symptoms are not severe, treatment is conservative. Quadriceps exercises are important. Analgesics are prescribed for pain, and warmth (e.g. radiant heat or short-wave diathermy) is soothing.

When the medial compartment alone is affected, and the joint is in varus, a realign-ment osteotomy of the tibia may redistribute weight to the lateral side of the joint. This is often effective in younger patients (those under 45). In older patients, where joint destruction is advanced, knee replacement is preferable. After operation, physiotherapy and continuous passive motion will help restore joint movement and muscle power.

Baker's cyst (popliteal cyst)

Patients with chronic arthritis of the knee sometimes develop a fluctuant swelling in the popliteal fossa. The misnamed 'cyst' is a synovial sac bulging from the back of the joint. It must be distinguished from a popliteal aneurysm which, of course, pulsates. Occasionally the synovial herniation leaks into the calf, causing pain and

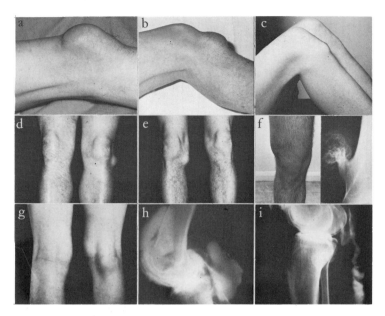

20.18 Lumps around the knee
In front: (a) prepatellar bursa; (b) infrapatellar bursa; (c) Osgood–Schlatter's disease.

On either side: (d) cyst of lateral meniscus; (e) cyst of medial meniscus; (f) cartilage-capped exostosis.

Behind: (g) semimembranosus bursa; (h) arthrogram of Baker's cyst; (i) leaking cyst.

swelling reminiscent of calf vein thrombosis. Treatment is directed to the underlying cause; in the short term joint aspiration and intra-articular injection of corticosteroid will reduce the effusion and relieve discomfort.

Bursitis

Prepatellar bursitis (housemaid's knee)

An uninfected bursitis is due to constant friction between skin and patella. It occurs in carpet layers and miners more often than in housemaids. The swelling lies directly over the patella, but the joint itself is normal. Treatment consists of firm bandaging, and kneeling is avoided; occasionally aspiration is needed. In chronic cases the lump is best excised.

Infrapatellar bursitis (clergyman's knee)

The swelling is superficial to the patellar ligament, distal to the patella; perhaps one who prays kneels more uprightly than one who scrubs. Treatment is similar to that for prepatellar bursitis.

Semimembranosus bursa

The bursa between the semimembranosus and the medial head of gastrocnemius may become enlarged. It presents usually as a painless lump behind the knee, in the medial part of the popliteal fossa. The lump is fluctuant but the fluid cannot be pushed into the joint, presumably because the muscles compress and obstruct the normal communication. The knee joint is normal. Occasionally the lump aches; if so, it may be excised.

Examination

Symptoms

The most common presenting symptoms are pain, deformity and swelling. It is important to know whether standing or walking provokes symptoms and whether shoe pressure is a factor.

Pain over a bony prominence or a joint is probably due to some local disorder. Pain across the forefoot (metatarsalgia) is less specific and is often associated with muscle fatigue.

Deformity may be in the ankle, the mid-foot or the toes. Parents often worry about their children who are 'flat-footed' or 'pigeon-toed'. Older patients may complain chiefly of having difficulty fitting shoes.

Swelling may be diffuse and bilateral, or localized. Swelling over the medial side of the first metatarsal head (a bunion) is common in older women.

Corns and callosities Often the main complaint is of shoe pressure on a tender corn over the joint or a callosity on the sole.

Numbness and paraesthesia may be felt in all the toes or in a circumscribed field served by a single nerve.

Signs with the patient standing and walking

Both legs and feet should be exposed, and ideally the trunk as well. The patient stands, first facing the surgeon and then with his back to him.

● LOOK

The legs, ankles, feet and toes are systematically inspected. Points to note are the colour of the skin and any swelling or deformity.

● FEEL

Palpation is postponed until the patient is sitting or lying.

● MOVE

The patient is asked to stand on tiptoes, then to walk normally and finally to walk on tiptoes. It is important to observe whether the gait is smooth and the foot well balanced, or whether the patient walks mainly on the inner or the outer border of the foot.

Signs with the patient sitting or lying

The patient is next examined lying on a couch, or it may be more convenient if he sits opposite the examiner and places his feet on the examiner's lap.

● LOOK

The heel is held square so that any foot deformity can be assessed. The toes and sole should be inspected for skin changes.

Thickening and keratosis over the proximal toe joints may form corns; the same changes on the sole are called callosities.

● FEEL

The skin temperature is assessed and the pulses are felt. If there is tenderness in the foot it must be precisely localized, for its site is often diagnostic. Any swelling, oedema or lumps must be examined. Sensation may be abnormal.

● MOVE

The foot can be regarded as a series of joints which should be examined methodically.

Ankle joint   With the heel grasped in the left hand and with the mid-foot in the right, dorsiflexion and plantarflexion are tested.

Subtalar joint   Grasping the heel alone, inversion and eversion are examined.

Mid-tarsal joint   The heel is held still with one hand while the other moves the tarsus up and down and from side to side.

Toes   Movements at the metatarsophalangeal and interphalangeal joints are tested.

Muscle power is tested by resisting active movement in each direction. Individual tendons may be palpated to establish whether they are intact and functioning.

● GENERAL EXAMINATION

If there is any sign of motor weakness or sensory change, a full neurological assessment and examination of the back are imperative. The shoes also should be examined; the pattern of wear may reflect abnormalities of weightbearing.

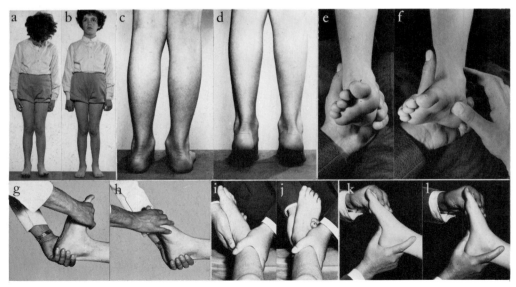

21.1 Examination   The patient examined standing, instinctively looks at her feet; this throws her off balance (a); she should look straight ahead (b). Next the feet are examined from behind (c) and on tiptoe (d); then held on the surgeon's lap with the heel square to see if the forefoot is varus (e), and to feel for tenderness (f). Ankle dorsiflexion (g) and plantarflexion (h) are examined; then subtalar inversion (i) and eversion (j). Finally (k, l) mid-tarsal and toe movements are tested.

● X-RAY

Anterioposterior and lateral views of the ankle and foot are the routine. Standing films, strain films and special views are sometimes needed. CT is useful for displaying the small intertarsal joints.

Deformities of the foot

Deformity may be due to: (1) congenital defects; (2) muscle imbalance; (3) ligamentous laxity; or (4) joint instability. Any deformity is aggravated by shoe pressure.

The normal foot is *plantigrade* – i.e. when the patient stands the sole is at right angles to the leg. *Equinus* (like a horse's foot) means that the hindfoot is fixed in plantarflexion. *Plantaris* looks similar, but the ankle is neutral and only the forefoot is plantarflexed. *Calcaneus* is fixed dorsiflexion at the ankle. A dorsiflexion deformity in the mid-foot produces a *rocker-bottom* foot.

Normally the medial border of the foot is slightly arched. If this arch is excessive, it produces a *cavus deformity*; if it is flattened out, a *valgus deformity* (flat-foot). Other common deformities are lateral deviation of the big toe (*hallux valgus*) and acute proximal interphalangeal flexion of one of the lesser toes (*hammer toe*).

Congenital club foot (talipes equinovarus)

This relatively common deformity shows a polygenic pattern of inheritance. Boys are affected twice as often as girls and the condition is bilateral in one-third of cases. Identical deformities occur with myelomeningocele and in arthrogryposis.

Pathological anatomy

The talus and calcaneum point downwards (equinus), whilst the navicular and the entire forefoot are shifted medially and rotated into supination (with the sole facing medially). The soft tissues of the calf and the medial side of the foot may be short and underdeveloped. If the condition is not corrected early, secondary growth changes occur in the bones; these are permanent.

Clinical features

The ankle is in equinus, and the foot is supinated and adducted; the sole faces medially. The heel may be small and high and the calf thin.

Gentle attempts at passive correction show the deformity to be fixed; in a normal baby with postural equinovarus the foot can be dorsiflexed and everted until the toes touch the front of the leg. The infant must

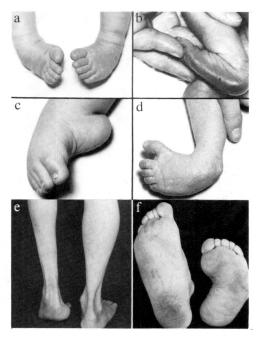

21.2 Talipes equinovarus (club foot) (a) True club foot is a fixed deformity, unlike (b) 'postural' talipes, which is easily correctible by gentle passive movement. (c) With true club foot the poorly developed heel is higher than the forefoot, which is also (d) varus. (e, f) The adult appearance when club foot has not been adequately corrected.

always be examined for associated disorders such as spinabifida or arthrogryposis.

X-RAYS showing the shape and position of the tarsal ossific centres are helpful in assessing progress after treatment.

Treatment

The objectives are: (1) to correct the deformity early; (2) to correct it fully; and (3) to hold the corrected position until the foot stops growing. Easy cases respond readily to stretching and splinting. Resistant cases respond poorly, relapse quickly and may tempt one to dangerously forceful manipulation; in them early operative correction is advisable so that manipulation and splintage can be gentle.

STRETCHING AND SPLINTING Treatment begins within 2 or 3 days of birth. Each component of the deformity is corrected in turn, and always in the following order: first the forefoot adduction, then the supination and finally the equinus. Attempts to overcome equinus first may 'break' the foot in the mid-tarsal region, creating a highly refractory 'rocker-bottom' deformity.

Without anaesthesia the foot is gently moulded towards the desired position and held there by adhesive strapping with felt pads protecting the skin at points of pressure. An alternative method is to apply a plaster cast over a protective layer of strapping. The process is repeated weekly for 6–8 weeks until the foot is not only corrected but *overcorrected*. Final correction must be confirmed by x-ray.

OPERATION In resistant cases operation at 8 weeks is less damaging than repeated, forceful manipulation. The tendo Achillis is lengthened and the tight invertors and plantarflexors are elongated or divided. The foot must be corrected fully and held in plaster.

TREATMENT AFTER CORRECTION Whether or not operation was needed, splintage continues; but now moulding and strapping need be repeated only at fortnightly or monthly intervals. This continues until the child starts walking; thereafter correction can be maintained by Denis Browne night splints and orthoses which permit walking in eversion. Splintage may need to be continued until puberty.

LATER OPERATIONS If the previous methods have failed and the child is less than 5 years old, open division of the contracted soft tissues is necessary for correction. Splintage is then resumed.

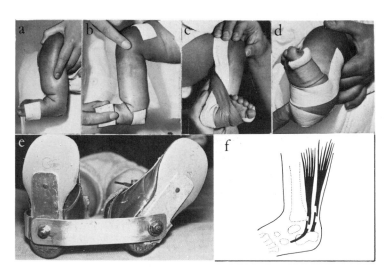

21.3 Treatment of congenital talipes (a–d) Manipuluation and strapping. (e) Denis Browne night shoes. (f) Very early operation.

Over the age of 5, correction of deformities is impossible without bone reshaping.

Over the age of 10 the best operation is probably a lateral wedge tarsectomy or, if the foot is mature, a triple arthrodesis.

Other varieties of talipes

Sometimes the only deformity is an *adducted forefoot*. This nearly always corrects with manipulation and splintage, and operation should not be considered below the age of 4 years. *Talipes calcaneus* (the foot dorsiflexed and valgus) usually corrects spontaneously, but if not, manipulation and splintage is always effective. Hip dislocation is sometimes associated and this should be excluded.

Flat foot (valgus foot; pes planus)

The medial arch of the foot may be normally low or normally high, but the term 'flat foot' implies that the arch has collapsed so that the medial border of the foot almost touches the ground.

Most little children are flat-footed when they first begin to walk; or rather they *seem* to be flat-footed, although often the appearance is created by a large medial fat pad. Only if the deformity persists, or recurs in adolescence, is it considered abnormal. The cause is unknown, but predisposing factors are generalized joint laxity, persistent knock knee and muscle weakness.

Acquired flat foot in later life may be due to paralysis (e.g. poliomyelitis), tendon rupture or joint erosion (e.g. rheumatoid arthritis).

Clinical features

In the common flexible flat foot there are no symptoms but the parents may notice that the feet are flat or that the shoes wear badly. Adults may develop 'foot strain' – a nagging ache in the feet after standing or walking.

The foot is examined with the patient standing (when the deformity will be obvious) and then with the patient sitting (to see if there is any tenderness and to test the range of movement).

The knees and hips should be examined for associated postural deformities, and

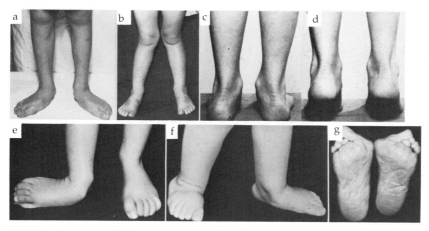

21.4 Flat foot – causal factors Flat foot may be associated with anatomical faults (upper row), or with physiological faults (lower row). (a) Tibial rotation; (b) knock knees; (c) a tight tendo Achillis – note that standing on tiptoe (d) restores the arch; (e) paralytic flat foot from old polio; (f) infantile flat foot; (g) middle-aged splay foot.

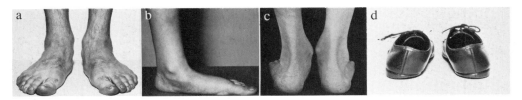

21.5 Flat foot − clinical features (a) prominent tuberosity of navicular; (b) flattening of the arch; (c) valgus heels, (d) deformed shoes.

general examination, including the spine, should be carried out to exclude any underlying disorder.

Rigid flat foot is seen in two rare conditions:

Congenital vertical talus The deformity is present at birth. The talus points downwards, the talonavicular joint is dislocated and the forefoot is pronated and valgus. Passive correction is extremely difficult.

Spasmodic flat foot This is usually seen in adolescents and young adults. The foot is painful and is held rigidly in eversion due to spasm of the peronei. X-ray or CT may show tarsal abnormalities or talocalcaneal erosion.

Treatment

Small children usually need no treatment; at most, the shoes may be altered to raise the inner side of the heel. Older children and young adults are sometimes helped by placing an arch support inside the shoe. Exercises will strengthen the muscles and reduce the likelihood of foot strain, but will do nothing to correct the deformity.

In cases that are clearly due to an underlying disorder (poliomyelitis or rheumatoid arthritis), operative correction and muscle rebalancing may be needed.

Congenital vertical talus usually needs operative correction.

Spasmodic flat foot is relieved by rest in a cast or a splint. If there is an abnormal tarsal bar or other bony irregularity, this may have to be removed or corrected by operation.

Pes cavus

In pes cavus the arch is higher than normal, the heel is in varus and often there is also clawing of the toes. The close resemblance to deformities seen in neurological disorders where the intrinsic muscles are weak or paralysed, suggests that idiopathic pes cavus is due to a similar type of muscle imbalance. The toes are drawn up into a 'clawed' position, the metatarsal heads are forced down into the sole and the arch at the midfoot is exaggerated.

Clinical features

Deformity may be noticed by the parents or the school doctor before there are any symptoms. There is often a family history, and as a rule both feet are affected. Pain may be felt under the metatarsal heads or over the toes where shoe pressure is most marked. Callosities appear at the same sites.

At first the deformities are mobile and can be corrected passively by pressure under the metatarsal heads; as the forefoot lifts, the toes flatten out automatically. Later the deformities become fixed.

Neurological disorders such as peroneal muscular atrophy and Friedreich's ataxia (page 85) must always be excluded.

Treatment

Often no treatment is required; apart from the difficulty of fitting shoes, the patient has no complaints. However, if deformities are marked yet still mobile, it may be considered

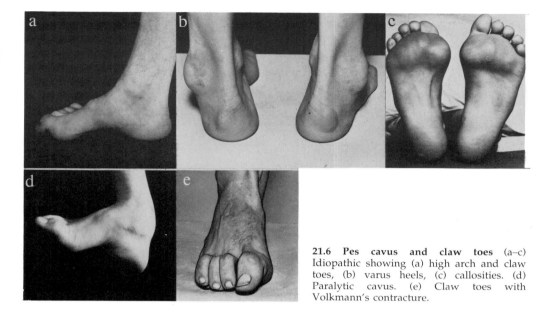

21.6 Pes cavus and claw toes (a–c) Idiopathic showing (a) high arch and claw toes, (b) varus heels, (c) callosities. (d) Paralytic cavus. (e) Claw toes with Volkmann's contracture.

wise to carry out a tendon rebalancing operation while the condition is still correctible; the long toe flexors are released and transplanted into the extensor expansions to pull the toes straight. Once deformities are fixed, they can be corrected only by arthrodesing the toe joints. More complex operations on the arch itself should be deferred until the age of 16. In adults, special shoes may be needed.

Hallux valgus

Hallux valgus is the commonest of the foot deformities (and probably of all musculoskeletal deformities). In people who have never worn shoes the big toe is in line with the first metatarsal, retaining the slightly fan-shaped appearance of the forefoot. In people who wear shoes the hallux assumes a valgus position; but only if the angulation is excessive is it referred to a 'hallux valgus'.

Splaying of the forefoot, with varus angulation of the first metatarsal, will predispose to lateral angulation of the big toe. Such metatarsus varus may be congenital, or it may result from loss of muscle tone in the forefoot in old people. Hallux valgus is also common in rheumatoid arthritis.

Pathological anatomy

The most obvious feature is prominence of the first metatarsal head. This is due to several factors: (1) increased width of the forefoot, with the first metatarsal shaft deviated medially away from the second (metatarsus primus varus); (2) the metatarsal head develops a protective bursa (bunion) where the shoe rubs; and (3) the big toe is inclined laterally towards the second toe, which is crowded and may become deformed. Often the big toe is also rotated, so that the nail faces medially.

Clinical features

Hallux valgus is usually bilateral, and is most common in the sixth decade and in females. There is a variety, strongly familial and by no means uncommon, which presents in adolescents.

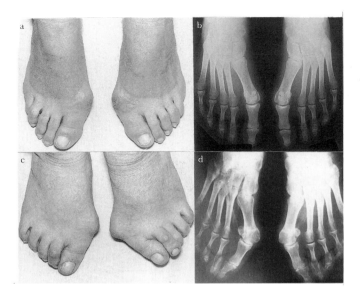

21.7 Hallux valgus (a, b) This girl's feet are well on the way to becoming as deformed as (c, d) those of her mother. Hallux valgus is not uncommonly familial.

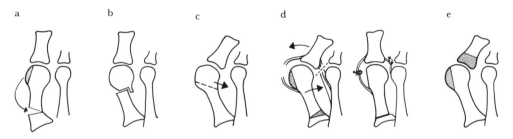

21.8 Hallux valgus – treatment (a) Basal osteotomy with bone graft inserted. (b) Mitchell's osteotomy. (c) Wilson's osteotomy. (d) Before and after basal osteotomy and capsulorrhaphy. (e) Keller's operation.

Often there are no symptoms, apart from the deformity. Pain, if present, may be due to (1) an inflamed bunion, (2) a hammer toe, (3) an associated wide splay foot with metatarsalgia and pain under the metatarsal heads, or (4) secondary osteoarthritis of the first metatarsophalangeal joint.

The deformity is obvious and the bunion is often swollen and inflamed. Hammer toe deformities may be present in the other digits. The metatarsophalangeal joints usually have good movement.

X-RAYS should be taken with the patient standing, to show the degree of metatarsal and hallux angulation. The first metatarso-phalangeal joint may be subluxated, or it may look osteoarthritic.

Treatment

ADOLESCENTS Deformity is usually the only symptom, but the mother is anxious to prevent it becoming as severe as her own. Nothing short of operation can prevent the deformity from increasing. This takes the form of a corrective osteotomy of the first metatarsal; once it is straight the big toe assumes a more normal position.

ADULTS All patients with hallux valgus can be made comfortable by careful attention

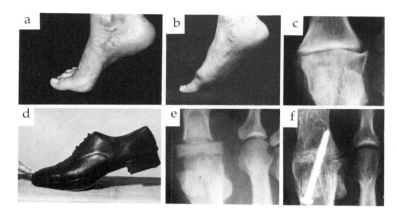

21.9 Hallux rigidus
(a) In normal walking the hallux dorsiflexes (extends) considerably. With rigidus (b), dorsiflexion is limited; (c) shows why the joint is rigid.

(d) A rocker sole relieves symptoms. Operations include joint replacement with a Silastic spacer (e) and arthrodesis (f).

to footwear. The shoe should be wide and the upper soft. Padding may be used to protect the bunion or a hammer toe. Foot exercises and an anterior platform type of support are useful when there is a splay foot with metatarsalgia.

In adults aged between 20 and 50, if deformity is not too severe, a tendon (adductor hallucis) release on the lateral side of the big toe, with trimming of the prominent metatarsal head and tightening of the medial capsule, may give adequate correction. For severe deformities, a metatarsal osteotomy will also be needed. In elderly patients the simplest solution is removal of the bunion and an excision arthroplasty in which the proximal part of the proximal phalanx is removed (Keller's operation).

NB: Corrective operations may produce a marked redistribution of stresses on weight-bearing and this can cause aching in the forefoot or – occasionally in elderly or osteoporotic individuals – stress fractures of the metatarsal bones.

Hallux rigidus

The 'rigidity' (joint stiffness) is due to osteoarthritis, the result of local trauma, osteochondritis dissecans of the first metatarsal head, gout or pseudogout. In marked contrast to hallux valgus, men are more commonly affected than women.

Clinical features

Pain on walking, especially on slopes or rough ground, is the predominant symptom. The hallux is straight and the metatarsophalangeal joint is knobbly; it feels enlarged and tender. Dorsiflexion is restricted and painful; plantarflexion is also limited, but less so.

X-RAY The changes are those of osteoarthritis: the joint space is narrowed, there is bone sclerosis and, often, large osteophytes.

Treatment

A rocker-soled shoe may abolish pain by allowing the foot to 'roll' without the necessity for dorsiflexion at the metatarsophalangeal joint.

If walking is painful despite this adjustment, an operation is advised. Joint replacement with a Silastic prosthesis effectively relieves pain and may increase the range of dorsiflexion. Arthrodesis also abolishes pain but the position should be tailored to the requirements of the individual patient.

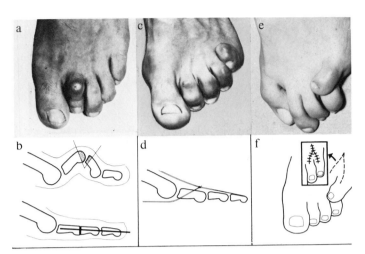

21.10 Disorders of the lesser toes (a) Hammer toe, and (b) treatment by excision-arthrodesis. (c) Curly toes and (d) treatment by flexor-to-extensor transfer. (e) Overlapping fifth toe, and (f) treatment by V/Y-plasty.

Claw toes

Flexion of the interphalangeal joints and hyperextension of the metatarsophalangeal joints constitute claw toes. This deformity is seen in neurological disorders (e.g. poliomyelitis and peroneal muscular atrophy) and in rheumatoid arthritis. Usually, however, no cause is found and the condition may be associated with idiopathic pes cavus; in such cases there is often a positive family history.

Clinical features

The patient complains of pain in the forefoot (metatarsalgia) and under the metatarsal heads. Usually the condition is bilateral and walking may be severely restricted. At first the joints are mobile and can be passively corrected; later the deformities become fixed and the metatarsophalangeal joints dislocated. Painful callosities may develop on the dorsum of the toes and under the metatarsal heads. In the most severe cases the skin ulcerates at the pressure sites.

Treatment

So long as the toes can be passively straightened, 'dynamic' correction is possible by transferring the long toe flexors to the extensors. When the deformity is fixed it may either be accepted and accommodated by special footwear, or treated by interphalangeal arthrodesis combined with tendon transfers.

Hammer toe

The proximal toe joint is fixed in flexion, whilst the distal joint and the metatarsophalangeal joint are extended. The second toe of one or both feet is commonly affected, and hyperextension of the metatarsophalangeal joint may go on to dorsal dislocation. Shoe pressure may produce painful corns or callosities on the dorsum of the toe and under the prominent metatarsal head.

Treatment

Operative correction is indicated for pain or for difficulty with shoes. The toe is shortened and straightened by excising the joint.

Rheumatoid arthritis

The ankle and foot are affected almost as often as the wrist and hand. During *stage 1*

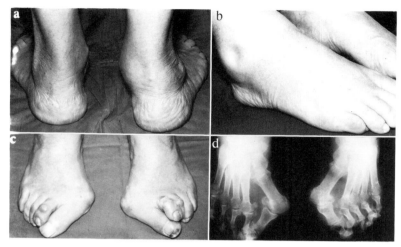

21.11 Rheumatoid arthritis Swelling of the hindfoot is more often due to tenosynovitis of tibialis posterior (a) or peronei (b) than to subtalar arthritis. If tendon rupture occurs, talar destruction and hindfoot deformity are inevitable. (c, d) Forefoot deformities are due primarily to progressive erosion of the metatarsophalangeal joints.

there is synovitis of the metatarsophalangeal, intertarsal and ankle joints, as well as of the sheathed tendons (usually the peronei and tibialis posterior). In *stage 2*, joint erosion and tendon dysfunction prepare the ground for the progressive deformities of *stage 3*.

The ankle and hindfoot

The earliest symptoms are pain and swelling around the ankle. Walking becomes increasingly difficult and, later, deformities appear. On examination, swelling and tenderness are usually localized to the back of the medial malleolus (tenosynovitis of tibialis posterior) or the lateral malleolus (tenosynovitis of the peronei). Less often the ankle swells (joint synovitis) and its movements are restricted. Inversion and eversion may be painful and limited. In the late stages the tibialis posterior may rupture, or become ineffectual due to progressive erosion of the tarsal joints,

and the foot gradually drifts into severe valgus deformity. *X-rays* show osteoporosis and, later, erosion of the tarsal and ankle joints. Soft-tissue swelling may be marked.

Treatment

In the stage of synovitis, splintage is essential (to allow inflammation to subside and to prevent deformity) while waiting for systemic treatment to control the disease. Initially tendon sheaths and joints may be injected with methylprednisolone, but this should not be repeated more than two or three times. A lightweight below-knee caliper with an inside supporting strap restores stability and may be worn almost indefinitely.

If the synovitis does not subside, operative synovectomy and (if necessary) tendon repair or transfer are advisable. In the very late stage, arthrodesis of the ankle and tarsal joints can still restore modest function and abolish pain.

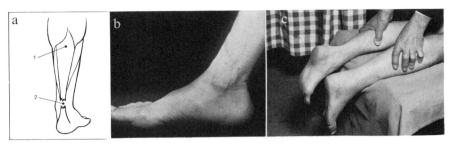

21.12 Tendo Achillis   (a) The soleus may tear at its musculotendinous junction (1) but the tendo Achillis itself ruptures 5 cm above its insertion (2). (b) The depression seen in this picture at the site of rupture later fills with blood. (c) Simmonds' test: both calves are being squeezed but only the left foot plantarflexes – the right tendon is ruptured.

The forefoot

Pain and swelling of the metatarsopha-langeal joints are among the earliest features of rheumatoid arthritis. Shoes feel uncomfortable and the patient walks less and less. Tenderness is at first localized to the metatarsophalangeal joints; later the entire forefoot is painful on pressing or squeezing. With increasing weakness of the intrinsic muscles and joint destruction, the characteristic deformities appear: a flattened anterior arch, claw toes and hallux valgus. Subcutaneous nodules are common and may ulcerate. Dorsal corns and plantar callosities also may break down and become infected. In the worst cases the toes are dislocated, inflamed, ulcerated and useless. *X-rays* show osteoporosis and periarticular erosion at the metatarsophalangeal joints.

Treatment

During the stage of synovitis, anti-inflammatory injections and attention to footwear may relieve symptoms. Once deformity is progressive, treatment is that of the claw toes and hallux valgus. Sometimes it is necessary to excise all the metatarsal heads in order to relieve pressure in the sole and to correct the toe deformities.

Ruptured tendo Achillis

Probably rupture occurs only if the tendon is degenerate. Consequently most patients are aged over 40. While pushing off (running or jumping), the calf muscle contracts; but the contraction is resisted by body weight and the tendon ruptures. The patient feels as if he has been struck just above the heel, and he is unable to tiptoe. Soon after the tear occurs, a gap can be seen and felt 5 cm above the insertion of the tendon. Plantarflexion of the foot is weak and is not accompanied by tautening of the tendon. Where doubt exists, Simmonds' test is helpful: with the patient prone, the calf is squeezed; if the tendon is intact, the foot is seen to plantarflex; if the tendon is ruptured the foot remains still.

Treatment

If the patient is seen early, the ends of the tendon may approximate when the foot is passively plantarflexed. If so, plaster is applied with the foot in equinus and is worn for 8 weeks. A shoe with a raised heel is worn for a further 6 weeks. Operative repair is probably safer, but an equinus plaster for 8 weeks and a heel raise for a further 6 weeks are still needed.

The diabetic foot

Foot disorders are common in diabetes and result from:

1. *Peripheral vascular disease* causing claudication, trophic changes, ulceration and even gangrene.
2. *Neuropathy* with sensory and/or motor impairment causing various foot deformities and possibly Charcot joints.
3. *Osteoporosis*, which may be severe enough to lead to fractures.
4. *Infection*, which is an ever-present danger in diabetes.

Treatment

The principles of treatment are:

1. Proper control of the diabetes.
2. Constant and careful attention to the skin and toenails to prevent infection.
3. Dry gangrene of the toe can be left to demarcate before amputation; wet gangrene and infection may call for immediate amputation.
4. Charcot joints causing instability may need splintage.
5. Osteoporotic fractures should be immobilized only until pain subsides; movement is important.

Gout

Swelling, redness, heat and exquisite tenderness of the metatarsophalangeal joint of the big toe ('podagra') is the epitome of gout. The condition may closely resemble septic arthritis, but the systemic features of infection are absent. The serum uric acid level may be raised.

Treatment with anti-inflammatory drugs will abort the attack; until the pain subsides the foot should be rested and protected from injury.

The painful foot

Pain is usually well localized to a single area: the heel, the mid-tarsal region or the forefoot.

The painful heel

In children the most likely cause is Sever's disease (apophysitis). It is not really a disease but a mild traction injury occurring in boys of about 10. Pain and tenderness are localized to the tendo Achillis insertion. The heel of the shoe should be raised a little and strenuous activities restricted for a few weeks.

In adolescent girls a calcaneal knob is common. The posterolateral portion of the calcaneum is too prominent and the shoe rubs on it, causing pain. If attention to footwear does not help, the knob is removed.

Young adults sometimes develop pain above the heel. The tendo Achillis is thickened and tender. It is common in athletes and is due to a peritendinitis. The acute form may be

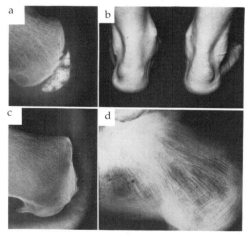

21.13 Heel disorders (a) Sever's disease – the apophysis is dense and fragmented. (b) Bilateral heel knobs. (c) 'Policeman's heel' – both heels had spurs but only one side was painful. (d) Paget's disease.

relieved by rest, ice-packs and strapping. The chronic form may need operation to divide the crural fascia; if there is a necrotic area in the tendon, this may need excision.

Pain under the heel and sharply localized tenderness, may occur in gout or in Reiter's disease. It is due to inflammation of the tough ligamentous tissue inserting into the calcaneum – a plantar fasciitis. The underlying disorder should be treated and the painful area protected from uneven pressure.

Older adults (40–60 years) may also develop a painful plantar fasciitis – usually less distressing than the acute disorder. It may be related to chronic stress ('policeman's heel'), but more often the cause is not apparent. A pressure-relieving pad, together with an arch support if there is flat foot, may help.

Painful tarsus

In children, osteochondritis of the navicular (Köhler's disease) may cause pain and tenderness over the dorsum of the mid-foot. If activities are restricted for a few weeks, the pain usually disappears.

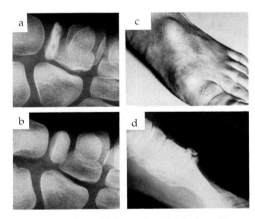

21.14 Painful tarsus (a) Köhler's disease compared with (b) the normal foot. (c, d) The 'overbone' (osteoarthritis at the first cuneiform-metatarsal joint).

In adults, pain in the same region is sometimes associated with a prominent ridge of bone. X-rays show osteophyte formation at the joint between the medial cuneiform and first metatarsal. If shoe adjustment fails to provide relief the lump may be bevelled off.

Painful forefoot (metatarsalgia)

Any foot abnormality which results in faulty weight distribution may cause nagging pain in the forefoot. It is therefore a common complaint in patients with hallux valgus, claw toes, pes cavus or flat foot. However, three specific disorders require special mention.

THE PAINFUL FOREFOOT

1. Foot strain
2. Freiberg's disease
3. Stress fracture
4. Morton's metatarsalgia
5. Gout
6. RA

Freiberg's disease This is a 'crushing' type of osteochondritis of the second metatarsal head (rarely the third). It affects young adults, usually women. A bony lump (the enlarged head) is palpable and tender; the joint is irritable. X-rays show the head to be wide and flat. If discomfort is marked the metatarsal head is excised.

Stress fracture, usually of the second or third metatarsal, occurs in young adults after unaccustomed activity. The affected shaft feels thick and tender. The x-ray appearance is at first normal, but later shows fusiform callus around a fine transverse fracture. Rest is all that is needed.

Morton's metatarsalgia The patient, usually a woman of 40–50 years, complains of sharp pain in the forefoot, radiating to the toes. Tenderness is localized to one of the interdigital spaces – usually the third – and

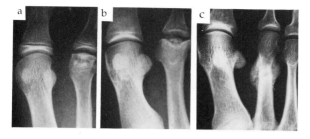

21.15 Metatarsalgia (a, b) Stages in the development of Freiberg's disease; (c) stress fracture of the second metatarsal.

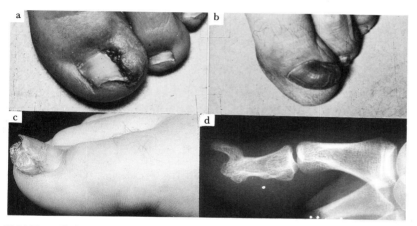

21.16 Toenail disorders (a) In-grown toenail. (b) Overgrown toenail (onychogryposis). (c) Undergrown toenail, caused by (d) a subungual exostosis.

sensation may be diminished in the cleft and adjacent toes. This is essentially an entrapment syndrome affecting one of the digital nerves, but secondary thickening of the nerve creates the impression of a 'neuroma'. If symptoms do not respond to protective padding the 'neuroma' is excised.

Toenail disorders

The toenail of the hallux may be ingrown, overgrown or undergrown.

INGROWN   The nail burrows into the nail groove; this ulcerates and its wall grows over the nail, so the term 'embedded toenail' would be better. The patient is taught to cut the nail square, to insert pledgets of wool under the ingrowing edges and always to keep the feet clean and dry. If these measures fail, the 'gutter' treatment is worth trying. A small wedge of soft tissue (where the nail digs in) is excised; a fine polythene tube is cut vertically in half and a segment inserted between nail and soft tissue. More radical measures include partial or complete removal of the nail, taking care to remove the germinal matrix.

OVERGROWN (ONYCHOGRYPOSIS) The nail is hard, thick and curved. A chiropodist can usually make the patient comfortable, but occasionally the nail may need excision.

UNDERGROWN   A subungual exostosis grows on the dorsum of the terminal phalanx and pushes the nail upwards. The exostosis should be removed.

Part 3   Fractures and Joint Injuries

The management of acute injuries 22

Trauma is the main cause of death in people under 40. Limb injuries are the commonest, head and visceral injuries are the most lethal: this simple observation determines the priorities in management.

Trauma mortality has a trimodal distribution. (1) Most deaths occur during the first hour after injury, before the patient reaches hospital. (2) A second peak in the death rate occurs between 1 and 4 hours after injury, when patients die mainly because of blood loss; this is the 'golden hour', during which death can and should be prevented by competent treatment. (3) A third peak occurs several weeks later when patients die of late complications and multiple organ failure.

The management of severe injuries proceeds in well-defined stages:

1. Emergency treatment immediately after the accident;
2. Resuscitation and evaluation in the hospital accident department;
3. Early treatment of visceral injuries and cardiorespiratory complications;
4. Treatment of musculoskeletal injuries;
5. Long-term rehabilitation.

Treatment at the scene of the accident

The first duty of a doctor arriving at the scene of a major accident is to introduce calm and order into the prevailing chaos. His actions should be swift yet unhurried, cautious yet purposeful. Messages are sent to the emergency services and the nearest accident centre is alerted.

Management of the injured follows a disciplined sequence: obtain access, free the airway, check ventilation, ensure haemostasis, combat shock, splint fractures, transport to hospital.

1. The patient's head and neck should be freed by removing the surrounding debris.
2. The upper airway is checked. If the patient is unconscious the jaw should be pulled forward; a finger in the mouth ensures that there is no mechanical obstruction.
3. If there is still difficulty with breathing, look for a chest wound. Administer oxygen if available.

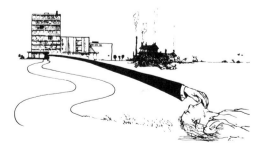

22.1 Severe injuries – emergency treatment The ABC of early management: Airway! Breathing! Circulation!

4. External bleeding should be staunched by direct pressure.

5. If facilities are available, intravenous fluids may be given for shock. Morphine is useful but should not be given to patients with abdominal or head injuries.

6. Injured limbs should be splinted as best possible, using whatever is available.

7. A collar should be applied and the spine held immobile lest there is an undetected fracture or dislocation.

8. The patient is then carefully lifted by at least two and preferably three people so that he can be transported with minimal physical manipulation.

Management in hospital

Initial assessment (primary survey)

The patient is stripped and examined rapidly from head to toe. The ABC of initial simultaneous evaluation and treatment is *AIRWAY, BREATHING* and *CIRCULATION*. If there are injuries around the head and face, damage to the cervical spine should be assumed and care should be taken not to flex or extend the neck until a cervical spine injury has been definitely excluded. Life-threatening conditions should be treated as they are identified.

The ABC of trauma management

Airway
Breathing
Circulation

Airway The upper airway is cleared and the jaw is pulled forward to dislodge any obstruction by the back of the tongue. If necessary, a pharyngeal airway is inserted; occasionally endotracheal intubation or cricolaryngotomy may be called for. During these manoeuvres the neck should be protected from movement.

Breathing If, despite a clear airway, ventilation is inadequate the chest should be carefully examined for atelectasis, pneumothorax or a flail segment. *Tension pneumothorax* is a life-threatening complication and should be treated by immediate decompression (see page 233). *Sucking chest wounds* must be closed and a *flail chest* may require endotracheal intubation and positive pressure ventilation. It is essential to give all severely injured patients supplemental oxygen and to take a blood sample for measurement of the arterial oxygen tension (Po_2) and carbon dioxide tension (Pco_2).

Circulation Any major external haemorrhage is controlled by direct pressure. The patient is assessed for signs of shock and blood specimens are taken for full blood count, estimation of electrolytes and cross-matching.

Consciousness The level of consciousness is assessed on the Glasgow Coma Scale (see page 231). All findings are carefully recorded and kept available for comparison with later assessment.

Resuscitation

Resuscitation has begun with the establishment of a clear airway and the restoration of breathing and ventilation. Equally important is to prevent hypovolaemia and treat shock. As a first measure a crystalloid solution such as Ringer's lactate is infused rapidly via one or two large-bore needles or venous cut-down. If the blood pressure does not stabilize after 2 litres of fluid, blood transfusion should be started.

If the blood pressure cannot be maintained by blood transfusion and cardiac embarrassment has been excluded, the source of continued bleeding must be sought and attended to. In severe shock, pneumatic anti-shock garments are sometimes used.

Secondary evaluation

Once the patient has been resuscitated a 'head to toe survey' is carried out. The back can be examined by gently 'log-rolling' the patient onto his side.

Further, definitive treatment will be decided by the findings during this review.

Shock

Shock is a generalized state of reduced tissue perfusion; if allowed to persist it will result in irreversible damage to the life-supporting organs. It may be caused by injury to the heart ('cardiogenic shock'). Usually, however, it is the result of haemorrhage and reduction of blood volume ('*hypovolaemic shock*'). Various compensatory mechanisms come into play, but if blood loss is too great they will fail: cardiac output falls, the blood pressure drops and decreased tissue perfusion leads to hypoxia, acidosis and progressive cell damage.

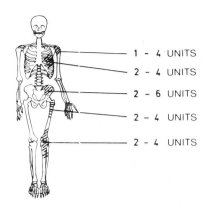

1 – 4 UNITS
2 – 4 UNITS
2 – 6 UNITS
2 – 4 UNITS
2 – 4 UNITS

22.2 Severe injuries – blood loss   Range of blood loss in closed fractures. The severely injured patient may lose more blood than you think!

Clinical features

The patient becomes apathetic and thirsty, his breathing shallow and rapid; the lips and skin are pale and the extremities feel cold and clammy. As compensation fails, the pulse becomes rapid and feeble while the blood pressure drops. Eventually renal function is impaired and urinary output falls.

Treatment

The treatment of hypovolaemic shock is urgent: the essentials are to arrest bleeding and to replace lost blood. Morphine may be of great value, but it should be given in small intravenous doses and must be completely withheld if there are head injuries or if abdominal injuries are suspected. Giving oxygen is important, even if the patient is not obviously dyspnoeic. Pneumatic antishock garments (military antishock trousers, or 'MAST' suits) are sometimes used; they work by compressing the capillary bed and increasing vascular resistance. If there are fractures, early reduction and splintage help to reduce the effects of shock.

The essential feature of treatment, however, is the early restoration of blood volume. A practical routine is to start with the rapid infusion of 2 litres of crystalloid solution such as Ringer's lactate; the patient's response is checked by measuring the heart rate, blood pressure and CVP, and, later on, urinary output and acid–base balance. If improvement is not sustained and other causes of cardiac embarrassment have been excluded, concealed haemorrhage into the chest or abdomen is probable and should be sought by investigations such as ultrasonography, CT and abdominal paracentesis or lavage.

If the patient does not respond quickly to intravenous crystalloids, or in any case if the haematocrit is less than 25%, blood transfusion will be necessary. In an emergency group O Rh-negative blood may be used until cross-matched blood is available.

It is important not only to give blood but also to give enough blood. Even with closed injuries there is far more bleeding into tissues than is commonly appreciated: two or three units may be lost with a single major limb fracture.

Adult respiratory distress syndrome (ARDS)

During the later stages of shock and septicaemia, endothelial cell damage and increased small-vessel permeability lead to the extravasation of haemorrhagic, protein-rich fluid into the pulmonary interstitial tissue and alveoli. Over a period of a few days the picture may change from pulmonary congestion to diffuse alveolar destruction. The early changes are reversible, but once diffuse alveolar damage occurs there is usually an inexorable progression to severe hypoxaemia, multiple organ failure and death.

Clinical features

About 36 hours after injury and hypovolaemic shock, the patient develops mild dyspnoea. Even before this, if blood gases are measured they may show a diminished Po_2. These changes are common after long-bone fractures, and fat embolism is often suspected. By the second or third day the clinical features are more obvious; the patient is restless, mildly cyanosed and shows signs of respiratory distress. X-rays may now show diffuse pulmonary infiltrates. Special lung function tests are required to show the full extent of the condition. In the most severe cases, pulmonary deterioration is inexorable and the outcome is fatal.

Treatment

The most important aspect of management is the early and effective treatment of shock. There is also evidence that, in patients with multiple injuries, the incidence of pulmonary dysfunction is reduced by early stabilization of fractures.

The treatment of established ARDS is supportive and aims to minimize further lung damage until recovery occurs, whilst optimizing oxygen delivery to the tissues. This requires highly specialized methods of artificial ventilation and continuous cardiopulmonary assessment.

Fat embolism

Circulating fat globules occur in most young adults after closed fractures of long bones;

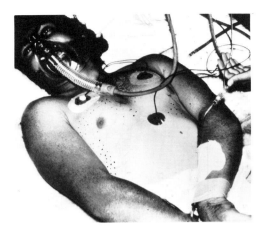

22.3 Fat embolism This man with bilateral femoral shaft fractures (closed) developed fat embolism. When this photograph was taken he was unconscious, his face was congested and he was on continuous oxygen with cardiac monitoring. The petechiae were smaller and fainter than shown here; they have been accentuated for clarity and to show their distribution.

fortunately, only a few develop the fat embolism syndrome, which is now thought to be part of the wider spectrum of acute post-traumatic respiratory distress.

The source of the fat emboli is probably the bone marrow, and the condition is more common in patients with multiple closed fractures; however, fat embolism has been reported in a variety of disorders other than skeletal trauma (e.g. burns, renal infarction and cardiopulmonary operations); the pathogenesis is still a matter of controversy.

The patient is usually a young adult with a closed long-bone fracture. Clinical features appear within 48 hours of injury (and often within 12 hours!); they include shortness of breath, restlessness and mild confusion, with a rise in temperature and pulse rate. In the worst cases the patient develops marked respiratory distress, followed by restlessness, coma and death. Clinical signs are few, but a careful search may reveal petechiae on the chest, in the axillae and in the conjunctival folds.

There is no infallible test for fat embolism, but a fairly constant finding is hypoxaemia;

the blood P_{O_2} should always be monitored during the first 72 hours of any major injury, and values below 8 kPa (60 mmHg) must be regarded with grave suspicion.

Treatment

There is no specific treatment for fat embolism; the most important measure is to counteract the hypoxaemia by giving oxygen, in mild cases by nasal catheter or oxygen mask and in severe cases by tracheal intubation and assisted ventilation: the blood P_{O_2} is carefully monitored and it should be maintained above 9.3 kPa (70 mmHg).

Supportive therapy includes blood and fluid replacement, with intravenous corticosteroids and heparin, which are thought to reduce pulmonary oedema and intravascular clotting.

Head injuries

Most head injuries result from a blow that causes either direct damage or intracerebral movement due to rapid acceleration or deceleration. Damage may consist of: (1) minor contusion causing transient loss of consciousness or amnesia; (2) severe contusion or laceration, due either to direct injury or to shearing forces; (3) localized intracranial bleeding; (4) fractures of the skull; (5) diffuse oedema and a rise in intracranial pressure.

Clinical assessment

The history may give important clues to the type and severity of the injury. Did the patient lose consciousness? If so, for how long? Was there a period of amnesia? Did the patient take drugs or alcohol? Is there a previous history of fits or neurological disorder? What other injuries are present?

There may be obvious swelling and/or bruising of the face. The scalp should be examined for cuts or localized swelling (haematoma); open wounds should be gently explored with a gloved finger to exclude underlying fractures. The nose and ears are examined for blood or CSF leakage; other signs of basal fracture are sub-conjunctival haemorrhage without a posterior margin, localized periorbital haematomas ('racoon eyes') and retromastoid bruising (Battle's sign).

The pupils are examined for asymmetrical dilatation and the light reflex is tested on each side. With increased intracranial pressure and tentorial herniation, compression of the IIIrd nerve results in dilatation of the pupil and a failure to react to light.

X-ray of the skull is mandatory and CT is needed for those with persistent subnormal consciousness, depressed skull fractures, penetrating injuries or focal neurological signs.

Throughout the examination great care must be exercised not to flex or extend the neck unless an associated cervical spine injury has been excluded.

The level of consciousness

The level of consciousness should be assessed according to the Glasgow Coma Scale (GCS). This is based on descending levels of eye opening and verbal and motor responses (Table 22.1). The maximum score, representing normality, is 15; a score of 8 or less implies severe head injury; absence of eye opening, speech and response to commands is indicative of coma. Persistent lack of response to painful stimuli (supraorbital or nail-bed pressure) suggests irrecoverable brain damage.

Repeated examination will show whether the patient's condition is improving or not. A deterioration of 2 points is highly significant and is an indication for CT.

Management

Most head injuries are fairly trivial and require no more than careful examination and reassurance. The indications for admission to hospital for observation and reassess-

Table 22.1 Glasgow Coma Scale

	Score
Eye-opening:	
Spontaneous	4
On command	3
On pain	2
Nil	1
Best motor response:	
Obeys	6
Localizes pain	5
Normal flexor	4
Abnormal flexor	3
Extensor	2
Nil	1
Verbal response:	
Orientated	5
Confused	4
Words	3
Sounds	2
Nil	1

ment are any of the following: (1) a diminished level of consciousness; (2) a history of transient loss of consciousness or amnesia; (3) a skull fracture; and (4) abnormal neurological signs.

In patients who appear to be comatose, drowsy, restless or merely confused it may be difficult to distinguish the effects of a head injury from those of hypoglycaemia, alcohol or drugs. All such patients, as well as those whose cerebral dysfunction may be due to shock or hypoxia, should be graded on the GCS and kept under observation until the diagnosis is clear.

Concussion Following a blow, there is a transient loss of consciousness, often associated with amnesia. The patient should be admitted to hospital and kept under observation for 24 hours.

Scalp wounds Scalp wounds can be sutured, provided there is no underlying depressed fracture.

Fractures A linear fracture may be quite harmless, but if there are associated neurological features a CT should be obtained to exclude intracranial damage or haematoma. If there is a CSF leak (otorrhoea or rhinorrhoea) the patient is given prophylactic benzyl penicillin. A depressed fracture requires exploration, elevation and clearance of damaged tissue.

Extradural haematoma The classic scenario is of a patient who has a head injury but seems to be perfectly well, is allowed to go home and then rapidly becomes unconscious. There may be a minor fracture which causes bleeding and cerebral compression. CT

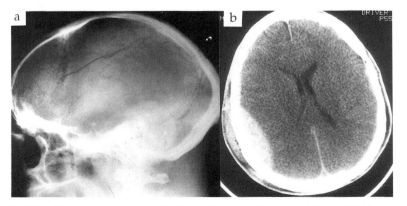

22.4 Head injuries – imaging (a) X-ray showing a fracture of the parietal bone. (b) A CT scan shows an extradural haematoma with distortion of the lateral ventricle on that side.

shows an extradural haematoma and a shift of the brain. This requires urgent treatment: burr holes and evacuation of the haematoma; if necessary, the middle meningeal artery is ligated.

Severe brain contusion Patients with severe head injuries (a GCS score of 8 or less) should be kept under continuous observation until they recover spontaneously, or develop signs calling for operative treatment, or ultimately show the features of 'brain death'. They are best managed by endotracheal intubation and artificial ventilation. The main indication for craniotomy is the development of an intracranial haematoma.

Chest injuries

Chest injuries may damage the rib cage or its contents. Remember that small wounds may hide serious complications.

Clinical assessment

The patient may have chest pain or show obvious signs of respiratory distress. The skin is inspected for bruising (a seat belt injury) and for open wounds (especially 'sucking' sounds, which communicate with the pleural cavity). The trachea is palpated to see if it is deviated and the chest is examined for signs of pulmonary collapse and mediastinal shift.

X-rays are essential: they may reveal fractures, pleural effusion, pneumothorax or lung collapse. Widening of the mediastinum suggests a ruptured aortic arch.

Management

1. *With all severe chest injuries*, three measures are important: blood replacement (but not with crystalloid fluids, which aggravate pulmonary congestion); the administration of oxygen; and adequate analgesics (but not respiratory depressants).

2. *Open wounds* that communicate with the pleural cavity cause a *sucking pneumothorax* and lung collapse. A moist swab strapped over the hole may suffice temporarily, but the wound should be securely stitched as soon as possible; an intercostal tube connected to an underwater seal allows the lung to expand.

3. *A simple closed pneumothorax* consists of an air leak into the pleural cavity. This is easily seen on an x-ray taken with the patient upright. Small collections require no treatment apart from breathing exercises. A large pneumothorax may need drainage (see below).

4. *A tension pneumothorax* occurs when a pleural tear acts like a valve, allowing air into the pleural cavity during inspiration but preventing it from escaping during expiration. The patient is distressed; chest movements are diminished, the mediastinum is shifted to the unaffected side and breath sounds are absent on the affected side. This is a lethal emergency; there may be only minutes in which to act before the patient dies. A large-bore needle should be inserted into the pleural

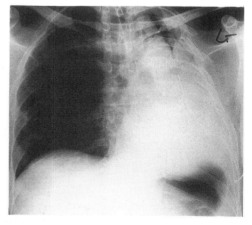

22.5 Tension pneumothorax This patient with rib fractures became increasingly distressed. The x-ray shows the 'black-out' of the right side of the chest, with the mediastinal contents shifted to the left.

cavity through the second intercostal space in the mid-clavicular line anteriorly. Once the emergency is over this is replaced by a thoracostomy tube which is inserted through the fourth intercostal space in the mid-axillary line and connected to an underwater seal; this is retained until the lung re-expands.

5. *Surgical emphysema* is the appearance of air under the skin, extending over the chest wall and into the neck. This happens when a lung perforation (or rupture) communicates with the subcutaneous tissues. If there is a tension pneumothorax it should be decompressed.

6. *Haemothorax* (from a torn lung or blood vessel) can be diagnosed by withdrawing blood through a needle. The blood is drained by an intercostal catheter through a low intercostal space. Breathing exercises are encouraged.

7. *Uncomplicated rib fractures* usually need no treatment other than analgesics. The patient with multiple fractures and extensive bruising should, however, be kept in hospital until complications have been positively excluded. If pain is marked, infiltration with local anaesthetic may be needed to facilitate breathing and prevent atelectasis and lung infection.

8. *A stove-in chest* has multiple fractures, often with underlying lung damage. Sometimes an entire section of the chest wall is isolated as a flail segment which is sucked inwards during inspiration and blown outwards during expiration. This so-called paradoxical respiration is useless for ventilating the lung and it may lead to respiratory failure (particularly if the lung is also damaged).

A stove-in chest with only moderate respiratory difficulty can be treated by strapping a large pack over the mobile segment and administering oxygen. More severe cases require endotracheal intubation and positive pressure ventilation; a chest drain connected to an underwater seal may be needed if there is lung damage. Positive pressure ventilation is maintained (if necessary by changing to a tracheostomy until the chest wall is stable).

9. *Severe lung damage* may lead to ARDS. This is discussed on page 229).

Abdominal injuries

A blow to the abdomen may rupture viscera or blood vessels. A ruptured spleen or liver may be deceptively 'silent', but it should be suspected if there are signs of continuing blood loss. An ultrasound scan may be helpful and abdominal paracentesis may show blood in the peritoneal cavity.

Stab wounds can be missed unless the abdomen is carefully examined. The size of the wound is no guide to the amount of damage; a sharpened bicycle spoke can perforate bowel, spleen, diaphragm and heart in a single blow.

If a serious injury is suspected, laparotomy is essential. A ruptured spleen is removed. Bleeding from a ruptured liver is difficult to control but an attempt should be made to suture or ligate injured vessels; if this fails, haemorrhage may be controlled by packing. A ruptured bowel can usually be repaired.

Pelvic injuries

Fractures of the pelvis are often associated with serious visceral injury and blood loss. This subject is dealt with in Chapter 29.

Crush syndrome

The crush syndrome may occur if a large bulk of muscle is crushed, as by fallen masonry, or if a tourniquet has been left on too long. When compression is released, acid myohaematin (cytochrome c) is carried to the kidney and blocks the tubules. An alternative explanation is that renal artery spasm leads to tubular necrosis.

Shock is profound. The released limb is pulseless and later becomes red, swollen and blistered; sensation and muscle power may be lost. Renal secretion diminishes and a low-output uraemia with acidosis develops. If renal secretion returns within a week the patient survives; most patients become increasingly drowsy and die within 14 days. Renal dialysis may be life saving.

To avert disaster, a limb crushed severely and for several hours should be amputated. Likewise, if a tourniquet has been left on for more than 6 hours the limb must be sacrificed. Amputation is carried out above the site of compression and before compression is released.

If compression has already been released, the limb must be cooled and the patient treated for shock and renal failure.

Tetanus

The tetanus organism flourishes only in dead tissue. It produces an exotoxin which passes to the central nervous system via the blood and the perineural lymphatics from the infected region. The toxin is fixed in the anterior horn cells and thereafter cannot be neutralized by antitoxin.

Established tetanus is characterized by tonic, and later clonic, contractions, especially of the muscles of the jaw and face (trismus, risus sardonicus), those near the wound itself, and later of the neck and trunk. Ultimately, the diaphragm and intercostal muscles may be fixed in spasm and the patient dies of asphyxia.

Prophylaxis

Active immunization of the whole population by tetanus toxoid is an attainable ideal. To the patient so immunized, booster doses of toxoid are given after all but trivial skin wounding. In non-immunized patients prompt and thorough wound toilet together with antibiotics may be adequate, but if the wound is contaminated, and particularly with delay before operation, then antitoxin is advisable. Horse serum carries a considerable risk of anaphylaxis, and human antitoxin (ATG) should be used. The opportunity is taken to initiate active immunization with toxoid at the same time.

Treatment

With established tetanus, intravenous antitoxin (again, human for choice) is advisable. Heavy sedation and muscle relaxant drugs may help; tracheal intubation and controlled respiration are employed for the patient with respiratory and swallowing embarrassment.

Gas gangrene

This terrifying condition is produced by clostridial infection (especially *C. welchii*). These are anaerobic organisms that can survive and multiply only in tissues with low oxygen tension; the prime site for infection, therefore, is a dirty wound with dead muscle which has been closed without adequate debridement. Toxins produced by the organisms destroy the cell wall and rapidly lead to tissue necrosis, thus promoting the spread of the disease.

Clinical features appear within 24 hours of the injury: the patient complains of intense pain and swelling around the wound and a brownish discharge may be seen; gas formation is usually not very marked. There is little or no pyrexia but the pulse rate is increased and a characteristic odour becomes evident. Rapidly the patient becomes toxaemic and may lapse into coma and die.

It is essential to distinguish gas gangrene, which is characterized by myonecrosis, from *anaerobic cellulitis*, in which superficial gas formation is abundant but toxaemia usually slight. Failure to recognize the difference may lead to unnecessary amputation for the non-lethal cellulitis.

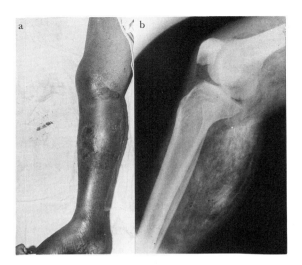

22.6 Gas gangrene   (a) Clinical picture of gas gangrene. (b) x-rays show diffuse gas in the muscles of the calf.

Prevention

Deep, penetrating wounds in muscular tissue are dangerous; they should be explored, all dead tissue should be carefully excised and, if there is the slightest doubt about tissue viability, the wound should be left open. Unhappily there is no effective antitoxin against *C. welchii*.

Treatment

The key to life-saving treatment is early diagnosis. General measures, such as fluid replacement and intravenous antibiotics, are started immediately. Hyperbaric oxygen has been used as a means of limiting the spread of gangrene. However, the mainstay of treatment is prompt decompression of the wound and removal of all dead tissue. In advanced cases, amputation may be essential.

Fracture pathology and diagnosis 23

A fracture is a break in the structural continuity of bone. It may be no more than a crack, a crumpling or a splintering of the cortex; more often the break is complete and the bone fragments are displaced. If the overlying skin remains intact it is a *closed* (or *'simple'*) *fracture*; if the skin or one of the body cavities is breached it is an *open* (or *'compound'*) *fracture*, liable to contamination and infection.

How fractures happen

Bone is relatively brittle, yet it has sufficient strength and resilience to withstand considerable stress. Fractures may follow: (1) a single traumatic incident; (2) repetitive stress; or (3) abnormal weakening of the bone.

Fractures due to a traumatic incident

Most fractures are caused by sudden and excessive force. They can result from (1) *direct violence* (e.g. a blow on the arm which shatters the ulna at the point of impact) or (2) *indirect violence*, such as bending and twisting of a long bone, or forcible traction by a tendon or ligament which literally pulls the bone apart.

COMPLETE FRACTURES The bone is completely broken into two or more fragments. If the fracture is *transverse*, the fragments usually remain in place after reduction; if it is *oblique* or *spiral*, they tend to slip and redisplace even if the bone is splinted. In an *impacted fracture* the fragments are jammed tightly together and the fracture line is indistinct. A *comminuted fracture* is one in which there are more than two fragments; because

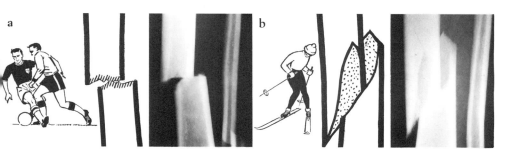

a   b

23.1 Mechanisms of injury (a) A direct blow causes a transverse fracture. (b) A twisting force causes a spiral fracture.

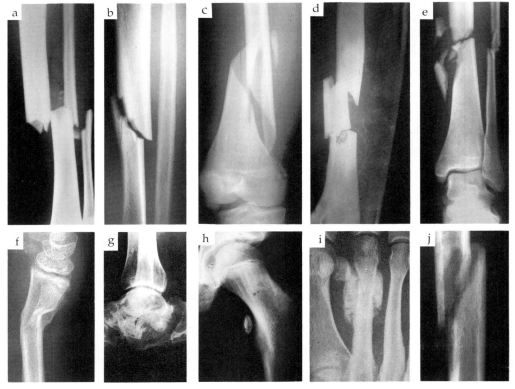

23.2 Common types of fractures   (a) Transverse; (b) oblique; (c) spiral; (d) segmental; (e) comminuted; (f) greenstick; (g) compression; (h) avulsion; (i) stress; (j) pathological.

there is poor interlocking of the fracture surfaces, these lesions are often unstable.

INCOMPLETE FRACTURES   Here the bone is incompletely divided and the periosteum remains in continuity. In a *greenstick fracture* the bone is buckled or bent (like snapping a green twig); this is seen in children, whose bones are more springy than those of adults. Reduction is usually easy and healing is quick. *Compression fractures* occur when cancellous bone is crumpled. This happens in adults, especially in the vertebral bodies. Complete reduction is impossible and some residual deformity is inevitable.

Fatigue or stress fractures

Cracks can occur in bone, as in metal and other materials, due to repetitive stress. This is most often seen in the tibia or fibula or metatarsals, especially in athletes, dancers and army recruits.

Pathological fractures

Fractures may occur even with normal stresses if the bone has been weakened (e.g. by osteoporosis or a tumour) or if it is excessively brittle (e.g. in Paget's disease).

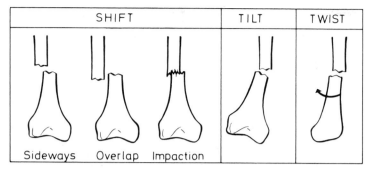

SHIFT			TILT	TWIST
Sideways	Overlap	Impaction		

23.3 Fracture displacements

How the fragments are displaced

After a complete fracture the fragments usually become displaced, partly by the force of the injury, partly by gravity and partly by the pull of muscles attached to them. Displacement is usually described in terms of apposition, angulation, rotation and altered length.

Apposition (shift) The fragments may be shifted sideways, backwards or forwards in relation to each other, so that the fracture surfaces lose contact. The fracture will usually unite even if apposition is imperfect, or indeed even if the bone ends lie side by side with the fracture surfaces making no contact at all.

Alignment (tilt)   The fragments may be tilted or angulated in relation to each other. Malalignment, if uncorrected, may lead to deformity of the limb.

Rotation (twist)   One of the fragments may be rotated on its longitudinal axis; the bone looks straight but the limb ends up with a rotational deformity.

Length   The fragments may be distracted and separated, or they may overlap, due to muscle spasm, causing shortening of the bone.

How fractures heal

The process of fracture repair varies according to the type of bone involved and the amount of movement at the fracture site. In a tubular bone, and in the absence of rigid fixation, healing proceeds in five stages.

1. Tissue death and haematoma formation Vessels are torn and a haematoma forms around and within the fracture. Bone at the fracture surfaces, deprived of a blood supply, dies back for a millimetre or two.

2. Inflammation and cellular proliferation Within 8 hours of the fracture there is an acute inflammatory reaction with proliferation of cells under the periosteum and within the breached medullary canal. The fragment ends are surrounded by cellular tissue, which bridges the fracture site. The clotted haematoma is slowly absorbed and fine new capillaries grow into the area.

3. Callus formation   The proliferating cells are potentially chondrogenic and osteogenic; given the right conditions, they will start forming bone and, in some cases, also cartilage. The cell population now also includes osteoclasts (probably derived from the new blood vessels) which begin to mop up dead bone. The thick cellular mass, with its islands of immature bone and cartilage, forms the callus or splint on the periosteal and endosteal surfaces. As the immature fibre bone (or

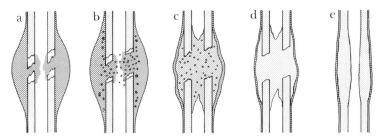

23.4 Fracture healing Five stages of healing. (a) *Haematoma*: there is tissue damage and bleeding at the fracture site; the bone ends die back for a few millimetres. (b) *Inflammation*: inflammatory cells appear in the haematoma. (c) *Callus*: the cell population changes to osteoblasts and osteoclasts; dead bone is mopped up and woven bone appears in the fracture callus. (d) *Consolidation*: woven bone is replaced by lamellar bone and the fracture is solidly united. (e) *Remodelling*: the new-formed bone is remodelled to resemble the normal structure.

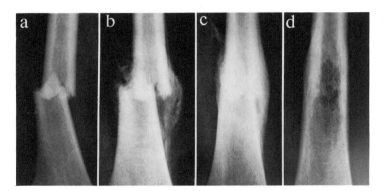

23.5 Fracture repair (a) Fracture; (b) union; (c) consolidation; (d) bone remodelling. The fracture must be protected until consolidated.

'woven' bone) becomes more densely mineralized, movement at the fracture site decreases progressively and the fracture unites.

4. Consolidation With continuing osteoclastic and osteoblastic activity the woven bone is transformed into lamellar bone. The system is now rigid enough to allow osteoclasts to burrow through the debris at the fracture line, and close behind them osteoblasts fill in the remaining gaps between the fragments with new bone. The bone is now strong enough to carry normal loads.

5. Remodelling The fracture has been bridged by a cuff of solid bone. Over a period of months, or even years, this crude 'weld' is reshaped by a continuous process of alternating bone resorption and formation. Thicker lamellae are laid down where the stresses are high; unwanted buttresses are carved away; the medullary cavity is reformed. Eventually, and especially in children, the bone reassumes something like its normal shape.

Healing by direct repair

Fractures of cancellous bone are fairly immobile from the start and the bone-forming surfaces are well apposed. New bone may be laid down directly across the fracture and callus formation is usually minimal. *Fractures treated by rigid internal fixation* also heal by direct repair. (The term 'primary' is sometimes

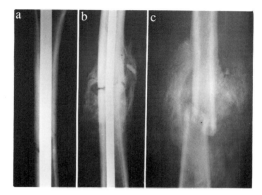

23.6 Callus and movement Three patients with femoral shaft fractures. (a) and (b) are both 6 weeks after fixation – in (a) the K-nail fitted tightly, preventing any movement, and there is no callus; in (b) the nail fitted loosely, permitting movement, so there is callus. (c) This patient had cerebral irritation and thrashed around wildly – at 3 weeks callus is excessive.

used but should not be taken to imply that it is better than indirect or 'secondary' healing by callus.) Osteoclasts appear at the fracture site and burrow through the bone debris; close behind them come osteoblasts, laying down new bone across the fracture. There is no callus and the new bone units, or osteons, depend on the metal implant for their integrity.

The time factor

Repair of a fracture is a continuous process and there are no specific events signifying a moment of 'union' or 'consolidation'. The ultimate test is the bone's ability to withstand the stresses placed upon it: fracture 'union' is incomplete repair and it is not safe to subject the unprotected bone to stress; 'consolidation' is also less than complete repair, but it allows unprotected function; only after remodelling and the restoration of normal bone density is the process of repair complete.

The rate of repair depends upon the *type of bone* involved (cancellous bone heals faster than cortical bone), the *type of fracture* (a

transverse fracture takes longer than a spiral fracture), the state of the *blood supply* (poor circulation means slow healing), the patient's *general constitution* (healthy bone heals faster) and, most of all, the patient's *age* (healing is almost twice as fast in children as in adults). The following serves as a rough guide for fractures of tubular bones in healthy adults.

	Upper limb	Lower limb
Callus visible	2–3 weeks	2–3 weeks
Union	4–6 weeks	8–12 weeks
Consolidation	6–8 weeks	12–16 weeks

Fractures that fail to unite

Sometimes the normal process of fracture repair is thwarted and the bone fails to unite. Causes of non-union are:

– distraction and separation of the fragments
– interposition of soft tissues between the fragments
– excessive movement at the fracture
– poor local blood supply.

In such cases cell proliferation is predominantly fibroblastic; the fracture gap is filled by fibrous tissue and the bone fragments remain mobile – rather like a false joint or pseudarthrosis. In *hypertrophic non-union* there is active osteogenesis and the bone ends are thickened (the 'elephant's foot' appearance); union is still possible provided the bone fragments are apposed and held immobile. In *atrophic non-union* bone formation peters out and the fragments are rounded or tapered (carrot-shaped); the fracture will never heal unless it is immobilized and grafted.

Clinical and radiological features

History

There is usually a history of *injury*, followed by *inability to use the injured limb*. But beware! The fracture is not always at the site of the injury: thus, a blow to the knee may fracture the patella, the femoral condyles, the shaft of the femur or even the acetabulum. If a fracture occurs with trivial trauma, suspect a pathological lesion. Children often sustain incomplete fractures which are easily missed. *Pain, bruising* and *swelling* are common symptoms, but they do not distinguish a fracture from a soft-tissue injury. *Deformity* is much more suggestive.

Always enquire about *symptoms of associated injuries*: numbness or weakness, skin pallor or cyanosis, blood in the urine, abdominal pain, transient loss of consciousness.

Ask about *previous injuries that might cause confusion when the x-ray is seen.*

Finally, a *general medical history* is important, in preparation for anaesthesia or operation.

Examination

General signs

A broken bone is part of a patient. It is important to look for evidence of: (1) shock or haemorrhage; (2) associated damage to brain, spinal cord or viscera; and (3) a predisposing cause (such as Paget's disease).

Local signs

Injured tissues must be handled gently. To elicit crepitus or abnormal movement is unnecessarily painful; x-ray diagnosis is painless. Nevertheless the familiar headings of clinical examination should always be considered, or damage to arteries and nerves may be overlooked.

● LOOK   Swelling, bruising and deformity may be obvious, but the important point is whether the skin is intact; if the skin is broken, and the wound communicates with the fracture, the injury is 'open' ('compound').

● FEEL   There is localized tenderness, but it is necessary also to examine distal to the fracture in order to feel the pulse and to test sensation. A vascular injury is a surgical emergency.

● MOVE   Crepitus and abnormal movement may be present, but it is more important to ask if the patient can move the joints distal to the injury.

X-ray

X-ray examination is mandatory. Certain pitfalls must be avoided, as follows.

Two views   A fracture or a dislocation may not be seen on a single x-ray film, and at least two views (anteroposterior and lateral) must be taken.

Two occasions   Soon after injury, a fracture (e.g. of the carpal scaphoid) may be difficult to see. If doubt exists, further examination must be carried out 10 days later, by which time bone resorption at the fracture site makes diagnosis easier.

Two joints   In the forearm or leg, one bone may be fractured and angulated. Angulation, however, is impossible unless the other bone also is broken, or a joint dislocated. The joints above and below the fracture must both be included on the x-ray films.

Two limbs   In x-rays of a child's elbow, normal epiphyses may confuse the diagnosis of a fracture, and films of the uninjured elbow are then helpful.

SPECIAL IMAGING   Sometimes the fracture – or the full extent of the fracture – is not apparent on the plain x-ray. *Tomography, CT* and *MRI* may be needed, especially with vertebral fractures; *radioisotope scanning* is helpful in diagnosing a suspected stress fracture.

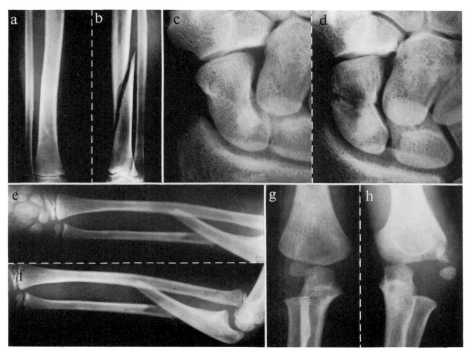

23.7 X-ray examination must be 'adequate'   (a, b) Two films of the same tibia: the anteroposterior view fails to show the fracture. (c) Fractured scaphoid not visible on the day of injury, but clearly seen (d) 2 weeks later. (e, f) Monteggia fracture-dislocation: failure to include both joints in forearm fractures (e) may result in a radiohumeral dislocation (f) being missed. (g, h) Fractured lateral condyle (h) – in a child, comparison with the uninjured side (g) is useful.

Spinal cord injury

With any fracture of the spine, however trivial it may appear to be, a meticulous neurological examination is essential, (1) to establish whether the spinal cord or nerve roots have been damaged, and (2) to obtain a baseline for later comparison if neurological signs should change.

Visceral injury

Fractures of the spine and pelvis may be associated with visceral injury. It is especially important to enquire about urinary function; if a urethral or bladder injury is suspected, diagnostic urethrography may be necessary.

Principles of fracture treatment

24

Closed fractures

The patient must be fully assessed and, if necessary, resuscitated before definitive treatment of any fracture is undertaken. The golden rule is 'treat the patient and not simply the part'.

In principle, fracture management consists of manipulation to improve the position of the fragments, followed by splintage to hold them together until they unite, while at all times preserving joint movement and overall function. Fracture healing is promoted by physiological loading of the bone, so muscle activity and early weight bearing are encouraged. These objectives are covered by three simple injunctions: REDUCE, HOLD, EXERCISE.

The problem is how to hold a fracture adequately and yet move the joints sufficiently: this is a conflict ('Hold v Move') which the surgeon seeks to resolve as rapidly as possible (e.g. by internal fixation); but it is important also to avoid unnecessary risks – and here is a second conflict ('Speed v Safety'). This dual conflict epitomizes the four factors that dominate fracture management.

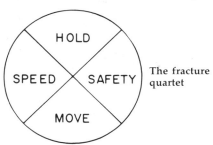

The fracture quartet

● Reduce

Although general treatment and resuscitation must always take precedence, there should be no undue delay in attending to the fracture; swelling of the soft parts during the first 12 hours makes reduction increasingly difficult. However, fractures that are undisplaced or only slightly displaced do not require reduction.

Alignment of the fragments is more important than apposition; provided normal alignment is obtained, overlap may be acceptable. The exception is a fracture involving an articular surface; this should be reduced as near to perfection as possible because any irregularity will predispose to degenerative arthritis.

There are two methods of reduction: closed and open.

Closed reduction

In general, closed reduction is used for all minimally displaced fractures and for most fractures in children.

Under appropriate anaesthesia and muscle relaxation, the fracture is reduced by a threefold manoeuvre: (1) the distal part of the limb is pulled in the line of the bone; (2) as the fragments disengage, they are repositioned (by reversing the original direction of force if this can be deduced); (3) alignment is adjusted in each plane. This is most effective when the soft tissues along one surface are intact; the soft-tissue strap prevents

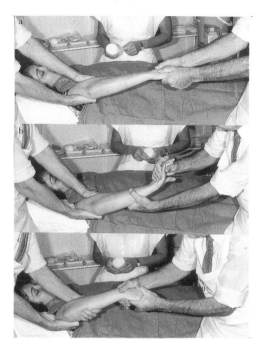

24.1 Closed reduction Reduction is carried out in three stages: (a) the surgeon pulls in the line of the bone while an assistant provides counter-traction; (b) the fragments are disimpacted, if necessary by increasing the angular deformity at the fracture; (c) the fragments are manipulated and pressed into position.

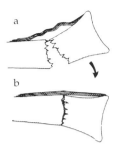

24.2 The soft-tissue strap (a) The soft tissues often remain intact on one side of the fracture. The tethering effect of this 'strap' can be used to facilitate reduction (b).

because of powerful muscle pull and may need prolonged traction.

Open reduction

Operative reduction of the fracture under direct vision is indicated: (1) when closed reduction fails, either because of difficulty in controlling the fragments or because soft tissues are interposed between them; (2) when there is a large articular fragment that needs accurate positioning; or (3) for avulsion fractures in which the fragments are held apart. As a rule, however, open reduction is merely the first step to internal fixation, the indications for which are discussed on page 249.

● Hold reduction

It is commonly supposed that, in order to unite, a fracture must be immobilized. This cannot be so since, with few exceptions,

over-reduction and stabilizes the fracture after it has been reduced.

Some fractures (e.g. of the femoral shaft) are difficult to reduce by manipulation

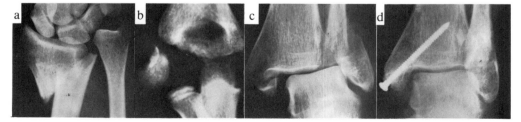

24.3 Indications for open reduction (a) This fracture could not be reduced by closed manipulation because the long proximal fragment had impaled the pronator quadratus muscle. (b) This lateral condyle had been pulled off the humerus and could not be reduced without operation. (c) This ankle fracture could not be reduced with the accuracy desirable at a joint surface, so open reduction (d) was performed.

fractures unite whether they are splinted or not. It is, however, naive to suppose that union would occur if a fracture were kept moving indefinitely; the bone ends must, at some stage, be brought to rest relative to one another. But it is not mandatory for the surgeon to impose this immobility artificially – Nature can do it, with callus; and callus forms in response to movement, not to splintage. *We splint most fractures, not to ensure union but (1) to alleviate pain and (2) to ensure that union takes place in good position.* Splintage also promotes soft-tissue healing and allows free movement of the unaffected parts. Remember – the objective is to splint the fracture, not the entire limb! The available methods are: (1) continuous traction; (2) cast splintage; (3) functional bracing; (4) internal fixation; and (5) external fixation.

Continuous traction

Traction is applied to the limb distal to the fracture, so as to exert a continuous pull in the long axis of the bone. This is particularly useful for shaft fractures of the femur or tibia, especially if they are oblique or spiral and easily displaced by muscle contraction.

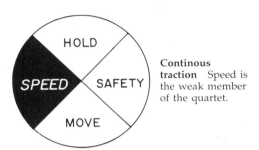

Continous traction Speed is the weak member of the quartet.

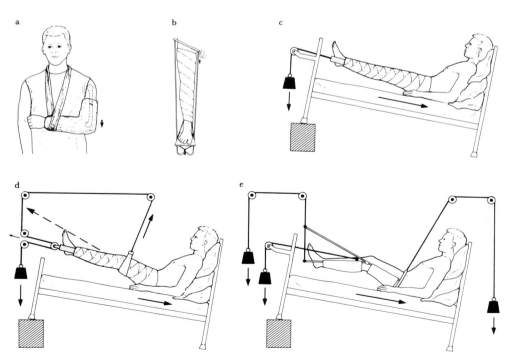

24.4 Methods of traction (a) Traction by gravity. (b)–(d) Skin traction: (b) fixed; (c) balanced; (d) Hamilton Russell. (e) Skeletal traction with a splint and a knee-flexion piece.

Traction cannot *hold* a fracture still, but it can pull a long bone straight and hold it out to length. And meanwhile the patient can *move* his joints and exercise his muscles.

Traction is *safe* enough, provided it is not excessive and care is taken when inserting the traction pin. The problem is *'Speed'*: not because the fracture unites slowly (it does not), but because lower limb traction keeps the patient in hospital. Consequently, as soon as the fracture is 'sticky' (deformable but not displaceable), traction should be replaced by cast splintage or functional bracing, if these methods are feasible.

TECHNIQUE   Traction *by gravity* alone is used for fractures of the humerus (the weight of the arm pulls the fragments into alignment). *Skin traction* can be used to produce a pull of up to 5 kg, which may be sufficient for some lower limb fractures. One-way stretch Elastoplast is stuck to the leg and held on with a bandage; traction is applied by cords or tapes. A more powerful pull (usually necessary for a fractured femur) can be obtained by *skeletal traction*. A wire or pin is inserted through the bone distal to the fracture and traction is applied via hooks or a stirrup.

COMPLICATIONS   There   are   two important complications of traction which should be guarded against.

Vascular insufficiency Traction tapes and circular bandages may constrict the circulation. This is particularly important in the very old and the very young. 'Gallows traction', in which the baby's legs are suspended from an overhead beam, should never be used for children over 12 kg in weight.

Nerve injury   Leg traction may predispose to peroneal nerve injury and a resultant drop foot; the limb should be checked repeatedly to see that it does not roll into external rotation.

Cast splintage

Plaster of Paris is still widely used as a splint, especially for distal limb fractures and

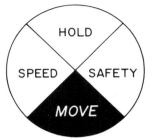

Plaster
With plaster, 'move' is the weak member of the quartet.

for most children's fractures. It is *safe* enough, so long as one is alert to the danger of a tight cast and provided pressure sores are prevented. The *speed* of union is neither greater nor less than with traction, but the patient can go home sooner. *Holding* reduction is usually no problem and patients with tibial fractures can bear weight on the cast. However, joints encased in plaster cannot *move* and are liable to stiffen; stiffness, which has earned the sobriquet 'fracture disease', is the main problem with plaster casts. Newer substitutes have some advantages over plaster (they are impervious to water, and also lighter) but as long as they are used as full casts the basic drawback is the same.

COMPLICATIONS   Plaster immobilization is safe, but only if care is taken to prevent certain complications. These are:

Tight cast   The cast may be put on too tightly, or it may become tight if the limb swells. The patient complains of diffuse pain; only later – sometimes much later – do the signs of *vascular compression* appear (see page 257). The limb should be elevated, but if pain persists the only safe course is to split the cast and ease it open (1) throughout its length and (2) through all the padding down to the skin. The split is down *to* skin – not *through* skin! Whenever swelling is anticipated the cast should be applied over thick padding and the plaster should be split before it sets so as to provide a firm but not absolutely rigid splint.

Pressure sores   Even a well-fitting cast may press upon the skin over a bony prominence (the patella, the heel, the elbow or the head

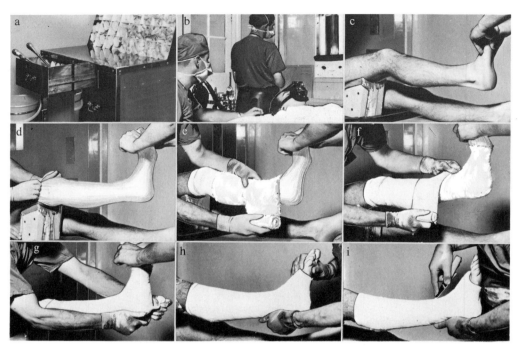

24.5 Plaster technique   Applying a well-fitting and effective plaster needs experience and attention to detail. (a) A well-equipped plaster trolley is invaluable. (b) Adequate anaesthesia and careful study of the x-ray films are both indispensable. (c) For a below-knee plaster the thigh is best supported on a padded block. (d) Stockinette is threaded smoothly onto the leg. (e) For a padded plaster the wool is rolled on and it must be even. (f) Plaster is next applied smoothly, taking a tuck with each turn and (g) smoothing each layer firmly onto the one beneath. (h) While still wet the cast is moulded away from the bony points. (i) With a recent injury the plaster is then split, so as to minimize the danger of compression due to swelling.

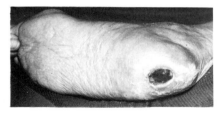

24.6 A complication of plaster   Pressure sores usually can be prevented – and every effort should be made to prevent them, because they are painful and very slow to heal.

of the ulna). The patient complains of localized pain precisely over the pressure spot. Such localized pain demands immediate inspection through a window in the cast. But pressure should have been prevented by adequately padding all prominent bony points before applying the cast.

Skin abrasion or laceration   This is really a complication of removing plasters, especially if an electric saw is used. Complaints of nipping or pinching during plaster removal should never be ignored; a ripped forearm invites litigation.

Functional bracing

Functional bracing, using either plaster of Paris of one of the lighter materials, is one way of overcoming the 'fracture disease' while still permitting fracture splintage and loading. Segments of a cast are applied only over the shafts of the bones, leaving the

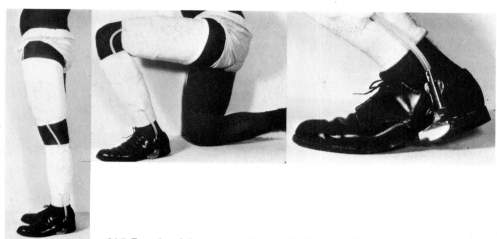

24.7 Functional bracing (cast-bracing) Despite plaster the patient has excellent joint movement (by courtesy of John A. Feagin MD). Note the polypropylene 'hinges' at the knee and ankle.

joints free; the cast segments are connected by metal or plastic hinges which allow movements in one plane. This is used most widely for fractures of the femur or tibia, but, since the brace is not very rigid, it is usually applied only when the fracture is beginning to unite, i.e. after 3–6 weeks of traction or conventional plaster. Used in this way, it comes out well on all four of the basic requirements: the fracture can be *held* reasonably well; the joints can be *moved*; the fracture joins at normal *speed* (or perhaps slightly quicker) without keeping the patient in hospital, and the method is *safe*.

Internal fixation

Bone fragments may be fixed with screws, transfixing pins or nails, a metal plate held by screws, a long intramedullary nail, circumferential bands, or a combination of these methods.

Properly applied, internal fixation *holds* a fracture so securely that *movements* can begin at once; with early movement the 'fracture disease' (stiffness) is abolished. As far as *speed* is concerned, the patient can leave hospital as soon as the wound allows, but he must remember that, even though the bone

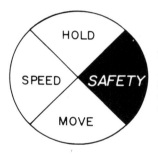

Internal fixation
With internal fixation, 'safety' is the weak member of the quartet.

moves in one piece, the fracture is not united – it is merely held by a metal bridge; weight-bearing is unsafe until the bone itself has united and this takes a considerable length of time. The greatest *danger*, however, is sepsis; if infection supervenes, all the manifest advantages of internal fixation (precise reduction, immediate stability and early movement) may be lost.

INDICATIONS   Internal fixation is never essential, but in adults it is often desirable. The chief indications are:

1. Fractures that cannot be reduced except by operation.
2. Fractures that are inherently unstable and prone to redisplacement after reduction

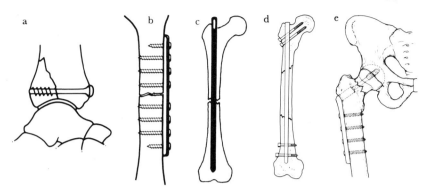

24.8 Internal fixation   The method used must be appropriate to the situation: (a) screws – interfragmentary compression; (b) plate and screws – most suitable in the forearm; (c) intramedullary nail – for the larger long bones; (d) interlocking nail and screws – ideal for the femur and tibia; (e) dynamic compression screw and plate – ideal for the proximal and distal ends of the femur.

(e.g. mid-shaft fractures of the forearm and fracture-subluxations of the ankle).

3. Fractures that unite poorly and take a long time to do so, principally fractures of the femoral neck.
4. Pathological fractures, in which bone disease may prevent healing.
5. Polytrauma, to minimize the risk of ARDS.
6. Fractures in patients who present nursing difficulties (paraplegics, those with multiple injuries and the very elderly).

COMPLICATIONS   Most of the complications of internal fixation are due to poor technique, poor equipment or poor operating conditions.

Infection.   Iatrogenic infection is now the most common cause of chronic osteitis; the metal does not predispose to infection but the operation does.

Non-union.   If the bones have been fixed rigidly with the ends apart, the fracture may fail to unite. This is more likely in the leg or the forearm if one bone is fractured and the other remains intact.

Implant failure.   Metal is subject to fatigue, and until some union of the fracture has occurred metal implants are precarious. Stress must therefore be avoided and a

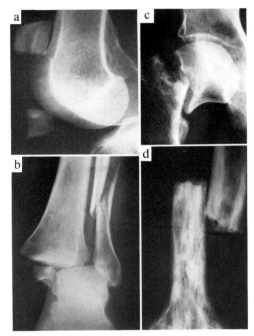

24.9 Indications for internal fixation   (a) This patella has been pulled apart and can be held together only by internal fixation. (b) Fracture-dislocation of the ankle is often unstable after reduction and usually requires fixation. (c) This patient was too ill for operation; her femoral neck fracture has failed to unite without rigid fixation. (d) Pathological fracture in Paget bone; without fixation, union is unlikely to occur.

patient with a plated tibia should walk with crutches and minimal weight-bearing for the first 3 months. Pain at the fracture site is a danger signal and must be investigated.

Refracture. It is important not to remove metal implants too soon, or the bone may refracture. A year is the minimum and 18 or 24 months safer; for several weeks after removal the bone is weak, and care or protection is needed.

External fixation

A fracture may be held by transfixing screws which pass through the bone above and below the fracture and are attached to an external frame. This is especially applicable to the tibia and the pelvis, but the method has also been used for fractures of the femur, the humerus and even the bones of the hand.

INDICATIONS External fixation is particularly useful for:

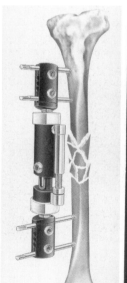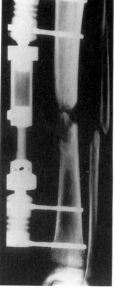

24.10 External fixation The bone is transfixed above and below the fracture. Stability is provided by the rigid external frame.

1. Fractures associated with severe soft-tissue damage where the wound can be left open for inspection, dressing or skin grafting.
2. Fractures associated with nerve or vessel damage.
3. Severely comminuted and unstable fractures, which can be held out to length until healing commences.
4. Fractures of the pelvis, which often cannot be controlled by any other method.
5. Infected fractures, for which internal fixation may be unwise.

COMPLICATIONS The main complications of external fixation are:

Pin-track infection This is particularly likely if the fixator is retained for more than 6 weeks. Regular cleaning of the pin entry sites is essential.

Delayed union Fracture healing may be delayed either because the fragments are held apart by the rigid fixator or because there is reduced load transmission through the bone (stress shielding). The risk is reduced by using a fixator that permits axial compression of the fragments or by removing the fixator after 6–8 weeks and replacing it by some alternative form of splintage that will allow bone loading.

● Exercise

More correctly: 'restore function' – not only to the injured parts but also to the patient as a whole. The objectives are to reduce oedema, preserve joint movement, restore muscle power and guide the patient back to normal activity.

Prevention of oedema Swelling is almost inevitable after a fracture and may cause skin stretching and blisters. Persistent oedema is an important cause of joint stiffness, especially in the hand; it should be prevented if possible and treated energetically if it is already present, by a combination of elevation and exercise. Not every

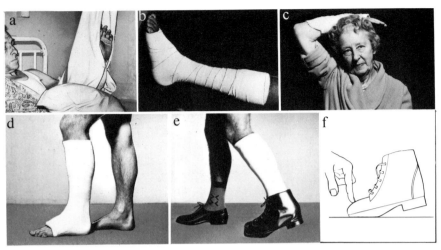

24.11 Some aspects of soft-tissue treatment   Swelling is minimized by (a) elevation and (b) firm support. Stiffness is minimized by exercises: this patient (c) with a Colles' fracture is in no danger of a stiff shoulder. To exercise muscles under a plaster is less easy – a walking plaster should be plantigrade (d); an over-boot with rocker action (e, f) facilitates normal walking and muscle activity.

patient needs admission to hospital, and less severe injuries of the upper limb are successfully managed by placing the arm in a sling; but it is then essential to encourage active use, with movement of all the joints that are free. With severe closed fractures, all open fractures and fractures treated by internal fixation it must be assumed that swelling will occur; the limb should be elevated and active exercises begun as soon as the patient will tolerate this. The essence of soft-tissue care may be summed up thus: elevate and exercise; never dangle, never force.

Active exercise   Active movement helps to pump away oedema fluid, stimulates the circulation, prevents soft-tissue adhesions and promotes fracture healing. A limb encased in plaster is still capable of isometric muscle contraction and the patient should be taught how to do this. When splintage is removed the joints are mobilized and muscle building exercises are steadily increased. Remember that the unaffected joints need exercising, too; it is all too easy to neglect a stiffening shoulder while caring for an injured wrist or hand.

Assisted movement   It has long been taught that passive movement can be deleterious, especially with injuries around the elbow where there is a high risk of developing myositis ossificans. Certainly forced movements should never be permitted, but gentle assistance during active exercises may help to retain function or regain movement after fractures involving the articular

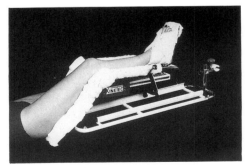

24.12 Continuous passive motion (CPM)   The platform on which the limb rests is motorized and provides passive flexion and extension of the knee.

surfaces. Nowadays this is done with machines that can be set to provide a specified range of movement ('continuous passive motion').

Functional activity   As the patient's mobility improves, an increasing amount of directed activity is included in the programme. He or she may need to be taught again how to perform everyday tasks such as walking, getting in and out of bed, bathing, dressing or handling eating utensils. Experience is the best teacher and the patient is encouraged to use the injured limb as much as possible. Those with very severe or extensive injuries may benefit from spending time in a special rehabilitation unit. But the best incentive to full recovery is the promise of re-entry into family life, recreational pursuits and meaningful work.

Open fractures

All open fractures must be assumed to be contaminated; the object of treatment is to ensure that they do not also become infected.

Emergency treatment

First aid and resuscitation are the same as for closed fractures. In addition, the wound should be covered by a sterile dressing or clean material.

Assessment

The entire limb, and the wound in particular, must be carefully examined in clean conditions. Ideally the wound should be photographed with a Polaroid camera, so that repeated uncovering is not needed. Four questions need to be answered: Is the circulation intact? Are the peripheral nerves intact? What is the state of the skin around the wound? Does the wound communicate with the fracture?; this should be assumed unless manifestly untrue. If it is thought necessary to insert a probe into the wound,

this should be done only in an operating theatre with sterile instruments.

Open fractures are usually classified as:

Grade I – a small, clean wound with little soft-tissue damage.

Grade II – a wound longer than 1 cm, but with only moderate soft-tissue damage.

Grade III – a large wound with severe soft-tissue damage and contamination. The risk of infection is less than 2% in Grade I and over 10% in Grade III. The worst injuries are those in which there is also arterial damage, often resulting in amputation.

Antibacterial prophylaxis

Antibiotics are given as soon as possible, no matter how small the wound, and are continued until the danger of infection has passed. In most cases a combination of benzyl penicillin and flucloxacillin, given 6-hourly for 48 hours, will suffice. If the wound is heavily contaminated, it is wise also to give gentamicin or metronidazole and to continue treatment for 4 or 5 days.

Tetanus prophylaxis is equally important: toxoid for those previously immunized, human antiserum for those who were not.

Treatment of the wound

Open fractures require early operation: (1) to cleanse the wound of foreign material; and (2) to remove devitalized tissue.

Under general anaesthesia the wound and the surrounding skin are cleaned with a mild detergent solution. A small, uncontaminated perforation-from-within may be treated by removing an ellipse of skin and then suturing the defect; the fracture can then be managed as for a closed injury. Larger wounds, penetrating wounds and all wounds that are likely to be contaminated require more extensive surgical toilet (debridement).

A thin margin of skin is excised and the wound extended proximally and distally to expose the underlying tissues. Bits of dirt and clothing are carefully removed and the entire wound is washed out with copious amounts of saline. Dead muscle can usually be recognized by its purplish discoloration, its mushy consistency, its failure to contract when stimulated and its failure to bleed when cut; all such tissue must be excised. Fragments of bone should be removed only if they are totally detached.

Bleeding vessels can usually be tied off, but if large vessels are damaged they may need suturing or grafting.

A cut nerve is best left undisturbed; it can be treated by suturing or grafting once the wound has healed.

To close or not to close the skin – this can be a difficult decision. Small (Grade I) wounds that are uncontaminated and operated on within a few hours of injury may, after debridement, be sutured (provided this can be done without tension) or skin grafted. All other wounds must be left open. The wound is lightly packed with sterile gauze and is inspected after 3–5 days: if it is clean, it is sutured or skin grafted ('delayed primary closure').

Grade III wounds may have to be debrided more than once and skin closure may call for advanced plastic surgery and the use of vascularized muscle flaps.

Treatment of the fracture

Grade I and Grade II injuries can be treated in the same way as closed injuries: the fracture is reduced and held in a plaster cast or by splintage and traction, with the limb elevated to reduce swelling; internal fixation may be used if there is a strong indication (see page 249) and provided a thorough debridement has been carried out. In Grade III injuries there is an even greater need for fracture stabilization. The safest way of achieving this is by external fixation. However, intramedullary nailing – preferably without preliminary reaming – has its advocates.

Open intra-articular fractures are treated by meticulous debridement and saline irrigation. The wound is left open and is inspected after 5 days; if it is clean, internal fixation may be used to obtain anatomical reduction. Early mobilization of the joint is encouraged.

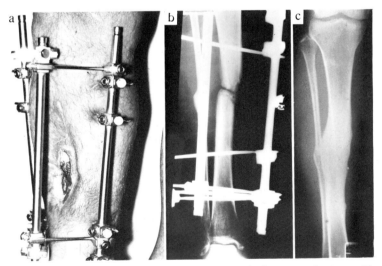

24.13 Open fracture – treatment (a, b) This patient had an open fracture with loss of skin. After debridement the fracture was held by external fixation; it went on to solid union (c).

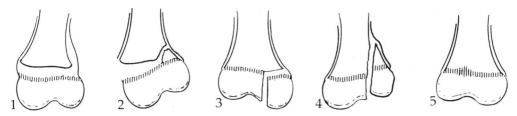

24.14 Physeal injuries Type 1 – separation of the epiphysis – usually occurs in infants but is also seen at puberty as a slipped femoral epiphysis. Type 2 – fracture through the physis and metaphysis – is the commonest; it occurs in older children and seldom results in abnormal growth. Type 3 – an intra-articular fracture of the epiphysis – needs accurate reduction to restore the joint surface. Type 4 – splitting of the physis and epiphysis – damages the articular surface and may also cause abnormal growth; if it is displaced it needs open reduction and fixation. Type 5 – crushing of the physis – may look benign but ends in arrested growth.

Injuries of the physis

Fractures in children may involve injury to the growth plate (or physis). They are a special problem because they can result in abnormal growth of the bone end. Salter and Harris' classification is useful (see fig. 24.14). Types 1 and 2 seldom cause any serious problem. However, in types 3, 4 and 5 the proliferative zone is inevitably damaged, resulting in early closure and cessation of growth, or asymmetrical growth and deformity.

Clinical features

The patient is usually a boy aged 10–12 years who falls and then complains of pain and tenderness near one of the larger joints. In infants the injury may be unsuspected.

X-rays The physis is radiolucent and the epiphysis may be incompletely ossified, making it difficult to discern the extent of the injury. Comparison with the normal side is a great help. Tell-tale features are widening of the physeal gap and tilting of the epiphysis. If the signs are dubious, re-x-ray 4 or 5 days later is essential.

Treatment

Undisplaced fractures are treated by cast splintage for 2–4 weeks; with types 3 and 4 check x-rays at 4 and 10 days are mandatory in order not to miss late displacement.

Displaced fractures are reduced as soon as possible. With types 1 and 2 this can usually be done closed; the part is then splinted for 3–6 weeks. Type 3 and 4 fractures demand perfect reduction, if necessary by open operation and internal fixation with Kirschner wires; the limb is then splinted for 4–6 weeks.

Complications

Premature fusion Type 3 and 4 injuries may result in a bony bridge across the growth plate. If the bridge is narrow it can be excised and replaced by a fat graft, with some prospect of preventing epiphyseal fusion.

Late deformity Asymmetrical growth or malunion of the fracture will result in deformity of the bone end. This may require corrective osteotomy. If there is severe shortening, bone lengthening may be needed.

Complications of fractures

25

The general complications of trauma are discussed in Chapter 22. In this chapter we describe only the local complications. *Early complications* affect mainly the soft tissues. *Late complications* occur months after the fracture and affect mainly the bones and joints.

Local complications

Early
1. Visceral injury
2. Vascular injury
3. Compartment syndrome
4. Nerve injury
5. Haemarthrosis
6. Infection

Late
1. Delayed union
2. Non-union
3. Malunion
4. Joint stiffness
5. Myositis ossificans
6. Avascular necrosis
7. Algodystrophy
8. Osteoarthritis

Visceral injury

Fractures around the trunk are often complicated by injuries to underlying viscera, the most important being penetration of the lung with life-threatening pneumothorax following rib fractures and rupture of the bladder or urethra in pelvic fractures. These injuries require emergency treatment.

Vascular injury

Fractures around the knee, the femoral shaft, the elbow and the humerus are the ones most commonly associated with damage to a major vessel. The artery may be cut, torn, compressed or contused, either by the initial injury or subsequently by jagged bone fragments. Even if its outward appearance is normal, the intima may be detached and the vessel blocked by thrombus, or a segment of artery may be in spasm. The effects vary from transient diminution of blood flow to profound ischaemia, tissue death and peripheral gangrene.

CLINICAL FEATURES The patient may complain of paraesthesia or numbness in the toes or the fingers. The injured limb is cold and pale, or slightly cyanosed, and the pulse is weak or absent.

X-ray will probably show one of the 'high-risk' fractures listed above. If a vascular injury is suspected an angiogram should immediately be performed; if it is positive, emergency treatment must be started.

TREATMENT All bandages and splints should be removed. If the fracture is displaced, it should be reduced. The circulation is then reassessed repeatedly over the next half hour. If there is no improvement, the vessels must be explored by operation – preferably with the benefit of preoperative or peroperative angiography. A torn vessel can be sutured, or a segment may be replaced by a vein graft; if it is thrombosed, endarterectomy may restore the blood flow. Where it is practicable, the fracture should be fixed internally.

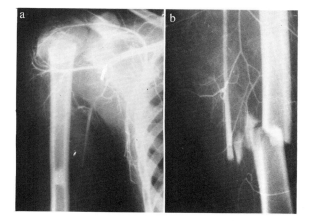

25.1 Vascular injury In both these patients the peripheral part of the limb was cold and pulseless; arteriography shows a cut-off of a major artery in association with (a) a fractured neck of humerus and (b) a fractured shaft of femur.

Compartment syndrome (Volkmann's ischaemia)

Fractures of the arm or leg can give rise to severe ischaemia even if there is no damage to a major vessel. Bleeding or oedema may increase the pressure within one of the osteofascial compartments; there is reduced capillary flow which results in muscle ischaemia, further oedema, still greater pressure and yet more profound ischaemia – a vicious circle that ends, after 12 hours or less, in necrosis of nerve and muscle within the compartment. Nerve is capable of regeneration but muscle, once infarcted, can never recover and is replaced by inelastic fibrous tissue (*Volkmann's ischaemic contracture*). A similar cascade of events may be caused by swelling of a limb inside a tight plaster cast.

CLINICAL FEATURES   'High-risk' injuries are fractures of the elbow, the forearm bones and the proximal third of the tibia. The classic features of ischaemia are the five Ps: Pain, Paraesthesia, Pallor, Paralysis and Pulselessness. Sometimes the skin is not pale, but cyanosed. But it is criminal to wait until all these features are present; the diagnosis can be made long before that. If the limb is unduly painful, swollen or tense, the muscles (which may be tender) should be tested by stretching them – when the toes or fingers are passively hyperextended there is increased pain in the calf or forearm. *The*

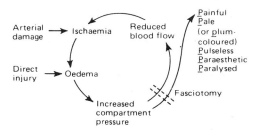

25.2 The vicious circle of Volkmann's ischaemia (Modified from the *Journal of Bone and Joint Surgery*, 1979, 61B, 298 by kind permission of Mr C.E. Holden and the Editor.)

presence of a pulse does not exclude the diagnosis.* In doubtful cases the intracompartmental pressure can be measured directly: if it is higher than 40 mmHg, urgent treatment is called for.

TREATMENT   The threatened compartment (or compartments) must be promptly decompressed by open fasciotomy. The wound should be left open and inspected 5

---

*If the fracture site is painful, or the skin is coloured plum;
If the radial pulse is absent, or the fingers feeling numb;
If the flexors don't like stretching, or the forearm feels too tense;
You must take off all the splints and ring the Medical Defence.
(with apologies to Rudyard Kipling)

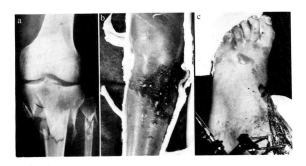

25.3 Compartment syndrome (a) A fracture at this level is always dangerous. This man was treated in plaster. Pain became intense and when the plaster was split (which should have been done immediately after its application), the leg was swollen and blistered (b). A tibial compartment decompression was performed – but too late; 2 days later (c) the foot became gangrenous.

days later: if there is some muscle necrosis, debridement can be done; if the tissues are healthy, the wound can be sutured (without tension), or skin-grafted or simply allowed to heal by secondary intention.

Nerve injury

Fractures are sometimes complicated by nerve injury; the tell-tale signs should be looked for during the initial examination (see Chapter 11). In closed injuries the nerve is seldom severed and spontaneous recovery should be awaited. If recovery has not begun by the expected time, the nerve should be explored; sometimes it is trapped between the fragments and occasionally it is found to be divided. In open fractures a complete lesion (neurotmesis) is more likely; the nerve is explored during wound debridement and repaired, either then or 3 weeks later.

Haemarthrosis

Fractures involving a joint may cause acute haemarthrosis. The joint is swollen and tense and the patient resists any attempt at moving it. The blood should be aspirated before dealing with the fracture.

Infection

Open fractures may become infected; closed fractures hardly ever do unless they are opened by operation.

Post-traumatic wound infection is now the most common cause of chronic osteomyelitis. This does not necessarily prevent the fracture from uniting, but union will be slow and the chance of refracturing is increased.

CLINICAL FEATURES The history is of an open fracture or an operation on a closed fracture. The wound becomes inflamed and starts draining seropurulent fluid, a sample of which will yield a growth of staphylococci or mixed bacteria.

TREATMENT All open fractures should be regarded as potentially infected and treated by giving antibiotics and meticulously excising all devitalized tissue. With acute infection, the tissues around the fracture should be opened and drained; the choice of antibiotic is dictated by bacterial sensitivity.

If chronic osteitis supervenes, the discharging sinus should be dressed daily and the fracture immobilized in an attempt to achieve union. External fixation is useful in such cases, but if an intramedullary nail has already been inserted this should not be removed; even worse than an infected fracture is one that is both infected and unstable.

The further treatment of chronic osteomyelitis is discussed on pages 15 and 16.

Delayed union

The timetable on page 241 is no more than a rough guide, but if those times are unduly

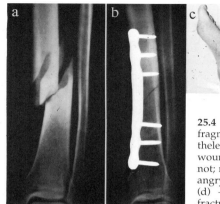
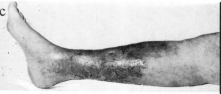
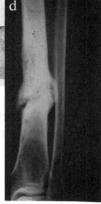

25.4 Infection (a) The upper tibial fragment had punctured the skin; nevertheless the fracture was plated (b). The wound healed rapidly, the fracture did not; months later the skin became red and angry (c). The plate was removed at 1 year (d) – the bone was still infected, the fracture still not consolidated.

prolonged the term 'delayed union' is used. Causes include severe soft-tissue damage, inadequate blood supply, infection, insufficient splintage and excessive traction. In the forearm and leg, fracture of only one bone often heals slowly because the intact bone acts like a spar holding the fragments apart.

Clinically the fracture site is usually tender, and is painful if subjected to stress. X-ray shows that the fracture line is still visible.

Treatment of the fracture must not be abandoned, but it should be reviewed to ensure that it is adequate. If there is no bridging callus by 3 months, internal fixation and bone grafting are indicated.

Non-union

Unless delayed union is properly treated, non-union is liable to follow. Other causes of non-union include: too large a gap (if part of the bone has been left at the scene of the accident, or if muscles have pulled fragments apart); and interposition of periosteum, muscle or cartilage between the fragments.

With delayed union the fracture site still looks as if it is healing, though slowly. With non-union it is clear that healing has stopped; the fracture gap is filled by fibrous tissue, producing a pseudarthrosis. There is painless movement at the fracture site and x-ray

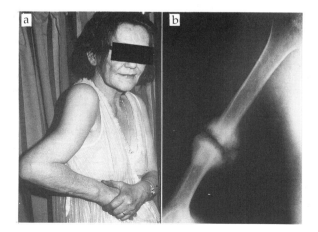

25.5 Non-union (a) Painless movement at the fracture site, the cardinal sign of (b) non-union.

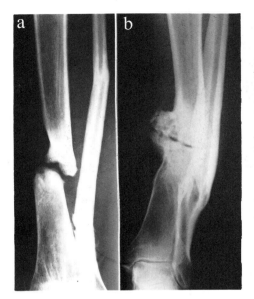

25.6 Non-union   (a) Atrophic non-union – bone grafting is needed. (b) Hypertrophic non-union – rigid fixation would probably suffice.

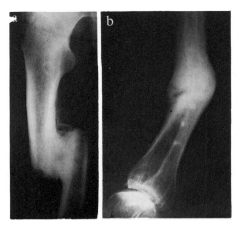

25.7 Malunion   (a) With overlap; (b) with angulation.

shows that the bone ends are smoothed off and sclerosed. In some cases the bone looks inactive, suggesting that the area is relatively avascular (atrophic non-union); in others, there is excessive bone formation on either side of the gap (hypertrophic non-union), as if healing might still occur once the bone ends are apposed and held immobile.

TREATMENT   Not all cases of non-union need treatment; an ununited scaphoid fracture is often asymptomatic. In a long bone with hypertrophic non-union, rigid fixation may be sufficient, but with atrophic non-union, fixation and bone grafting are needed.

Malunion

When the fragments join in an unsatisfactory position the fracture is said to be malunited. Causes are failure to reduce a fracture adequately and failure to hold reduction while healing proceeds.

TREATMENT   Angulation in a long bone of more than 15 degrees, or a marked rotational deformity, may need correction by osteotomy and internal fixation. Shortening of more than 3 cm in one of the lower limbs will need attention: either a raised boot or a bone operation to equalize the length of the limbs (see page 98).

Growth disturbance

In children, damage to the epiphyseal growth plate (or physis) may lead to abnormal growth and deformity (see page 255).

Joint stiffness

Joint stiffness after a fracture commonly occurs in the knee, the elbow, the shoulder and (worst of all) in the small joints of the hand. Sometimes the joint itself has been injured; a haemarthrosis forms and goes on to synovial adhesions. More often the stiffness is due to oedema and fibrosis of the capsule, the ligaments and the muscles around the joint, or adhesion of the soft tissues to each other or to the underlying bone. All these conditions are made worse by prolonged immobilization.

TREATMENT The best treatment is prevention – by exercises that keep the joints mobile from the outset (see page 251). If a joint has to be splinted, make sure that it is held in the correct position (see page 294). Joints that are already stiff take time to mobilize, but prolonged and patient physiotherapy can work wonders. If the stiffness is due to intra-articular adhesions, gentle manipulation under anaesthesia followed by continuous passive motion may free the joint.

Occasionally, adherent or contracted tissues need to be released by operation (e.g. when knee flexion is prevented by adhesion of the quadriceps).

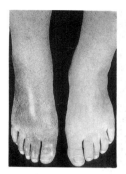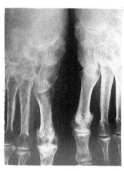

25.8 Sudeck's atrophy The right foot is somewhat swollen and the skin is dusky, smooth and shiny. X-rays show a typically patchy osteoporosis.

Myositis ossificans

Heterotopic ossification in the muscles sometimes occurs after an injury, particularly dislocation of the elbow or a blow to the brachialis, the deltoid or the quadriceps. It is thought to be due to muscle damage, but it also occurs without a local injury in unconscious or paraplegic patients.

Soon after the injury, the patient (usually a fit young man) complains of pain; there is local swelling and soft-tissue tenderness. X-ray is normal but a bone scan may show increased activity. Over the next 2–3 weeks the pain gradually subsides, but joint movement is limited; x-ray may show fluffy calcification of the soft tissues. By 8 weeks the bony mass is easily palpable and is clearly defined in the x-ray.

TREATMENT The worst treatment is to attack an injured and stiffish elbow with vigorous muscle-stretching exercises; this is liable to precipitate or aggravate the condition. The joint should be rested in the position of function until pain subsides; gentle active movements are then begun. Anti-inflammatory drugs may reduce stiffness.

Months later, when the condition has stabilized, it may be helpful to excise the bony mass.

Algodystrophy (Sudeck's atrophy)

Sudeck's atrophy is a form of reflex sympathetic dystrophy usually seen in the foot or the hand, often after relatively trivial injury. The patient complains of continuous, burning pain; at first there is local swelling, redness and warmth but as the weeks go by the skin becomes pale and atrophic. Movements are grossly restricted and x-rays show patchy rarefaction of the bones.

With prolonged physiotherapy (elevation and graduated exercises) there is usually slow but steady recovery, especially if treatment is begun early. If this fails, sympathetic block or sympatholytic drugs such as intravenous guanethidine may bring relief.

Avascular necrosis (see also Chapter 6)

Certain regions are notorious for their propensity to develop ischaemia and bone necrosis after injury. They are: (1) the head of the femur (after fracture of the femoral neck or dislocation of the hip); (2) the proximal part of the scaphoid (after fracture through its waist); and (3) the body of the talus (after fracture of its neck).

There are no symptoms associated with avascular necrosis, but if the fracture fails to

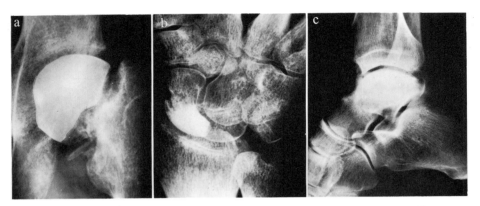

25.9 Avascular necrosis If the fracture cuts off the blood supply to part of the bone the avascular part appears dense on x-ray. Three common sites are: (a) head of femur, (b) proximal portion of scaphoid, (c) posterior half of talus.

unite or if the bone collapses the patient may complain of pain. X-ray shows the characteristic increase in bone density and, later, collapse of the avascular segment.

TREATMENT   Treatment usually becomes necessary when joint function is threatened. In old people with necrosis of the femoral head an arthroplasty is the obvious choice; in younger people, realignment osteotomy (or even arthrodesis) may be wiser. Avascular necrosis in the scaphoid or talus may need no more than symptomatic treatment, but arthrodesis of the wrist or ankle is sometimes needed.

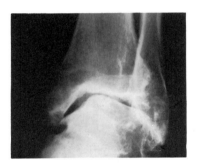

25.10   Osteoarthritis Secondary   osteoarthritis following fracture-dislocation of the ankle.

Osteoarthritis

A fracture involving a joint may severely damage the articular cartilage and give rise to post-traumatic osteoarthritis within a period of months. Even if the cartilage heals, irregularity of the joint surface may cause localized stress and so predispose to secondary osteoarthritis years later. Little can be done to prevent this once the fracture has united.

Malunion of a shaft fracture may radically alter the mechanics of a nearby joint and this, too, can give rise to secondary osteoarthritis. Residual angulation of more than 15 degrees in a lower limb bone should be carefully assessed for its effect on joint function and, if necessary, corrected by osteotomy.

Stress fractures and pathological fractures

26

Stress fractures

A stress or fatigue fracture is one occurring in the apparently normal bone of a healthy person. It is caused, not by a single traumatic incident, but by repetitive minor stress.

Sites affected

These include the shaft of the humerus (in adolescent cricketers); the femoral shaft (in footballers); the tibia and fibula ('runner's fracture'); the metatarsals ('march fracture'); and the pars interarticularis of the fifth lumbar vertebra (in gymnasts).

Fatigue fractures occur even more easily in abnormal bone (e.g. in osteoporosis, osteo-malacia or Paget's disease) but these are more properly regarded as pathological fractures or 'insufficiency' fractures.

Clinical features

There is usually a history of unaccustomed and repeated activity. A common sequence of events is: pain after exercise – pain during exercise – pain without exercise. The affected site may be slightly swollen and warm. The bone feels tender and, sometimes, palpably thickened.

X-ray

Early on, the fracture is difficult to detect, but a bone scan will show increased activity at the painful spot. A few weeks later one may see a small transverse defect in the cortex and, later still, localized periosteal

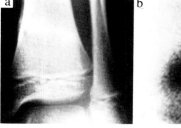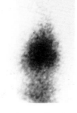

26.1 Stress fractures (a) The stress fracture of this tibia is only just visible, but it had already been diagnosed 2 weeks earlier when the scan (b) showed a hot spot above the ankle.

new bone formation. These appearances can be mistaken for those of an osteosarcoma, a horrifying trap for the unwary.

Treatment

Most stress fractures need no treatment other than an elastic bandage or a short splint and avoidance of the painful activity until the lesion heals. Surprisingly, this can take many months and the forced inactivity is not easily accepted by the hard-driving athlete or dancer.

Pathological fractures

When abnormal bone gives way this is referred to as a pathological fracture (sometimes called an insufficiency fracture). Under the age of 20 the common causes are benign bone tumours and cysts. Over the age of 40 the common causes are metabolic bone disease, myelomatosis, secondary carcinoma and Paget's disease.

CAUSES OF PATHOLOGICAL FRACTURE

Congenital

Osteogenesis imperfecta
Fibrous dysplasia

Infection

Osteomyelitis

Metabolic

Osteomalacia
Osteoporosis
Paget's disease

Benign tumours

Bone cysts
Chondroma

Malignant tumours

Primary bone tumours
Myeloma
Metastatic disease

Clinical features

Bone that fractures spontaneously, or after trivial injury, must be regarded as abnormal until proved otherwise. In older patients one should always ask about previous illnesses or operations: a malignant tumour, no matter how long ago it occurred, may be the source of a late metastatic lesion; a history of gastrectomy, intestinal malabsorption, chronic alcoholism or prolonged drug therapy (especially with corticosteroids) should suggest a metabolic bone disorder.

Local signs of bone disease (an infected sinus, an old scar, swelling or deformity) should not be missed. *Generalized features* can be equally informative: Paget's disease, Cushing's syndrome and congenital dysplasias all have characteristic appearances.

X-rays

Understandably, the fracture itself attracts most attention. But the surrounding bone must also be examined, and features such as cyst formation, cortical erosion, abnormal trabeculation and periosteal thickening should be sought. The type of fracture, too, is important: vertebral compression fractures may be due to severe osteoporosis or osteomalacia, but they can also be caused by skeletal metastases or myeloma.

Biopsy

Some lesions are so typical that a biopsy is unnecessary (solitary cyst, fibrous cortical defect, Paget's disease). Others are more obscure and a biopsy is essential for diagnosis. If open reduction of the fracture is indicated, the biopsy can be done at the same time; otherwise a definitive procedure should be arranged.

Treatment

The principles of fracture treatment remain the same: reduce, hold, exercise. But the choice of method is influenced by the condition of the bone; and the underlying pathological disorder may need treatment in its own right.

Generalized bone disease In most of these conditions (including Paget's disease) the bones fracture more easily, but they heal quite well provided the fracture is properly immobilized. Internal fixation is therefore advisable (and for Paget's disease almost essential). Patients with osteomalacia, hyperparathyroidism, renal osteodystrophy and Paget's disease may need systemic treatment as well.

Local benign conditions Fractures through benign cyst-like lesions usually heal quite well and they should be allowed to do so before tackling the local lesion. Treatment is

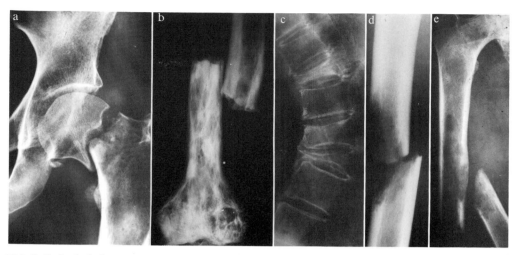

26.2 Pathological fractures Fractures associated with (a) osteoporosis, (b) Paget's disease, (c, d) secondary deposits and (e) myelomatosis.

therefore the same as for ordinary fractures in the same area, although in some cases it will be necessary to take a biopsy before immobilizing the fracture. When the bone has healed, the tumour can be dealt with by curettage or local excision.

Primary malignant tumours The fracture may need splinting but this is merely a prelude to definitive treatment of the tumour, which by now will have spread to the surrounding soft tissues. The prognosis is almost always very poor.

Metastatic tumours Fractures through metastatic lesions heal poorly (and some do not heal at all). To spare the patient the agony of spending the remaining months in bed, and often in pain, internal fixation is the treatment of choice. If there is much bone destruction, metal fixation can be supplemented by packing the area with methylmethacrylate cement. This is followed by local irradiation of the bone.

Usually the primary malignant tumour will have been diagnosed (and treated)

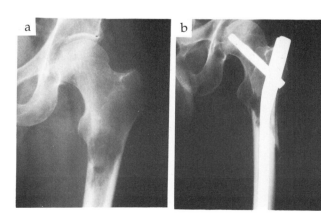

26.3 Pathological fractures – treatment (a) This patient with a secondary deposit below the lesser trochanter was advised to have prophylactic nailing. While she was being prepared she sustained an undisplaced fracture. This was securely fixed (b) and was followed by radiotherapy.

before. If not, certain basic investigations should be carried out to exclude myelomatosis and primary carcinomas of the breast, lung, kidney, thyroid and prostate. A bone scan should also be performed, to disclose other skeletal lesions.

Prophylactic fixation   If a metastatic focus is found in an intact long bone and the x-ray shows that it is a destructive lesion, prophylactic internal fixation should be carried out (preferably without exposing the lesion). This is then followed by local irradiation.

Joints are usually injured by twisting or tilting forces that stretch the ligaments and capsule. If the force is great enough the ligaments may tear, or the bone to which they are attached may be pulled off. The articular cartilage, too, may be damaged if the joint surfaces are compressed or if there is a fracture into the joint.

As a rule, forceful angulation will tear the ligaments rather than crush the bone, but in older people with porotic bone the ligaments may hold and the bone on the opposite side of the joint is crushed instead.

Torn ligaments heal by fibrous scarring. If the separated ends are tightly sutured, scarring will be minimal and the tensile strength of the ligament will approach normality. If the ends are left apart, or are imperfectly sutured, the gap will be filled by fibrous tissue which inevitably stretches under tension.

Strained ligament

Only some of the fibres in the ligament are torn and the joint remains stable. This always follows an injury in which the joint is momentarily twisted or bent into an abnormal position. The joint is painful and swollen, and the tissues may be bruised. Tenderness is localized to the injured ligament and tensing the tissues on this side causes a sharp increase in pain.

Treatment

The joint should be firmly strapped and rested until the acute pain subsides. Thereafter active movements are encouraged, and exercises practised to strengthen the muscles.

Ruptured ligament

The ligament is completely torn and the joint is unstable. Sometimes the ligament holds and the bone to which it is attached is avulsed; this is effectively the same lesion but easier to deal with because the bone fragment can be securely reattached.

As with a strain, the joint is suddenly forced into an abnormal position; sometimes the patient actually hears a snap. The joints most likely to be affected are the ones that are least well protected by surrounding muscles: the knee, the ankle and the finger joints.

Pain is severe and there may be considerable bleeding under the skin; if the joint is swollen, this is probably due to a haemarthrosis. The patient is unlikely to permit a more searching examination, but under general anaesthesia the instability can be demonstrated; it is this that distinguishes the lesion from a strain. X-ray may show a detached flake of bone where the ligament is inserted.

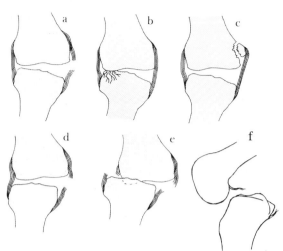

27.1 Joint injuries Severe stress may cause various types of injury. (a) A ligament may rupture, leaving the bone intact. If the soft tissues hold, the bone on the opposite side may be crushed (b), or a fragment may be pulled off by the taut ligament (c). Subluxation (d) means the articular surfaces are partially displaced; dislocation (e,f) refers to complete displacement of the joint.

Treatment

A torn ligament will heal spontaneously by fibrosis if it is held without tension for 4–6 weeks. In the past this formed the basis of treatment for most ligament injuries and it is still acceptable (1) when surgical repair is particularly difficult or unrewarding, and (2) when joint instability is not very marked, especially (3) in elderly patients who will make only light demands on the joint. After a period of immobilization, movement and exercise are encouraged while avoiding tension on the ligament.

In younger individuals, and in most cases where instability is marked, surgical repair is the treatment of choice – and the sooner the better, for once the tissues retract it may be impossible to appose them by suturing. Postoperatively the joint is immobilized to take tension off the ligament; after 3 or 4 weeks, movements are begun but the joint is protected for another 4–6 weeks.

Dislocation and subluxation

Dislocation means that the joint surfaces are completely displaced and are no longer in contact; subluxation implies a lesser degree of displacement, such that the articular surfaces are still partly apposed.

Clinical features

Following an injury the joint is painful and the patient tries at all costs not to move it. The shape of the joint is abnormal and the bony landmarks may be displaced. The limb is often held in a characteristic position; movement is painful and restricted. X-rays will usually clinch the diagnosis; they will also show whether there is an associated bony injury affecting joint stability – i.e. a fracture-dislocation.

The apprehension test   If the dislocation is reduced by the time the patient is seen, the joint can be tested by stressing it in such a way as almost to reproduce the suspected dislocation: the patient develops a sense of impending disaster and forcefully resists further manipulation.

Recurrent dislocation   If the ligaments and joint margins are damaged, repeated dislocation may occur. This is seen especially in the shoulder and the patellofemoral joint.

Habitual   (voluntary)   dislocation   Some patients acquire the knack of dislocating (or subluxating) the joint by voluntary muscle contraction. Ligamentous laxity may make this easier, but the habit often betrays a manipulative and neurotic personality. It is important to recognize this because such patients are seldom helped by operation.

Treatment

The dislocation must be reduced as soon as possible; usually a general anaesthetic is required, and sometimes a muscle relaxant as well. The joint is then rested or immobilized until soft-tissue healing occurs –

usually after 3–4 weeks. If ligaments have been torn, they may have to be repaired (see page 330).

Complications

Many of the complications of fractures are seen also after dislocations: vascular injury, nerve injury, avascular necrosis of bone, heterotopic ossification, joint stiffness and secondary osteoarthritis. The principles of diagnosis and management of these conditions have been discussed (Chapter 25).

Injuries of the upper limb

The great bugbear of upper limb injuries is stiffness – particularly of the shoulder, but sometimes of the elbow and hand as well. In elderly patients especially, it is as important to preserve movement as it is to treat the fracture.

Fractured clavicle

A fall on the shoulder or the outstretched hand breaks the clavicle; the outer fragment is pulled down by the weight of the arm and the inner half is held up by the sternomastoid muscle.

Special features

A lump is usually obvious, and occasionally a sharp fragment threatens the skin. Vascular complications are rare.

X-RAY The fracture is usually in the middle third of the bone and the outer fragment lies below the inner.

Treatment

Accurate reduction is neither possible nor essential. All that is needed is to support the arm in a sling until the pain subsides (usually 2–3 weeks). Thereafter active shoulder exercises should be encouraged; this is particularly important in older patients.

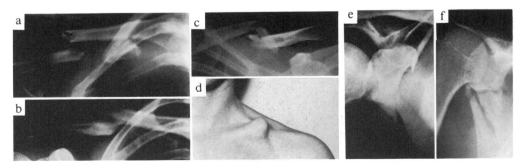

28.1 Shoulder girdle injuries (1) Fractured clavicle: (a) the common site; (b) union in the usual slightly faulty position. (c) Comminuted fracture which united leaving (d) a large lump. Fractured scapula: (e) neck; (f) body.

Complications

Malunion is inevitable; in children the bone is soon remodelled but in adults the slight deformity has to be accepted.

Fractured scapula

The *body of the scapula* is fractured by a crushing force, which usually also fractures ribs and may dislocate the sternoclavicular joint. The *neck of the scapula* may be fractured by a blow or by a fall on the shoulder.

Special features

Shoulder movements are painful but possible. If breathing also is painful, thoracic injury must be excluded.

X-RAY   The films may show a comminuted fracture of the body of the scapula, or a fractured scapular neck with the outer fragment pulled downwards by the weight of the arm. Occasionally a crack is seen in the acromion or the coracoid process.

Treatment

Reduction is usually unnecessary. The patient wears a sling for comfort and from the start practises active exercises of the shoulder, elbow and fingers. With fracture dislocation of the shoulder, a large glenoid fragment may need to be fixed with a screw.

Acromioclavicular joint injuries

A fall on the shoulder tears the acromioclavicular ligaments, and upward subluxation of the clavicle may occur; more severe injury also tears the coracoclavicular ligaments and results in complete dislocation of the joint.

Special features

The patient can usually point to the site of injury. If there is tenderness but no deformity, it is probably a strain or a subluxation. With dislocation the patient is in more pain and a prominent 'step' can be seen and felt.

X-RAY   The films show either a subluxation with only slight elevation of the clavicle, or dislocation with considerable separation. A stress view, taken with the patient holding a 5 kg weight in each hand, may reveal the displacement more clearly.

Treatment

Subluxation does not affect function and does not require any special treatment; the arm is rested in a sling until pain subsides (usually no more than a week) and shoulder exercises are then begun.

Dislocation is poorly controlled by padding and strapping. In a physically active person, operative reduction is preferable: either a screw driven across the acromioclavicular

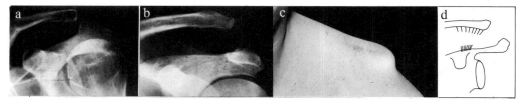

28.2 Acromioclavicular joint   With subluxation (a) deformity is slight. With complete dislocation (b, c) displacement is marked; (d) the conoid and trapezoid ligaments are torn.

joint, or one passed from the clavicle downwards into the coracoid process. The shoulder is rested for 3 weeks and exercises are then encouraged. In physically less demanding patients the injury should be treated as for a subluxation; although the 'bump' persists, disability is usually mild.

A late complication is osteoarthritis of the acromioclavicular joint; this can usually be managed conservatively, but if pain is marked the outer end of the clavicle can be excised.

Sternoclavicular dislocation

This uncommon injury is caused by a fall on the shoulder. The inner end of the clavicle is usually displaced anteriorly, producing a visible and palpable prominence.

Treatment by splintage is unsatisfactory and internal fixation carries unnecessary risks. The patient should be persuaded to accept the slight deformity and mild discomfort during strenuous activity.

Anterior dislocation of the shoulder

This common injury is caused either by a fall on the backward-stretching hand or by forced abduction and external rotation of the shoulder. The head of the humerus is driven forward, tearing the capsule or avulsing the glenoid labrum, and usually ends up just below the coracoid process. There may be an associated fracture of the proximal end of the humerus.

Special features

Pain is severe. The patient supports the arm with the opposite hand and is loth to permit any kind of examination. The lateral outline of the shoulder is flattened and a small bulge may be seen and felt just below the clavicle. The arm must always be examined for nerve and vessel injury.

X-RAY   This will show the overlapping shadows of the humeral head and glenoid fossa, with the head usually lying below and medial to the socket.

Treatment

Reduction is most easily carried out under general anaesthesia and full relaxation, so as to minimize the risk of further damage. The simplest method is to pull on the arm in slight abduction while the body is stabilized in counter-traction. If anaesthesia is contraindicated, the prone position with the arm hanging may facilitate reduction.

Kocher's method is sometimes used. The elbow is bent to 90 degrees and held close to

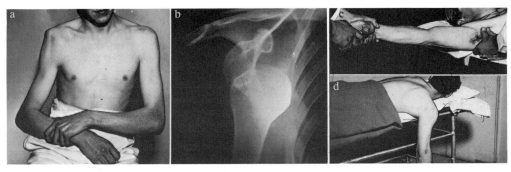

28.3 Shoulder dislocations – anterior   (a, b) Anterior dislocation of the shoulder. (c, d) Two methods of reduction.

the body; no traction should be applied. The arm is slowly rotated 75 degrees laterally, then the point of the elbow is lifted forwards and adducted, and finally the arm is rotated medially.

An x-ray is taken to confirm reduction and exclude a fracture. When the patient is fully awake, active abduction is gently tested to exclude an axillary nerve injury.

The arm is rested in a sling for a week or two and active movements are then begun, but combined abduction and lateral rotation must be avoided for at least 3 weeks.

Complications

Nerve injury The axillary nerve may be injured; the patient is unable to contract the deltoid muscle and there may be a small patch of anaesthesia over the muscle. The lesion is usually a neurapraxia which recovers spontaneously after a few weeks.

Occasionally the posterior cord of the brachial plexus is injured. This is alarming, but usually recovers with time.

Vascular injury The axillary artery may be damaged. The limb should always be examined for signs of ischaemia. Management is described on page 256.

Fracture-dislocation If there is an associated fracture of the proximal humerus, open reduction and internal fixation will be necessary.

Recurrent dislocation If the glenoid labrum has been damaged or detached, recurrent dislocation is likely.

Posterior dislocation of the shoulder

This commonly missed injury is not a complete dislocation but a fracture-subluxation. It is usually caused by forced internal rotation of the abducted arm or by a direct blow on the front of the shoulder. It should always be suspected after an epileptic fit or an electric shock.

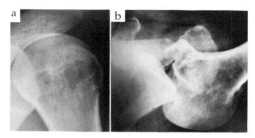

28.4 Posterior shoulder dislocation (a) The anteroposterior view may look almost normal, but the humeral head is globe-shaped; (b) the lateral view shows obvious subluxation.

Special features

The diagnosis is frequently missed because, in the anteroposterior x-ray, the humeral head may seem to be in contact with the glenoid. But clinically the condition is unmistakable because the arm is held in medial rotation and is locked in that position.

X-RAY In the anteroposterior projection the humeral head, because it is medially rotated, looks somewhat globular. A lateral film is essential; it shows posterior subluxation and, sometimes, indentation of the humeral head.

Treatment

The arm is pulled and rotated laterally, while the head of the humerus is pushed forwards. After reduction the management is the same as for anterior dislocation.

Recurrent dislocation of the shoulder (see also page 121)

Once a shoulder has been dislocated, this may happen repeatedly – and with increasing ease – over the ensuing months or years. In these cases the capsule and labrum may have been stripped from the margin of the glenoid and the humeral head may be indented. In the vast majority of cases recurrence is anterior, but occasionally it is posterior; the distinction is not as easy as it may seem, because often by the time the patient is seen the head is back in the socket and there is only the history to go by.

With recurrent anterior dislocation, the patient complains that the shoulder 'slips out' when the arm is lifted into abduction and lateral rotation, as in swimming or dressing or reaching backwards and upwards. At first it has to be 'put back' by someone; as time goes by, reduction becomes easier and often the patient may learn to do it himself. The 'apprehension test' is positive: if the shoulder is passively manipulated into abduction, extension and lateral rotation, the patient tenses up and anxiously resists further movement.

X-RAY   An anteroposterior view with the shoulder in internal rotation will often show a posterolateral defect of the humeral head where the bone has been damaged by the rim of the glenoid fossa. CT may show the damaged glenoid labrum.

Treatment

If the patient is disabled, an operation will be needed: for anterior dislocation, some form of anterior capsular reconstruction is usually successful; recurrent posterior dislocation is more difficult and may require soft-tissue reconstruction combined with a bone operation to block abnormal movement at the back of the shoulder.

Fractures of the proximal humerus

Fractures of the proximal humerus usually occur after middle age and are most common in osteoporotic individuals. The patient falls on the outstretched hand, fracturing the surgical neck; one or both tuberosities may also be fractured.

Special features

Pain may not be very severe because the fracture is often firmly impacted. However, the appearance of a large bruise in the upper part of the arm is very suspicious.

X-RAY   In the elderly, a transverse fracture extends across the surgical neck, and often the greater tuberosity also is fractured. The shaft is usually impacted into the head in an abducted position.

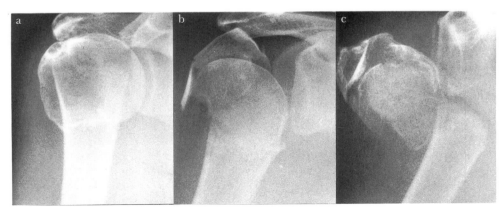

28.5 Fractures of the upper humerus   Classification is all very well, but x-rays are more difficult to interpret than line drawings. (a) Two-part fracture. (b) Three-part fracture involving the neck and the greater tuberosity. (c) Four-part fracture.

In younger patients, the proximal end of the humerus may be broken into several pieces. According to Neer's classification, a *one-part fracture* is one in which the fragments are undisplaced or firmly impacted, i.e. the humerus appears to be 'in one piece'; if the neck fracture is displaced, it is a *two-part fracture*; and if one or both tuberosities are fractured and displaced, it appears as a *three-part* or *four-part fracture*.

Treatment

Impacted or minimally displaced fractures need no treatment apart from a short period of rest with the arm in a sling. Once the fracture has united (usually after 6 weeks), active exercises are encouraged.

Two-part fractures can usually be reduced closed; the arm is then bandaged to the chest for 4 weeks, after which shoulder exercises are commenced (the elbow and hand are, of course, exercised throughout).

Three-part fractures usually require open reduction and internal fixation; and four-part fractures may need prosthetic replacement.

Complications

Shoulder dislocation Combined fracture and dislocation of the shoulder is difficult to manage. The dislocation should be reduced (this may require an operation) and the fracture can then be tackled in the usual way.

Vascular and nerve injuries These may occur with three and four-part fractures and should be sought at the initial examination.

Stiffness Shoulder stiffness is common. It can be minimized by starting exercises as early as possible.

Fractured shaft of humerus

A fall on the hand may twist the humerus, causing a spiral fracture. A fall on the elbow with the arm abducted may hinge the bone, causing an oblique or transverse fracture. A direct blow to the arm causes a fracture which is either transverse or comminuted. A fracture of the shaft in an elderly patient may be through a metastasis.

Special features

The arm is painful, bruised and swollen. Active extension of the fingers should be tested because the radial nerve is occasionally damaged.

X-RAY The possibility that the fracture may be pathological should be remembered.

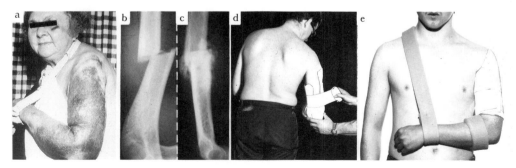

28.6 Fractured shaft of humerus (a) The telltale bruise. (b, c) Transverse fracture with only moderate displacement. (d) A U-slab of plaster (after a few days in a shoulder-to-wrist hanging cast) is usually adequate, though (e) a ready-made functional brace is simpler and probably better.

Treatment

Fractures of the humerus require neither perfect reduction nor total immobilization; the weight of the arm with an external cast is usually enough to pull the fragments into alignment. The cast is applied from the shoulder to the wrist; after 2–3 weeks it may be replaced by a shorter cast (shoulder to elbow) or by a removable brace. Exercises of the shoulder can be started within a week, but abduction is avoided until the fracture has united.

If the fracture is very unstable and difficult to control, fixation is preferable – a plate and screws, or a long intramedullary nail, or an external fixator.

Complications

Nerve injury   Radial nerve palsy (wrist drop and paralysis of the metacarpophalangeal extensors) may occur with shaft fractures. In closed injuries the nerve is very seldom divided, so there is no hurry to operate. A 'lively' splint is used to support the wrist and hand while recovery is awaited. If there is no sign of this by 6 weeks, the nerve should be explored. In complete lesions (neurotmesis), nerve suture is often unsatisfactory, but function can be largely restored by tendon transfers.

Non-union   Mid-shaft fractures sometimes fail to unite. This is treated by bone grafting and internal fixation.

Supracondylar fracture

This is a childhood fracture – in fact, one of the most common of all fractures in children. It is caused by a fall on the outstretched hand. The humerus breaks just above the condyles and the distal fragment is pushed and tilted backwards.

Special features

The child is in pain and the elbow is swollen. It is essential to feel the pulse and check the circulation.

X-RAY   In the lateral view of the elbow, the distal fragment is tilted and shifted posteriorly; sometimes it is completely displaced. Very rarely, displacement is anterior.

Treatment

If the fracture is displaced it must be reduced as soon as possible, under general anaesthesia. First the uninjured elbow is examined in full extension, to assess the normal carrying angle and rotational movement. Then the fracture is reduced in a methodical, stepwise manoeuvre: (1) traction for 2–3 minutes in the length of the arm with countertraction above the elbow; (2) correction of any sideways tilt and shift; (3) gradual flexion of the elbow while traction is maintained; (4) pressure behind the distal fragment to correct posterior tilt. THEN

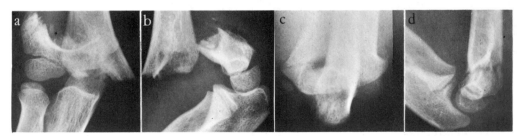

28.7 Supracondylar fractures (1)   (a, b) This considerably displaced fracture was reduced (c, d) by the method shown in Fig. 28.8. Note that the anteroposterior view in (c) is taken with the elbow flexed.

FEEL THE PULSE; if it is absent, relax the amount of elbow flexion until it reappears. X-rays are taken to confirm the reduction and ensure that there is no residual angulation or rotational deformity.

The arm is held in a collar and cuff, continuously, for 3 weeks. After that, active elbow flexion is permitted but the arm is supported in a sling and extension is avoided for another 3 weeks.

Complications

Vascular injury The great danger of supracondylar fracture is injury to the brachial artery. Peripheral ischaemia may be immediate and severe; more commonly forearm oedema and a mounting compartment syndrome lead to necrosis of the muscle and nerve (see page 257).

Nerve injury The median nerve may be injured but loss of function is usually temporary and recovery can be expected in 6–8 weeks.

Malunion Sideways or backward shift of the distal fragment is gradually obscured by remodelling. But malrotation or sideways angulation will result in permanent deformity of the elbow – usually cubitus varus. If

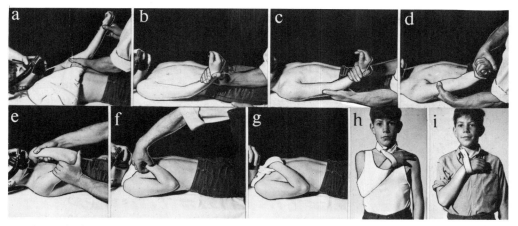

28.8 Supracondylar fractures (2) – treatment of displaced fracture (a) The uninjured arm is examined first; (b) traction on the fractured arm; (c) correcting lateral shift and tilt; (d) correcting rotation; (e) correcting backward shift and tilt; (f) feeling the pulse; (g) the elbow is kept well flexed while x-ray films are taken; (h) for the first 3 weeks the arm is kept under the vest; after this (i) is it outside the vest.

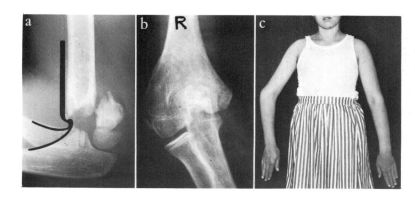

28.9 Supracondylar fractures (3) – complications The most serious complication is arterial damage (a) leading to Volkmann's ischaemia. (b, c) Varus deformity of the right elbow following poor reduction.

the deformity is marked, it will need correction by supracondylar osteotomy.

Fracture-separation of the humeral epiphyses

The distal humeral epiphyses begin to ossify at the age of about 3 and fuse with the shaft at about 16; between these ages they may be sheared off or avulsed by a fall on the hand. Only two of these injuries are at all common: separation of the epicondyle on the medial side and fracture-separation of the entire condyle on the lateral side.

Separation of the medial epicondyle

If the wrist is forced into extension, the medial epicondylar epiphysis is avulsed by the attached wrist flexors; if the elbow opens up on the medial side, the epicondylar fragment may be pulled into the joint. The inner side of the elbow is swollen and acutely tender; the x-ray has to be studied very carefully to detect the epicondylar fragment.

Treatment Minor displacement may be disregarded but an epicondyle trapped in the joint must be freed. Manipulation with the elbow in valgus and the wrist hyperextended (to pull on the flexor muscles) may be successful; if it fails, the joint must be opened and the fragment retrieved and sutured back in position.

Fracture-separation of the lateral condyle

If the child falls with the elbow stressed in varus, a large fragment including the lateral condyle is avulsed by the attached wrist extensors. The extent of this injury is often not appreciated. Because the capitellar epiphysis is largely cartilaginous, the bone fragment may look deceptively small on x-ray. Displacement can be quite marked due to muscle pull. The fracture is important for two reasons: (1) it may damage the growth plate; and (2) it always involves the joint, thus making accurate reduction desirable.

Treatment An undisplaced fracture can be treated by splinting the elbow for 2 weeks

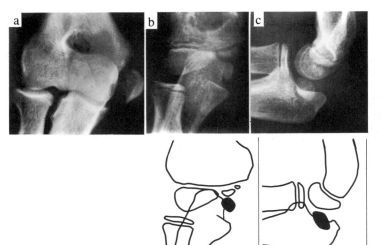

28.10 Fractured medial epicondyle (a) Avulsion of the medial epicondyle following valgus strain. Sometimes the epicondylar fragment is trapped in the joint (b, c); the serious nature of the injury in this particular case is liable to be missed unless the surgeon specifically looks for the trapped fragment.

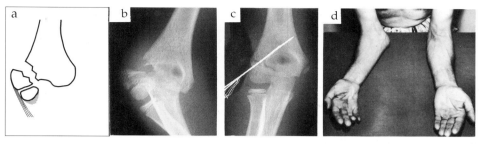

28.11 Fractured lateral condyle   (a, b) A large fragment of bone and cartilage is avulsed; even with reasonable reduction, union is not assured and open reduction with fixation (c) is often wise. If non-union occurs, there is a risk of valgus deformity and delayed ulnar palsy (d).

and then starting exercises. A displaced fracture may be reduced by manipulation, but if this fails operative reduction must be carried out and the fragment fixed in position with a screw or Kirschner wires.

Complications The important complication of lateral condyle fracture is deformity of the elbow, due to: (1) malunion of the fracture; (2) non-union, with upward displacement of the fragment; or (3) damage to the lateral part of the growth plate. The elbow is deviated laterally (cubitus valgus) and this, in turn, may stretch the ulnar nerve and cause delayed ulnar palsy. If deformity is marked it should be corrected by osteotomy of the humerus.

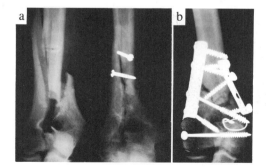

28.12 T-shaped and Y-shaped fractures (a) Y-shaped fracture fixed with two screws – an excellent range was obtained; (b) surgical virtuosity is sometimes rewarding, but not always – this ended up with a stiff elbow.

Fracture of the capitulum

In adults, a fall on the hand with the elbow straight may cause a fracture of the capitulum; sometimes the fracture passes through the notch of the trochlea.

The fracture can be difficult to reduce. If closed manipulation fails, operation is essential: the joint is opened from the lateral side and the separated fragment of bone (usually larger than expected) is replaced or removed.

Bicondylar fractures

A fall on the point of the elbow drives the olecranon process upwards, splitting the condyles apart.

Special features

Swelling is often considerable and the arm is held immobile.

X-RAY The fracture extends from the lower humerus into the elbow joint; it may be T-shaped, Y-shaped or comminuted. Often the condyles are separated, and either may be tilted in any direction.

Treatment

Whatever the treatment, the elbow is likely to end up somewhat stiff.

One method is to disregard the x-ray and concentrate on joint mobility; as soon as pain permits, active movements are encouraged and this sometimes moulds the fragments into reasonable position; the final range is usually better than expected. A modification of conservative treatment is to apply skeletal traction through a pin in the olecranon; the patient remains in bed with the humerus vertical and the elbow bent, but elbow movements are encouraged from the outset.

The alternative is to operate and piece the fragments together using Kirschner wires or plates and screws for internal fixation; the x-ray may look better but function is often disappointing.

Complications

Vascular injury Vigilance is required to make the diagnosis and institute treatment as early as possible.

Nerve injury There may be damage to either the median or the ulnar nerve. It is vital to examine the hand and record the findings before treatment is commenced.

Myositis ossificans Severe soft-tissue damage may lead to heterotopic ossification. Forced movement should be avoided.

Stiffness Comminuted intercondylar fractures always result in some degree of stiffness. The disability may be reduced by encouraging an energetic exercise programme. Late operations to improve elbow movement are usually unrewarding.

Fractured upper end of radius

A fall on the outstretched hand forces the elbow into valgus and pushes the radial head against the capitulum. In adults the radial head may be split or broken; in children the bone is more likely to fracture through the neck of the radius. In addition, the articular cartilage of the capitulum may be bruised or chipped; this cannot be seen on x-ray but is an important complication.

Special features

This fracture is sometimes missed, but painful rotation of the forearm and tenderness on the lateral side of the elbow should suggest the diagnosis.

X-RAY The typical adult fracture is an undisplaced split through the radial head, which may easily be missed on a single x-ray; less often there is a marginal fragment, and sometimes the head is crushed or badly comminuted. In children the fracture is through the neck, and the proximal end of the radius may be displaced.

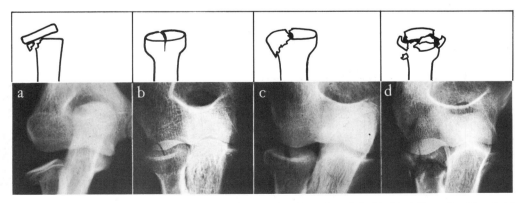

28.13 Fractured upper radius   In the child (a) fractured neck. In the adult (b) chisel-like split of head, (c) marginal fracture, (d) comminuted fracture.

Treatment

Treatment differs substantially in adults and children.

Adults   With an undisplaced split the arm is held in a collar and cuff for 3 weeks; active flexion and extension may be encouraged, but rotation should be left to return by itself.

A single large fragment may be pinned back with a Kirschner wire.

A severe fracture is best treated by excising the radial head, or replacing it with a Silastic prosthesis. The elbow is splinted for 2 weeks and then exercises are begun.

Children   Up to about 20 degrees of tilt is acceptable. Beyond that, reduction is needed. The arm is pulled into extension and slight varus. With his thumb the surgeon pushes the displaced radial fragment into position. If this fails, open reduction is performed. The head of the radius must never be excised in children because this will interfere with the synchronous growth of radius and ulna.

Complications

Joint stiffness   In adults especially, the elbow may be slow to regain full mobility, but persistent physiotherapy (and the avoidance of forced manipulation) will usually restore satisfactory function.

Osteoarthritis   If the articular surfaces are damaged, secondary osteoarthritis may ensue.

Fractured olecranon

Two types of injury are seen: (1) a comminuted fracture which is due to a direct blow or a fall on the elbow; and (2) a clean transverse break, which is a traction lesion that occurs when the patient falls onto the hand while the triceps muscle is contracted.

Special features

A graze or bruise over the elbow suggests a comminuted fracture; the triceps is intact and the elbow can be extended against resistance. With a transverse fracture there may be a palpable gap and the patient is unable to extend the elbow against resistance.

Treatment

A *comminuted fracture* leaves the extensor mechanism in continuity; it is treated by rest

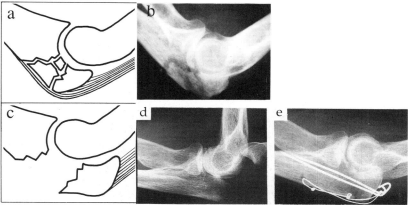

28.14 Fractured olecranon   (a, b) Comminuted fracture – best treated by activity. (c, d) Gap fracture – the extensor mechanism is not intact: treatment by tension-band wiring (e).

until acute pain subsides and then active movements are encouraged. For a *transverse fracture*, if there is no displacement at all the elbow is immobilized by a cast for 2–3 weeks and then exercises are begun. But if there is any displacement, closed treatment is useless and the extensor mechanism should be repaired operatively; the fracture is reduced and held with a screw or by tension-band wiring.

Complications

Non-union Non-union sometimes occurs after inadequate reduction and fixation of a transverse fracture. If elbow function is good, it can be ignored; if not, rigid internal fixation will be needed.

Osteoarthritis The fracture involves the elbow joint, so secondary osteoarthritis may occur if reduction is less than perfect.

Dislocation of the elbow

A fall on the hand may dislocate the elbow. The forearm is pushed backwards and the elbow dislocates posteriorly or posterolaterally.

Special features

Deformity is usually obvious and the elbow is held immobile. It is important to exclude damage to vessels or nerves.

X-RAY   An x-ray should always be taken to exclude an associated fracture.

Treatment

The patient should be fully relaxed under anaesthesia. The surgeon pulls on the forearm while the elbow is slightly flexed. With one hand, sideways displacement is corrected, then the elbow is further flexed while the olecranon process is pushed forward. Reduction should always be checked by x-ray.

The arm is held in a collar and cuff with the elbow flexed above 90 degrees. After 1 week the patient gently exercises his elbow; at 3 weeks the collar and cuff can be discarded.

Complications

Complications are fairly common, and some are potentially so serious that the patient with a dislocation or a fracture-dislocation of the elbow must be observed with the closest attention.

Vascular injury The brachial artery may be damaged. The management of forearm ischaemia is described on page 256).

Nerve injury Occasionally the median or ulnar nerve is injured (see page 258).

Elbow stiffness The elbow reacts unkindly to injury and stiffness is quite common. Physiotherapy is important but passive movements and forceful manipulation should be avoided.

Myositis ossificans The elbow is the most common site for acute post-traumatic soft-tissue ossification. Persistent or recurrent pain and increasing stiffness are the danger signals. The diagnosis and management are described on page 261.

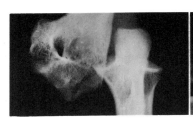
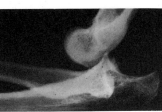

28.15 Elbow dislocations
Lateral and posterior displacement

Dislocation of the radial head

Isolated dislocation of the radial head is rare and one should always suspect a concurrent fracture of the ulna (see page 285) or shortening of the ulna due to bone dysplasia.

If the ulna is normal, traumatic dislocation can be reduced by supination and direct pressure over the radial head; the arm is held supine in plaster for 6 weeks.

If there is concomitant shortening of the ulna (e.g. in diaphyseal aclasis), reduction will be impossible, and the abnormality must be accepted.

Pulled elbow

In young children the elbow may be injured by pulling on the arm; the orbicular ligament slips up over the head of the radius into the radiocapitellar joint.

A child aged 3 or 4 years is brought with a painful, dangling arm: there is usually a history of the child being jerked by the arm and crying out in pain. The forearm is held in pronation and any attempt to supinate it is resisted. There are no x-ray changes.

Spontaneous recovery sometimes occurs if the arm is rested in a sling for a few days. A more dramatic cure can be achieved by forcefully supinating and then flexing the elbow; the ligament slips back with a snap.

Fractured radius and ulna

A twisting force (commonly a fall on the hand) causes a spiral fracture with the bones broken at different levels; a direct blow or an angulating force causes transverse fractures at the same level.

Special features

Deformity is usually obvious. The hand must be examined for circulatory and neurological abnormality.

X-RAY   In children the fracture is often greenstick. In adults the fragments may be severely displaced, partly because of the rotational pull of the forearm muscles.

Treatment

In children, closed reduction is usually successful and the fragments can be held in

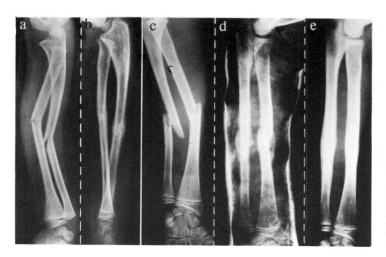

28.16 Fractured radius and ulna in children Greenstick fractures (a) only need correction of angulation (b), and plaster. Complete fractures (c) are harder to reduce: but, provided alignment is corrected and held in plaster (d), slight lateral shift remodels with growth (e).

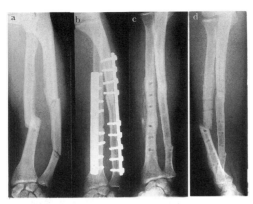

28.17 Fractured radius and ulna in adults (a, b) These fractures are usually treated by internal fixation with sturdy plates and screws. However, removal of the implants is not without risk. (c, d) In this case the radius fractured through one of the screw holes.

a full-length cast, from axilla to metacarpal shafts; this is applied with the elbow at 90 degrees and the forearm in neutral rotation. The position is checked by x-ray at 2 weeks and, if it is satisfactory, splintage is retained until both fractures are united (usually 6–8 weeks).

In adults, unless the fragments are in close apposition, reduction is difficult and redisplacement in a cast almost invariable. Most surgeons opt for open reduction and internal fixation from the outset. The fragments are held by plates and screws or intramedullary rods. In most cases a full-length cast will still be necessary, at least for the first 6 weeks, to protect against rotatory strains. Fracture consolidation is not hastened by internal fixation and the bones still take about 12 weeks to attain strong union.

Complications

Compartment syndrome (see page 257). Fractures of the forearm bones are always associated with swelling of the soft tissues, with the attendant risk of a compartment syndrome. The threat is even greater, and the diagnosis more difficult, if the forearm

is wrapped up in plaster. The byword is 'watchfulness'; if there are any symptoms or signs of circulatory embarrassment, treatment must be prompt and uncompromising.

Delayed union and non-union Delayed union of one or other bone (usually the ulna) is not uncommon; immobilization may have to be continued beyond the usual time. Non-union will require bone grafting and internal fixation.

Malunion With closed reduction there is always a risk of malunion. If pronation or supination is severely restricted, and there is no cross-union, mobility may be improved by excising the distal end of the ulna.

Fracture of a single forearm bone

Fracture of the radius alone or of the ulna alone is uncommon. It is important for two reasons: (1) an associated dislocation may be undiagnosed; if only one forearm bone is broken and there is displacement, one or other radioulnar joint must be dislocated (*see* below); (2) non-union is liable to occur unless it is realized that one bone takes just as long to consolidate as two.

Special features

Ulnar fractures are easily missed – even on x-ray. If there is local tenderness, a further x-ray a few days later is wise.

X-RAY   Always look for the dislocation – of either the proximal or the distal radioulnar joint. A full-length x-ray of the forearm is essential.

Treatment

Ulnar fractures are rarely displaced. With radial fractures there may be rotary displacement; to achieve reduction the forearm usually needs to be supinated for upper

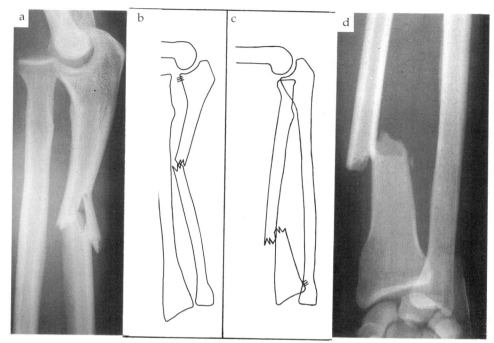

28.18 Fracture dislocations (a, b) Monteggia – the ulna is fractured and the head of the radius dislocated; (c, d) Galleazzi – the radius is fractured and the head of the ulna is dislocated.

third fractures, neutral for middle third fractures, and pronated for lower third fractures.

A complete plaster is applied, to include the elbow and wrist joints, exactly as though both forearm bones were broken. It may be 12 weeks before consolidation is complete.

NOTE Because one bone is intact, the ends of the broken bone may be slightly sprung apart and union is liable to be delayed; for this reason many surgeons prefer internal fixation for single bone fractures.

Fracture-dislocations

When a single forearm bone is fractured, there is liable to be a dislocation of either the proximal or the distal radioulnar joint. These two types of injury are best known by their Italian eponyms, Monteggia and Galeazzi.

Special features

Monteggia The upper half of the ulna is fractured, angulated and shortened; the radial head is dislocated and lies in front of the capitulum, but a good lateral x-ray is required to show this.

Galeazzi Here it is the radius that is fractured in its lower half; the inferior radioulnar joint is dislocated and the head of the ulna stands out prominently on the back of the wrist.

Treatment

The clue to successful treatment is to restore the length of the fractured bone; only then can the dislocated joint be fully reduced. In children it is sometimes possible to do this by manipulation, but in adults Monteggia and Galeazzi fractures are best treated open, plating the fracture and making sure (by further x-rays) that the dislocation is reduced. The arm is held in plaster until union occurs.

Complications

Unreduced dislocation The diagnosis is sometimes missed because x-rays do not include the wrist and elbow. Persistent dislocation may require excision of the proximal radius or distal ulna.

Colles' fracture

The injury which Abraham Colles described in 1814 is a transverse fracture of the radius just above the wrist, with dorsal displacement of the distal fragment. It is the most common of all fractures in older people, the high incidence being related to the onset of postmenopausal osteoporosis. Thus the patient is usually a woman who has fallen on her outstretched hand.

Special features

If the fracture is displaced, there is a characteristic 'dinner-fork' deformity of the wrist: the lower end of the forearm is bent and shifted backwards and over to the radial side.

X-RAY   The fracture runs transversely across the radius about 2 cm from the wrist, and often the ulnar styloid process is broken off. The radial fragment is (1) tilted and shifted backwards, (2) tilted and shifted radially, and (3) impacted.

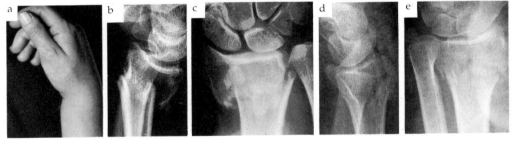

28.19 Colles' fracture (1)   (a) Dinner-fork deformity. (b, c) The chief displacements are backwards and radially. (d, e) After reduction.

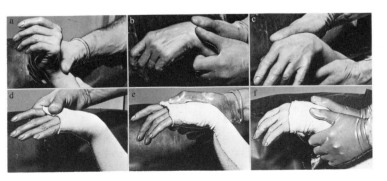

28.20 Colles' fracture (2) Reduction: after preliminary traction (a) disimpaction (not always necessary), (b) pronation and forward shift, (c) ulnar deviation.

Splintage: (d) stockinette, (e) wet plaster slab, (f) slab bandaged on and reduction held till plaster set.

Treatment

If the fracture is undisplaced (or only very slightly displaced), it is splinted in a plaster slab that is wrapped around the dorsum of the forearm and wrist and bandaged firmly in position. *Displaced fractures* must be reduced under anaesthesia. The hand is firmly grasped and traction is applied in the length of the bone to disimpact the fragments; the distal fragment is then pushed into place by pressing firmly on the back of the wrist with the thumbs while holding the front of the forearm with the fingers. The position is checked by x-ray.

A cast (or well-fitting dorsal slab) is applied from just below the elbow to the palm of the hand, with the wrist in the neutral position or slightly flexed.

It is essential to check the position again by x-ray 10 days later. Often the fracture redisplaces in the cast and if this happens re-manipulation may be needed.

The plaster is worn for 6 weeks and during this time active movements and exercises of the fingers, elbow and shoulder are encouraged.

Complications

Malunion Redisplacement and malunion are common, but in most cases the deformity and disability are accepted rather than subject an elderly person to another anaesthetic and a bone operation.

Subluxation of the radioulnar joint With displacement of the distal fragment, the radioulnar joint may be disrupted. The head of the ulna is unduly prominent and rotation of the wrist may be impaired. If the disability is marked, the distal end of the ulna can be excised.

Tendon rupture The tendon of extensor pollicis longus occasionally ruptures a few weeks after the fracture. The frayed fibres cannot easily be sutured; a tendon transfer is carried out, using one of the extensors of the index finger.

Stiffness The shoulder or fingers are often allowed to become stiff – from neglect. This can nearly always be avoided by encouraging active use.

Sudeck's atrophy This is an extremely disabling condition. The hand becomes painful, stiff and hypersensitive, resisting all forms of treatment for months (see page 261).

Smith's fracture

Smith (a Dubliner, like Colles) described a similar fracture about 20 years later. However, in this injury the distal fragment is displaced *anteriorly* (which is why it is sometimes called a 'reversed Colles'). It is caused by a fall on the back of the hand.

Treatment is usually by manipulation and splintage with the wrist extended; an above-elbow cast is needed and is retained for 6 weeks.

Barton's fracture

This injury may look like any other uncomplicated distal radial fracture, but it is fundamentally different: (1) the fracture line runs into the wrist joint; and (2) the fragment is displaced anteriorly, carrying the carpus with it. It is, therefore, a fracture-dislocation of the wrist and it is inherently unstable.

Treatment The fracture can be easily reduced; but it is just as easily redisplaced. Internal fixation, using a small anterior plate, is therefore recommended.

Fractured radial styloid

This injury is caused by forced radial deviation of the wrist and may occur after a fall. The fracture line is transverse, extending

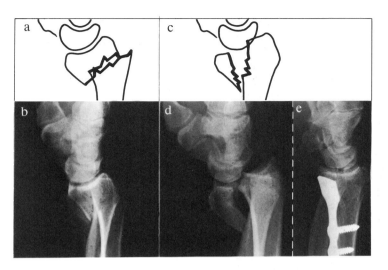

28.21 Fractures with forward displacement (a, b) Smith's fracture. (c, d) Fracture-dislocation (Barton's fracture), reduced and held (e) with a small anterior plate.

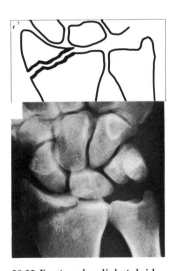

28.22 Fractured radial styloid

across the base of the styloid process; the fragment is often undisplaced.

Treatment

If the fragment is displaced, it should be reduced and held with a screw or Kirschner wires

Comminuted fractures

Instead of the radius breaking cleanly, the distal end of the bone may be fragmented; the x-ray shows several fracture lines, some of which enter the wrist joint.

Treatment

Accurate reduction is seldom possible, but an attempt should be made to restore the length and alignment of the lower forearm. In younger and more active patients, external fixation is applied, with pins through the radius proximally and the metacarpals distally. If a Pennig fixator is used, movements can begin at 3 weeks with the fixator still in place. Once the fracture is firm (usually by 6–8 weeks) the fixator is removed.

Fracture of the distal radius in children

The break – often a greenstick injury – occurs more proximally than a Colles' fracture. The distal fragment is usually tilted backwards and the radioulnar joint may be injured.

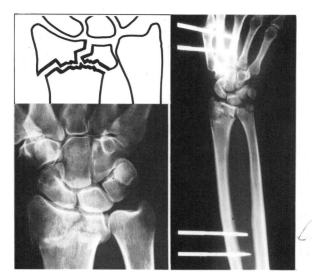

28.23 Comminuted fractures of the lower radius A severely comminuted fracture of the lower radius can be reduced by powerful traction using an external fixator; pins passed through the second metacarpal and the proximal radius are connected by an external rod.

Treatment

Reduction may seem misleadingly simple, but if the fragments are caught in the pronator quadratus muscle, this can be an embarrassing exercise. Fortunately, some residual angulation can be accepted in children under 10 years, as remodelling will ultimately efface the deformity.

Fracture-separation of the distal radial epiphysis

The force which in an older person causes a Colles' fracture may, in a child, cause a fracture-separation of the lower radial epiphysis. The epiphysis is shifted and tilted backwards and may also be shifted and tilted radially. As it displaces, it carries with it a triangular fragment of the radial metaphysis. The fracture is reduced and held in the same way as a Colles' fracture. The injury usually does not cause any disturbance of bone growth.

Fractured carpal scaphoid

A fall on the dorsiflexed hand may fracture the scaphoid. Probably the force is a combination of dorsiflexion and radial deviation. The deviation occurs between the two rows of carpal bones; the scaphoid, lying partly in each row, fractures across its waist. The injury is rare in children and in the elderly.

Special features

The appearance may be deceptively normal, but the astute observer can usually detect fullness in the anatomical snuffbox; precisely localized tenderness in the same situation is an important diagnostic feature.

X-RAY Anteroposterior, lateral and oblique views are all essential; even then the fracture may not be seen in the first few days after the injury. Two to 3 weeks later the break is often much clearer; it is usually transverse and through the narrowest part of the bone (waist), but it may be more proximally situated (proximal pole fracture) or more distal.

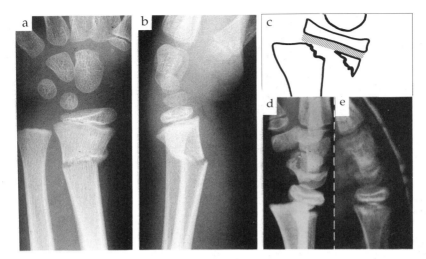

28.24 Fractures in children (a, b) Greenstick fracture of the distal radius. (c, d, e) Fracture separation of the distal radial epiphysis, before and after reduction.

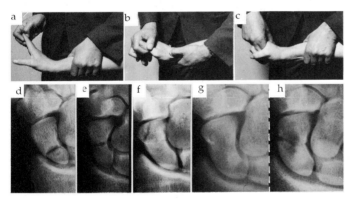

28.25   Scaphoid   fractures
Clinical signs: (a) pain on dorsi-flexion, (b) localized tender-ness, (c) pain on gripping.

X-ray signs. Fracture may be through (d) the proximal pole, (e) the waist, or (f) the tubercle. Even when no fracture is seen at first (g), a repeat film at 2 weeks (h) shows it clearly.

Diagnosis

Sprains of the wrist are rare; any patient who has injured the wrist and is tender in the region of the scaphoid should be treated as for a scaphoid fracture until this is disproved by further x-rays 2 weeks later.

Treatment

Displacement is not common, but when it is present an attempt should be made to reduce it by manipulation under anaesthesia.

A complete plaster is applied from the upper forearm to just short of the metacar-pophalangeal joints of the fingers, but incor-porating the proximal phalanx of the thumb. The wrist is held dorsiflexed and the thumb forwards in the 'glass-holding' position. After 6 weeks the plaster is removed and an x-ray is taken; if the fracture is still visible the plaster is reapplied and retained for a further 6 weeks. Beyond this point one should regard it as a case of delayed union and operation is then indicated – usually a

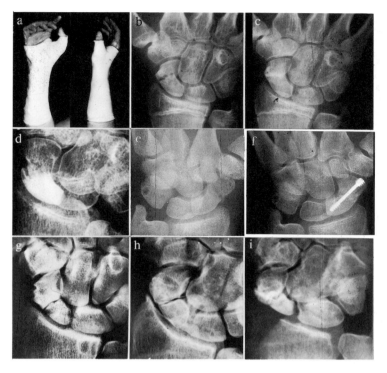

28.26 Scaphoid fractures – treatment and complications (a) Scaphoid plaster – position and extent. (b, c) Before and after treatment: in this case radiological union was visible at 10 weeks.

(d) Avascular necrosis of proximal half; (e) early non-union, treated successfully by (f) inserting a screw.

(g) Established non-union with sclerosis; (h) non-union with localized osteoarthritic changes; (i) osteoarthritis treated by excising the radial styloid.

compression screw or bone grafting procedure, followed by another 6 weeks in plaster.

Complications

Avascular necrosis The proximal fragment may die, especially with proximal pole fractures, and then at 2–3 months it appears dense on x-ray. Treatment is needed if there is persistent pain and weakness of the wrist; the dead fragment and the radial styloid should be excised.

Early non-union It may be apparent in 3–6 months that the bone ends at the fracture are becoming sclerosed. The fracture may be fixed in compression with a screw, or a bone graft inserted. Plaster is worn for 2 months.

Established non-union A patient may be seen because of a recent injury, but x-rays show an old, un-united fracture with sclerosed edges. He may recall a previous 'sprain' which was in reality an undiagnosed scaphoid fracture. The wrist soon became painless, fortifying both patient and doctor in their error. Provided avascular necrosis has not occurred, non-union of the scaphoid does not necessarily cause symptoms, but there is an increased likelihood of pain following overuse or further injury. In most cases the patient can be persuaded to accept the disability, at least until osteoarthritis supervenes.

Osteoarthritis Avascular necrosis, or an ununited fracture, may lead to osteoarthritis of the wrist. If symptoms and signs are confined to the radial side, pain may be relieved by excising the radial styloid. If the entire wrist joint is involved, arthrodesis may be the only answer.

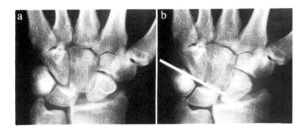

28.27 Scapholunate separation After a fall this patient had pain and tenderness in the anatomical snuff-box. The scaphoid is intact but (a) there is an obvious gap between the lunate and scaphoid. After open reduction the scaphoid was held in position with a K-wire (b) until capsular healing was complete.

Scapholunate separation

Injury to the wrist may cause tilting or subluxation of the scaphoid and disruption of the ligaments between scaphoid and lunate. There is persistent tenderness over the dorsum of the wrist. The diagnosis should not be long in doubt because the x-ray appearance is pathognomonic; in the AP view the scaphoid is foreshortened and there is an unnatural gap between scaphoid and lunate; in the lateral view the lunate may be tilted somewhat out of its normal axis.

If closed manipulation fails, the bones should be repositioned by open operation and held in place with a Kirschner wire; the wrist is immobilized in plaster for 3 weeks.

Chronic carpal instability Carpal subluxation is often missed and the injury is diagnosed as a 'sprained wrist'. The patient goes on complaining of pain and weakness of grip (see page 135).

Carpal dislocation

A fall with the hand forced into dorsiflexion may tear the tough ligaments that normally bind the carpal bones. The lunate usually remains attached to the radius and the rest of the carpus is displaced backwards (*perilunar dislocation*). Sometimes the hand immediately snaps forwards again but, as it does so, the lunate may be levered out of position to be displaced anteriorly (*lunate dislocation*). Sometimes the scaphoid remains attached to the radius and the force of the perilunar dislocation causes it to fracture through the waist (*trans-scaphoid perilunar dislocation*).

Special features

The wrist is painful and swollen and is held immobile. If the carpal tunnel is compressed there may be paraesthesia or blunting of sensation in the territory of the median nerve and difficulty in flexing the fingers actively.

X-RAY Most dislocations are perilunar. The carpus is diminished in height and the bone shadows overlap abnormally in the anteroposterior view; displacement may be more obvious in the lateral view. One or more of the carpal bones may be fractured (usually the scaphoid). If the lunate is dislocated, it has a characteristic triangular shape in the anteroposterior x-ray.

Treatment

Closed reduction may be successful; this is done by a combination of traction and manipulation of the wrist, with thumb pressure applied to the displaced bones. If closed reduction fails, open reduction and decompression of the carpal tunnel is imperative; if the scaphoid is fractured it should be fixed with a screw at the same time.

After reduction, the wrist is held in plaster for 4–6 weeks; exercises are then encouraged. In severe carpal injuries, full function is seldom regained.

Complications

Nerve injury The median nerve may be compressed in the carpal tunnel. This

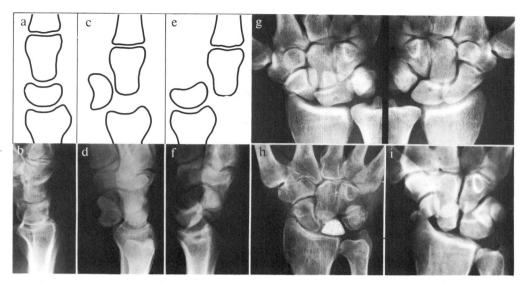

28.28 Lunate and perilunar dislocations   (a, b) Lateral view of normal wrist; (c, d) lunate dislocation; (e, f) perilunar dislocation. (g) Anteroposterior view of both wrists with dislocated left lunate – compare the 'triangular' appearance on the left with the 'square' appearance on the right. (h) Avascular necrosis following reduction. (i) Associated fracture of scaphoid.

usually improves after reduction but it may still be necessary to divide the transverse carpal ligament in order to decompress the nerve.

Avascular necrosis   The lunate may be detached from its blood supply and undergo necrosis. There are no helpful signs until the x-ray shows increased bone density. Treatment is required only if the bone collapses or if secondary osteoarthritis ensues. If wrist movement is good, excision of the lunate and replacement by a Silastic prosthesis is advised; if the wrist is painful and stiff, arthrodesis may be preferable.

Hand injuries

Hand injuries are important out of all proportion to their apparent severity, because of the need for perfect function. Local oedema and stiffness of the joints – common accompaniments of all injuries – are

more threatening in the hand than anywhere else. Fractures may heal and joints re-stabilize, and yet the patient may still be left with a useless hand because of insufficient attention to splintage, the prevention of swelling and rehabilitation.

The patient should be examined in a clean environment with the hand displayed on sterile drapes. The history should include details of the accident, as well as the patient's age, occupation and 'handedness'. Examination should establish (1) the degree of mutilation, (2) the presence of any deformity, (3) the state of the circulation, (4) nerve function and (5) tendon function.

Closed injuries and small wounds can often be treated under regional block anaesthesia. Large wounds and multiple fractures are better dealt with under general anaesthesia.

SPLINTAGE   Splintage must be kept to a minimum. If only one finger is injured, it alone should be splinted – either by strapping it to its neighbour so that both move as

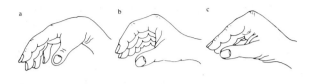

28.29 Three positions of the hand The hand in (a) the position of relaxation, (b) the position of function ('ready for action') and (c) the position of safety ('ligaments taut'). **Hands should never be splinted with the metacarpophalangeal joints extended.**

one ('buddy-strapping'), or by fashioning a splint that does not impede movement in the uninjured fingers. If the whole hand is splinted or bandaged, this must always be in the 'position of safety' – with the knuckle joints flexed at least 70 degrees and the finger joints almost straight. That way the ligaments are at full stretch, so if they do become adherent it is still possible to regain movement with physiotherapy.

SWELLING   Swelling must be controlled by elevating the hand and by early and repeated active exercises.

REHABILITATION   Long term physiotherapy and rehabilitation are best carried out in a special Hand Therapy Unit under the supervision of both physiotherapists and occupational therapists.

Open injuries

The spectrum of open injuries embraces tidy or 'clean' cuts, lacerations, crushing and injection injuries, burns and pulp defects. Examination should be gentle and painstaking. Skin damage is important, but it should be remembered that even a tiny, clean cut may conceal nerve or tendon damage. Sensation is tested and retested. Active movements are elicited to assess tendon damage, but if this is too painful the resting attitude of the fingers is a useful guide.

X-ray examination may show fractures or foreign bodies.

TREATMENT   Antibiotics, if indicated, are given as soon as possible, and suitable prophylactics against tetanus and gas gangrene. Under anaesthesia the hand is thoroughly cleaned. Only obviously dead skin should be removed; for adequate

exposure the wound may need enlarging.

Extensor tendons   Primary repair is easy and safe; the only contraindication is a dirty wound.

Flexor tendons   Division of the superficialis tendon alone causes little deformity and does not need repair. All other lacerations of one or both tendons at any level should ideally be treated by primary suture – but only if the cut is clean, operation is early and the surgeon sufficiently expert. Otherwise only cuts proximal to the flexor sheath or distal to the superficialis insertion should be sutured directly; those within the flexor sheath (between the distal palmar crease and the proximal interphalangeal joint) are liable to form adhesions if sutured, and are therefore best left alone; the wound is closed and secondary suture or grafting carried out 3–6 weeks later.

POSTOPERATIVE MANAGEMENT
Function is paramount; the most skilful surgery is wasted if the fingers are allowed to get stiff. In all cases the hand should be well padded with gauze and wool and bandaged *with the fingers in the 'position of safety'*. Oedema and swelling are minimized by keeping the hand elevated and starting exercises as soon as possible.

Secondary operations may be needed weeks or even months later, to replace unhealthy skin or repair a tendon or nerve. Bone and joint injuries may require late reconstructive surgery.

Fractured metacarpals

The metacarpal bones are vulnerable to blows and falls upon the hand, or the longi-

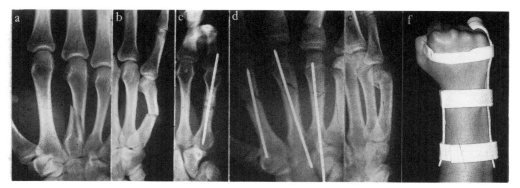

28.30 Metacarpal fractures (a) A spiral fracture of a single metacarpal (especially an 'inboard' one) is adequately held by neighbouring bones and muscles; (b) a displaced fracture (especially an 'outboard' one) is often best held by a wire (c). With several adjacent metacarpals fractured (d), internal fixation may be the only safe way to avoid stiffness. (e) Fractured metacarpal neck. If splintage is used (f), only the damaged ray should be immobilized.

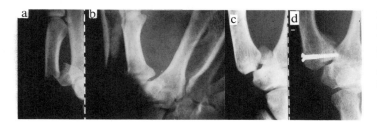

28.31 Fractures of the first metacarpal base A transverse fracture (a) can be reduced and held in plaster (b). Bennett's fracture-dislocation (c) is best held with a small screw (d).

tudinal force of the boxer's punch. The bones may fracture at their base, in the shaft or through the neck.

Special features

If the fragments are displaced (which is unusual) there may be a bump on the back of the hand, or one of the knuckles may be flattened. There is considerable swelling and local tenderness.

X-RAY Fractures of the base of the metacarpal are usually impacted. Fractures of the shaft are either transverse or oblique; there may be shortening or angulation of the fragments. Fractures of the metacarpal neck may result in forward tilting of the distal fragment.

Bennett's fracture-subluxation A special case is Bennett's fracture of the base of the thumb metacarpal. The oblique fracture extends into the first carpometacarpal joint; the large distal fragment may displace proximally, producing, in effect, a fracture-subluxation which is difficult to control.

Treatment

Skin damage demands wound toilet followed by suture or skin grafting. Treatment of the wound takes precedence over treatment of the fracture.

Undisplaced fractures Fractures that are undisplaced (or only slightly displaced) require no reduction. A firm crepe bandage is worn for 2 or 3 weeks but this should not be allowed to interfere with active movements of the fingers, which must be practised assiduously.

Displaced fractures With fractures of the metacarpal neck, angulation of up to 20 degrees can be accepted. All other displaced metacarpal fractures should be reduced by traction and pressure. Reduction can be held by a plaster slab extending from the forearm over the fingers (only the damaged ones). The slab is maintained for 3 weeks and the undamaged fingers are exercised.

If a displaced fracture cannot be reduced by manipulation, or if reduction cannot be held, it should be treated by open reduction and internal fixation. A Kirschner wire can be run up the shaft of the bone, or the fragments can be transfixed with wires running cross-wise into the adjacent bones. It is important always to correct rotation, otherwise the finger will go awry during flexion. A useful guide is to remember that in flexion every finger points towards the scaphoid.

Bennett's fracture The fracture is easily reduced by pulling on the thumb, abducting it and extending it. An attempt can be made to hold the position with a plaster cast, which is then worn for 4 weeks. However, if x-ray shows that a perfect position is not maintained, the fracture should be fixed with a small screw or Kirschner wire; the wrist is held in a plaster slab for 3 weeks.

Complications

Malunion Angulation may result in a visible bump or a flattened knuckle, but function is usually good. Rotational deformity is much more serious because the patient cannot properly close the fist. This may need correction by osteotomy.

Osteoarthritis of the first carpometacarpal joint In Bennett's fracture, if the joint is seriously damaged or subluxed, osteoarthritis may ensue. Treatment is usually conservative, but if pain becomes intolerable an operation may be needed – either arthrodesis of the joint or excision of the trapezium.

Stiffness of the hand Metacarpal fractures invariably unite and even if angulation persists, malunion is less disabling than stiffness. The principles of preventive treatment are discussed on pages 293–294.

Fractured phalanges

Phalangeal fractures usually result from direct violence and therefore any part of the bone may be broken; sometimes the flexor tendon sheath is damaged as well.

Treatment

Open wounds should always be treated first. Skin must be preserved and carefully

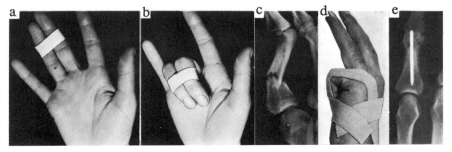

28.32 Phalangeal fractures   An undisplaced fracture is splinted by strapping the finger to its neighbour (a, b). A displaced fracture (c) needs more extensive strapping (d) or internal fixation (e).

sutured, and wound healing must not be jeopardized by the treatment of the fractures.

Undisplaced fractures need the minimum of splintage. Strapping the finger to its uninjured neighbour will relieve pain and allow movement. After 2 weeks the strapping can be removed.

Displaced fractures The bone should be straightened under general anaesthesia, carefully avoiding malrotation, and then splinted with the joints partially flexed. This is most simply achieved by placing a rolled bandage in the palm and holding the flexed finger over it with a firm crepe bandage. After 3 weeks, splintage should be discarded and movement begun. Occasionally a displaced fracture can be held more easily with an intramedullary Kirschner wire.

Fractures of the distal phalanx are usually due to crushing injuries or a blow from a hammer. The soft-tissue damage is more important than the fracture.

NOTE   As in all hand injuries, the danger of stiffness is ever present, and a stiff finger can be worse than no finger. The principles of soft-tissue care should never be neglected: *elevate, keep splintage to a minimum, move, exercise.*

Dislocations

Carpometacarpal

This dislocation is caused by forceful dorsiflexion of the wrist combined with a longitudinal impact. Thus it is seen typically in boxers and in motorcyclists.

The dislocation is reduced by traction, manipulation and thumb pressure. A protective slab is worn for 6 weeks. If reduction is unstable (usually in the thumb carpometacarpal joint), it may need to be held with a Kirschner wire until the soft tissues heal.

Metacarpophalangeal

Usually the thumb is affected, sometimes the fifth finger and rarely the other fingers. A hyperextension force may dislocate the phalanx backwards, and the capsule and muscle insertions in front of the joint may be torn. If the metacarpal head has been forced like a button through the hole, closed reduction may be impossible.

Closed reduction is attempted by pulling on the thumb and levering the phalanx forwards. If this fails, the joint is exposed

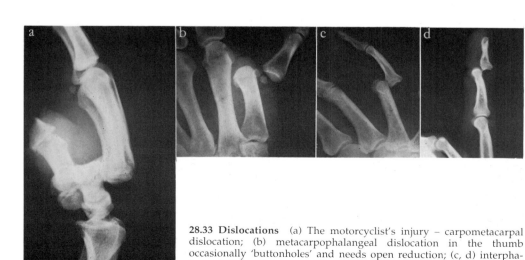

28.33 Dislocations   (a) The motorcyclist's injury – carpometacarpal dislocation; (b) metacarpophalangeal dislocation in the thumb occasionally 'buttonholes' and needs open reduction; (c, d) interphalangeal dislocations are easily missed if not x-rayed.

from the dorsum and, while strong traction is applied, the metacarpal head is levered into place. The joint is then strapped in the flexed position for 1 week.

Interphalangeal

Backward dislocation at the distal joint is common and is easily reduced by pulling. The joint should be strapped flexed for a few days.

Sprains of the finger joints

Partial or complete tears of the ligaments are common and usually due to forced angulation at the joint. Healing is often slow and the joint remains slightly thickened for months.

Milder injuries require no treatment; with more severe strains the finger should be splinted for a week or two. But the patient should be warned that the joint is likely to remain swollen and slightly painful for 6–12 months.

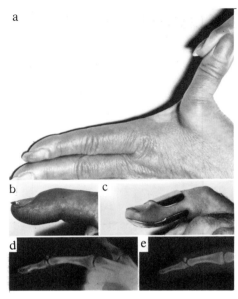

28.34 Soft-tissue injuries (a) 'Game-keeper's thumb' – a tear of the ulnar collateral ligament of the metacarpophalangeal joint. (b) Mallet finger treated by a splint (c); this is adequate when the bony fragment (if any) is small (d), but a large fragment (e) needs fixation.

'Gamekeeper's thumb' (or 'skier's thumb')

In former years, gamekeepers who twisted the necks of little animals ran the risk of tearing the ulnar collateral ligament of the thumb metacarpophalangeal joint. Nowadays this injury is seen in skiers who fall onto the extended thumb, forcing it into hyperabduction. A small flake of bone may be pulled off at the same time.

If the ligament is completely torn, immediate operative repair is advised. A partial tear can be treated by plaster splintage for 2 or 3 weeks.

Mallet finger

If the fingertip is forcibly bent during active extension, the extensor tendon may rupture or a flake of bone may be avulsed from the base of the distal phalanx. This sometimes occurs when the finger is stubbed in making a bed or catching a ball.

A pure soft-tissue injury can be treated by splinting the distal joint in extension for 6 weeks. If there is a large flake of bone it should be repositioned with a Kirschner wire.

The spine

Spinal injuries carry a double threat: damage to the vertebral column and damage to the neural tissues. There is the ever present fear that movement may harm the cord; hence the importance of defining these injuries as stable and unstable.

A *stable injury* is one in which progressive displacement is unlikely; if the cord is not injured, there is little risk of later damage. With an *unstable injury* progressive displacement may cause damage (or further damage) to the cord.

Stability depends largely on the integrity of the ligaments, particularly the posterior ligament complex consisting of the supraspinous ligament, the interspinous ligaments and the capsules of the facet joints. Generally speaking, it requires damage to both the ligaments and the bony column to produce an unstable spine. Fortunately, only 10 per cent of spinal injuries are unstable and less than 5 per cent are associated with cord damage.

Healing is usually slow. In fracture-dislocations new bone formation may lead to fusion of the damaged vertebrae; thus the spine will eventually stabilize itself. However, in pure ligamentous injuries some degree of instability may persist.

Mechanism of injury

Injuries usually occur when the spinal column collapses in its vertical axis – typically, in a fall from a height or when someone is trapped under a cave-in; the direction of force at any level of the spine is determined by the position of the vertebral column at the moment of impact. The flexible cervical and lumbar segments may also be injured by violent free movements of the neck or trunk. The important types of displacement are (1) hyperextension; (2) flexion; (3) flexion combined with rotation; and (4) axial displacement ('compression').

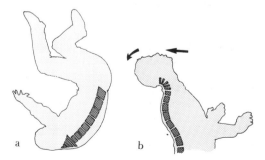

a   b

29.1 Mechanism of injury The spine is usually injured in one of two ways: (a) a fall onto the head or the back of the neck; and (b) a blow on the forehead, which forces the neck into hyperextension.

Hyperextension

Hyperextension is rare in the thoracolumbar region but quite common in the neck; a blow on the face or the forehead forces the head backwards and there is nothing to restrain the occiput until it strikes the upper part of the back. The anterior ligaments and the disc may be damaged or the neural arch may be fractured. Usually the injury is stable, but fracture of the pedicle of C2 ('hangman's fracture') is often unstable.

Flexion

If the posterior ligaments remain intact, forced flexion will crush the vertebral body into a wedge; this is a stable injury and is by far the most common type of vertebral fracture. If the posterior ligaments are torn, the upper vertebral body may tilt forward on the one below; this type of subluxation is often missed in the neck because by the time an x-ray is taken the vertebrae have fallen back into place. If the ligaments are torn and the vertebral body is also fractured, the lesion is unstable.

Flexion-rotation

Most serious injuries of the spine are due to a combination of flexion and rotation. The ligaments and joint capsules are strained to the limit; they may tear, the facets may fracture or the top of one vertebra may be sliced off. The result is a forward shift or dislocation of the vertebra above, with or without bone damage. All fracture-dislocations are unstable.

Axial displacement

A vertical force acting on a straight segment of the cervical or lumbar spine will compress the vertebral body and may cause a comminuted (or 'burst') fracture. A large fragment may be driven backwards into the spinal canal. It is this that makes these fractures dangerous; there is a high incidence of neurological damage.

Diagnosis

Every patient who has suffered a major accident should be fully examined for spinal injury. Any complaint of pain or stiffness in the neck or back should be taken seriously, even if the patient is walking or moving without apparent difficulty. Enquire about numbness, paraesthesia or weakness in the limbs. With an unconscious patient, awareness is everything.

The history of the accident may contain important clues: a fall from a height, a diving injury, head-on collisions, a cave-in or a ceiling collapsing on the patient, or a sudden jerk of the neck following a rear-end collision (whiplash injury) – these are all common causes of spinal damage.

- LOOK   Bruising of the face, or a superficial abrasion of the forehead, should suggest a hyperextension force. The neck may be held skew, or the patient may be supporting the head with his hands. With the patient supine, the chest and abdomen can be examined for associated injuries. Next the limbs are quickly examined for evidence of neurological damage. To examine the back, the patient is log-rolled onto one side with extreme care. Bruising indicates the probable level of injury.

- FEEL   The spinous processes are carefully palpated. Sometimes a gap can be felt where ligaments are torn. A haematoma over the spine is a sinister feature. The bones and soft tissues are gently tested for tenderness.

- MOVE   Movement of the spine can be dangerous – it may imperil the cord – so it is avoided until a diagnosis has been made. If there is a suggestion of cord injury, a painstaking neurological examination is essential.

- IMAGING   The x-ray examination is crucial. It should be carried out with the least possible manipulation of the neck or back, yet it must be complete enough to provide the essential information. *Lateral views of the cervical spine must include all the vertebrae from C1 to T1, otherwise a low injury will be missed.*

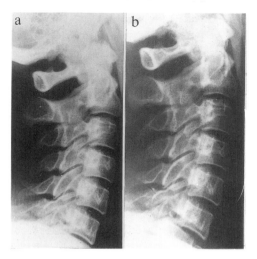

29.2 Spine injuries – x-ray diagnosis (1) (a) Following a traffic accident this patient had a painful neck and consulted her doctor three times; on each occasion she was told 'the x-rays are normal'. But count the vertebrae! There are only six in this film. (b) When a strenuous effort was made to show the entire cervical spine a dislocation of C6 on C7 could be seen at the very bottom of the film.

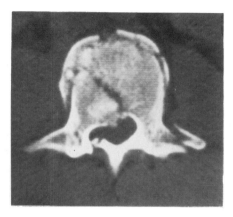

29.3 Spine injuries – x-ray diagnosis (2) The plain x-ray showed the fracture but gave little indication of the amount of fragmentation and displacement. This CT scan revealed that one large fragment was encroaching dangerously on the spinal canal.

Anteroposterior views must include the odontoid process. Oblique views also may be necessary. CT is invaluable for showing fractures of the vertebral body and neural arch or encroachment of the spinal canal.

MRI is helpful in displaying the soft tissues (intervertebral discs and ligamentum flavum) and lesions in the cord. It is especially indicated in patients with deteriorating neurological signs.

Principles of management

First aid

The first priority is to ensure that the airway is free and the patient can breathe.

Patients with suspected spinal injuries should be moved as little as possible, and then only 'in one piece' so that there is no intervertebral movement. The neck should be supported during transport.

Early management in hospital

General assessment is carried out. Often there are severe associated injuries. If the patient needs resuscitation or tracheal intubation, beware the danger of flexing or extending the neck! Ventilation must be ensured, and shock and haemorrhage are treated. The patient is carefully assessed for spinal injury and a neurological examination is carried out; this will serve as an important baseline in future management. X-rays are taken.

The neck and back are held in the anatomical position with pillows and supports, and definitive treatment of the spinal injury is deferred until a full diagnosis has been made. The clinical examination is repeated some hours after admission; the signs may have changed!

General care of the face, the tracheal tube (if there is one), the chest, the abdomen, the bladder and the skin is important. Other fractures are splinted until the priorities have been decided.

Patients with cord damage need special attention to prevent pressure sores and bladder complications.

Definitive treatment

1. Patients with no bony damage and only mild soft-tissue injuries may be dealt with in the accident department and sent home, with instructions to return for assessment a week later.
2. Severely injured patients should be nursed, unclothed, on a firm mattress. If there are neurological changes, special attention should be paid to the skin and bladder. Analgesics are given but narcotic drugs should be avoided.
3. Stable fractures can be left as they are and treated by supporting the spine in a position that will cause no further strain.
4. Dislocations and subluxations must be reduced, whether by adjusting the posture, by traction or by open operation.
5. Unstable fractures should be held secure until the tissues heal and the spine becomes stable. In the cervical spine this can be done (and should be done as soon as possible after admission) by traction. If this proves ineffectual or unduly irksome, internal or external fixation may be used.

6. Complete neurological lesions are usually established at the time of admission and there is rarely any chance of improving them by decompressing the cord; the fracture should be stabilized and rehabilitation commenced as soon as possible. The main indication for surgical decompression is incomplete neurological damage associated with radiologically demonstrable cord or nerve root compression.
7. A NOTE ON TRACTION In the cervical spine, 'traction' means skeletal traction – either by tongs or by a halo device attached to the skull. If the halo is fitted to a body cast it can be used as an external fixator for prolonged immobilization.

Cervical spine injuries

The patient may complain of neck pain and stiffness, or paraesthesia in the upper limbs. A skew neck is an ominous sign. Movements should be tested with the greatest care, or better still postponed until after the neck has been x-rayed.

Avulsion fractures

Fracture of the seventh cervical spinous process may occur with severe muscle

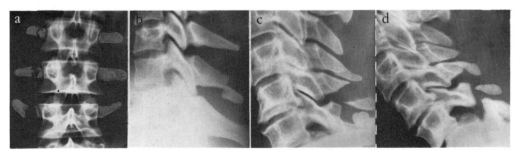

29.4 Avulsions (a) Fractured lumbar transverse processes; (b) clay-shoveller's fracture. (c) This patient was at first thought to have a simple avulsion, but a subsequent flexion film (d) showed the serious nature of the injury – a severe fracture-dislocation.

contraction ('clay-shoveller's fracture'). This is painful but harmless. As soon as symptoms permit, neck exercises are encouraged.

Cervical strain ('whiplash')

The imaginative term 'whiplash' is applied to a soft-tissue injury that occurs when the neck is suddenly jerked into hyperextension. Usually this follows a rear-end collision; the body is thrown forwards and the head falls backwards. There is disagreement about the exact pathology but it is likely that the anterior longitudinal ligament is strained or torn and the disc may be damaged as well.

Patients complain of pain and stiffness in the neck, which may be quite intractable and persist for a year or longer. This is often accompanied by other, more ill-defined, symptoms such as headache, dizziness, depression, blurring of vision and numbness or paraesthesia in the arms. There are usually no physical signs, and x-rays show only minor postural changes. No form of treatment has been shown to be of much value. Analgesics will relieve pain and physiotherapy is soothing. Patients need to be encouraged to bear the discomfort until the symptoms subside. However, be warned: over 10 per cent of patients have some residual discomfort lasting indefinitely.

Fracture of C1

A blow to the top of the head may cause a 'bursting' force which fractures the ring of the atlas (Jefferson's fracture). There is no encroachment on the neural canal and, usually, no neurological damage. X-rays – and CT even better – will show the fracture. If it is undisplaced, the injury is stable and the patient needs only a rigid collar. If there is sideways spreading of the lateral masses, the injury is unstable and should be treated by 6 weeks' skull traction followed by a further 6 weeks in a firm collar; alternatively the skull traction can be discontinued once the acute pain subsides, and replaced by a halo-body orthosis for 6 weeks followed by another 6 weeks in a collar.

Fractured odontoid

This results from high-velocity accidents or severe falls. A displaced fracture is really a

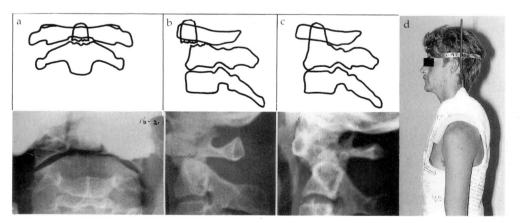

29.5 Odontoid fractures   (a, b) Fractured base of odontoid peg, permitting forward shift of the atlas and skull. (c) Similar forward shift follows rupture of the transverse ligament. The safest treatment is (d) immobilization in a halo–body cast.

fracture-dislocation of the atlantoaxial joint in which the atlas is shifted forwards or backwards, taking the odontoid process with it. Cord damage is rarely seen – perhaps because only the fortunate patients without damage survive! The patient complains of pain and a feeling as if 'my head is falling off'.

Undisplaced fractures can be treated with a well-fitting cervical brace, which is worn for 12 weeks. Displaced fractures should be reduced by traction and immobilized by applying a halo-body orthosis. The patient is allowed up, and if, at 12 weeks, the fracture is still unstable, posterior fusion of C1 to C2 is advisable.

Fracture of the pedicle of C2

The 'hangman's fracture' is seen in civilian life in motor accidents where the head strikes the windshield, forcing the neck into hyperextension. It is potentially dangerous (as the sinister name implies!) and is best treated by immobilization in a halo-body cast for 12 weeks.

Wedge compression fracture

Wedge compression is a flexion injury; the posterior ligaments remain intact and the front of the body is crushed, but the fracture is stable. No reduction is needed. A collar is worn for 6–8 weeks, mainly to prevent progressive kyphosis.

Vertical compression fracture

Central compression of the vertebral body may follow a direct blow to the top of the head (e.g. in a diving accident). If the vertebral body remains intact the fracture is stable and neurological injury is rare; a rigid collar or halo-body orthosis is worn for 6–8 weeks. If the vertebral body is fragmented – a 'burst' fracture – bone fragments may be driven backwards (this is best shown on CT)

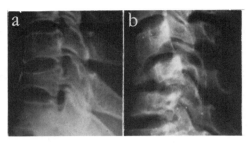

29.6 'Compression' fractures of the cervical spine A true wedge-compression fracture (a) is stable because the posterior ligaments remain intact. A comminuted fracture (b) is best regarded as unstable because the large posterior part of the vertebral body can be displaced backwards.

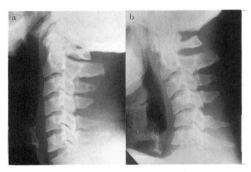

29.7 Cervical spine subluxation (a) The film taken in extension shows no displacement of the vertebral bodies, but there is an unduly large gap between the spinous processes of C4 and 5. (b) With the neck slightly flexed the subluxation is obvious.

and there is a risk of neurological complications. The fracture is treated by skull traction for 6–8 weeks, followed by a rigid collar or halo-body orthosis for a similar period. Patients with neurological damage may require anterior decompression and posterior fusion.

Cervical subluxation

This is a pure flexion injury; the bones are intact but the posterior ligaments are torn. A vertebra tilts forward on the one below,

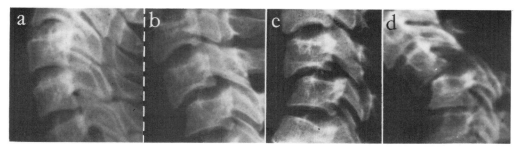

29.8 Subluxation and dislocation   In (a) the cervical spine looks normal, but the film in flexion (b) shows forward subluxation – the posterior ligaments are torn. (c) Fracture-dislocation with moderate forward shift, signifying a unilateral facet dislocation. (d) Another fracture-dislocation with severe forward shift; this is an unstable injury with a high incidence of cord damage.

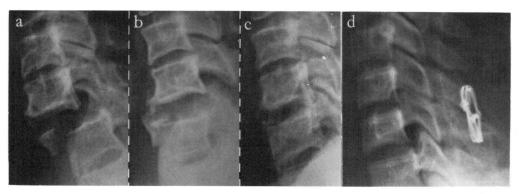

29.9 Treatment of fracture-dislocation   (a–c) Stages in the reduction of a fracture-dislocation by skull traction; (d) subsequent wiring to ensure stability.

opening up the interspinous space posteriorly. X-ray shows the increased gap between the spines. A collar for 6 weeks is usually adequate, but if flexion and extension x-rays show persistent instability, a posterior spinal fusion may be necessary.

Dislocations between C3 and T1

These are flexion-rotation injuries in which the articular facets ride forward over the facets below. Usually one or both of the articular masses is fractured but sometimes there is a pure dislocation ('jumped facets'). The posterior ligaments are ruptured and the spine is unstable. Often there is cord damage. X-ray shows the marked forward displacement of a vertebra on the one below.

Initial treatment   The displacement must be reduced. This can usually be achieved by heavy skull traction (10–15 kg) for several hours. If this fails (usually because of locked facets), gentle manipulation with relaxation may succeed. If this, too, is unsuccessful, open reduction from the back is essential.

Subsequent treatment   Once the displacement is reduced there is a choice of further management. The easiest is simply to continue with traction (reduced to 5 kg) for 6 weeks and then a rigid collar for a further

6 weeks. More convenient for the patient is to immobilize the neck in a halo-body orthosis for 12 weeks. The third method, most applicable when open reduction is required, is to carry out a posterior fusion straight away; the patient is allowed up in a cervical brace which is worn for 6–8 weeks.

Unilateral facet dislocation

This, too, is a flexion-rotation injury but only one articular facet is dislocated. On x-ray the vertebral body appears to be partially displaced (less than one-third of its width) and the upper segment of spine is slightly rotated on the lower. Cord damage is unusual.

Reduction may occur spontaneously while the neck is being positioned for traction. In most cases, skull traction will unlock the single facet and reduce the dislocation. Traction is continued for a further 3 weeks; the patient is then allowed up in a rigid collar, which is worn for a further 6 weeks.

Thoracolumbar injuries

Wedge compression fracture

This is by far the most common vertebral fracture and is due to spinal flexion with the posterior ligaments remaining intact. The front of the vertebra is crushed. Pain is usually quite marked but the fracture is stable. If the loss of anterior vertebral height is less than 50 per cent the best treatment is activity. The patient is kept in bed for a week or two until pain subsides but spinal exercises are encouraged from the outset. Once the patient gets up, a corset may lend additional comfort and security.

If loss of vertebral height is greater than 50 per cent, progressive collapse may occur. A well-fitting plaster jacket is applied with the patient's back extended and is retained for 12–16 weeks. An alternative approach, provided the facilities are available, is to attempt reduction by operative distraction and internal fixation.

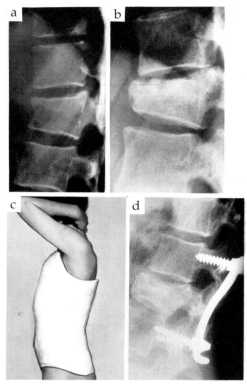

29.10 Wedge compression   (a) With 20 per cent loss of height and (b) with 50 per cent loss of height. (c) Both of these could be treated in a plaster jacket. (d) Progressive collapse can be prevented by internal fixation.

Vertical compression fracture

Minimally displaced compression fractures are stable; the injury is treated by bed rest until the pain subsides, followed by exercises. If the fracture is comminuted or displaced (a 'burst' fracture), CT may show that the posterior portion of the vertebral body is perilously close to the dura and nerve roots. If there is no marked retropulsion of bone or neurological damage, the injury can be treated by immobilization in a plaster jacket, which is applied not with the spine hyperextended but in the neutral position. After 6 weeks it can be replaced by a polyethylene brace.

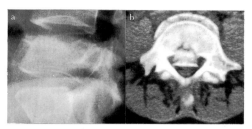

29.11 Lumbar burst fracture Severe compression may cause retropulsion of the vertebral body (a). The extent of spinal canal encroachment is best shown by CT (b).

If there is neurological damage, or the CT suggests that the neural structures are in peril from displaced bone or discal fragments, decompression and stabilization are needed.

Dislocation and fracture-dislocation

In these severe flexion-rotation injuries the posterior ligaments are completely torn and one vertebra is markedly displaced upon the one below. The articular processes are usually fractured and the vertebral bodies may be damaged, too. The injury most commonly occurs at the thoracolumbar junction and is usually associated with damage to the lowermost part of the cord or to the cauda equina. The fracture is always unstable.

The patient should be nursed with the greatest care so as not to jeopardize the cord or the nerve roots any further. Pelvic traction is applied while the patient's condition is assessed. Further treatment depends on the nature of the injury.

Fractures with paraplegia Traction alone may achieve reduction; with suitable facilities for nursing, these patients can be treated conservatively. They require frequent turning (to prevent pressure sores), but the body must be moved in one piece ('log-rolling') and this requires a lot of assistance. The skin and soft tissues need constant attention. After 6–8 weeks the patient can be slowly mobilized out of bed; a spinal brace is usually necessary. In dedicated units it has been shown that 95 per cent of paraplegic patients can be managed in this way; operation is reserved for the few who have locked facets or in

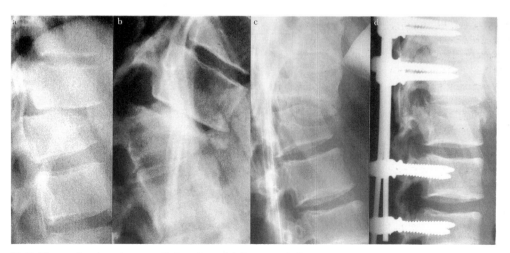

29.12 Thoracolumbar fracture-dislocation (a) Fracture-dislocation at T11/12 in a 32-year-old woman who was a passenger in a truck that overturned. She was completely paraplegic and operation was not thought worthwhile. (b) Four weeks later the deformity has increased, leaving her with a marked gibbus. (c, d) A similar injury in a 17-year-old man, treated by open reduction and internal fixation.

whom the fracture-dislocation cannot be reduced for other reasons.

The alternative approach is to operate without delay and fix the unstable spine with plates or metal rods. Nursing is made much easier, the patients often feel more comfortable and the period in bed can be significantly shortened.

Fractures without paraplegia These are definitely the minority. The unstable dislocation threatens to damage the cord, which has so far escaped injury. If the articular processes are fractured, the dislocation can usually be reduced by traction in extension; the spine is then immobilized, either by a well-fitting plaster jacket or by internal fixation.

If the articular processes are locked, reduction will be difficult and operation is advisable. The bones are carefully unlocked and the spine is fixed with plates or metal rods. A well-fitting brace is worn for at least 3 months.

Traumatic paraplegia

Injuries of the spine may be complicated by damage to the spinal cord or cauda equina. The injuries most likely to do this are 'burst' fractures and fracture-dislocations of the thoracolumbar region or the lower cervical spine.

Complete transection of the cord results in either paraplegia (thoracic and lumbar lesions) or quadriplegia (cervical lesions). Initially there is complete paralysis and anaesthesia, with loss of the anal reflex (spinal shock). At this stage, and for the first 48 hours, the diagnosis cannot be absolutely certain. However, if the anal reflex returns and the neural deficit persists, the cord lesion is complete. Gradually the features of an upper motor neuron lesion appear, with spastic paralysis and exaggerated reflexes.

Incomplete transection results in partial sensory and motor loss below the level of the lesion. Signs vary according to which part of the cord is damaged.

Cauda equina injury, which is a lower motor neuron lesion, causes flaccid paralysis.

Management

Decompression of the cord seems a tempting possibility, but laminectomy alone has proved a failure; its only effect is to make an already unstable spine even more so. Anterior decompression has been used with some success, but the procedure is still not widely accepted. Operation simply to fix an unstable injury may facilitate nursing and speed rehabilitation.

No matter whether the paraplegia is complete or partial, temporary or permanent, it is the overall management which is important, and especially the management in the first 24 hours. The patient must be transported with great care to avoid further damage, and preferably taken to a spinal centre. The strategy is outlined below.

Skin

Within a few hours skin which is anaesthetic may develop pressure sores; these must be prevented by meticulous nursing. Immediate fixation of the spine enables these essential nursing procedures to be carried out much more easily and without discomfort to the patient. Creases in the sheets and crumbs in the bed are not permitted. Every 2 hours the patient is gently rolled onto his side and his back is carefully washed (without rubbing), dried and powdered. After a few weeks the skin becomes a little more tolerant and the patient can turn himself. Later he should be taught how to relieve skin pressure intermittently during periods of sitting. If sores have been allowed to develop, they may never heal without excision and skin grafting.

Bladder and bowel

For the first 24 hours the bladder distends only slowly, but if the distension is allowed to progress, overflow incontinence occurs and infection is probable. In special centres it is usual to manage the patient from the outset by intermittent catheterization under sterile conditions. If early transfer to a paraplegia centre is not possible, continuous drainage through a fine Silastic catheter is advised. If infection supervenes, antibiotics are given.

As the local reflexes gradually return, automatic emptying of the bladder may occur whenever it becomes distended. If the cauda equina is damaged, this reflex is lost and bladder emptying has to be initiated by manual suprapubic pressure. Bladder training is begun as soon as possible and the patient learns to manage this function himself.

Bowel training is somewhat easier and is helped by the use of enemas and aperients.

Muscles and joints

The paralysed muscles, if not treated, may develop severe flexion contractures. These are usually preventable by moving the joints passively through their full range twice daily.

With lesions below the cervical cord, the patient should be up within 3 months; standing and walking are valuable in preventing contractures. Calipers are usually necessary to keep the knees straight and the feet plantigrade. The calipers are removed at intervals during the day while the patient lies prone, and while he is having physiotherapy. The upper limbs must be trained until they develop sufficient power to enable the patient to use crutches and a wheelchair.

If flexion contractures have been allowed to develop, tenotomies may be necessary. Painful flexor spasms are rare unless skin or bladder infection occurs. They can sometimes be relieved by tenotomies, neurectomies, rhizotomies or the intrathecal injection of alcohol.

Heterotopic ossification may restrict or abolish movement, especially at the hip. It is doubtful whether ossification can be prevented, but once the new bone is mature it can safely be excised.

Morale

The morale of a paraplegic patient is liable to reach a low ebb, and the restoration of self-confidence is an important part of treatment. Constant enthusiasm and encouragement by doctors, physiotherapists and nurses are essential. The earlier the patient gets up the better, and training for a new job should be carried out as soon as possible.

The thorax

Rib fractures

Rib fractures are almost always due to direct injury. However, in osteoporotic patients ribs may fracture with minor stresses such as coughing or sneezing.

The patient complains of a sharp pain in the chest. This is markedly aggravated by deep breathing or coughing, or by anteroposterior compression of the chest wall. X-ray shows one or more fractures, usually near the rib angle.

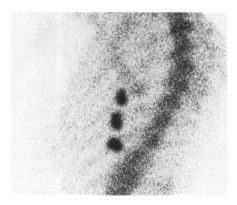

29.13 Rib fractures   Undisplaced rib fractures are often difficult to see on the x-ray; a week later they show up clearly on the radionuclide scan.

Treatment

In most cases treatment is needed only for pain; an injection of local anaesthetic will bring immediate relief. Breathing exercises are encouraged.

Fracture of the sternum

The sternum may be fractured by a direct blow to the chest, or indirectly during a flexion injury of the spine.

If displacement is minimal, no treatment is needed. If the sternum is severely displaced, it should be lifted forwards (under general anaesthesia) with the aid of a bone-hook.

NOTE: Complex thoracic injuries are discussed on page 233.

The pelvis

Fractures of the pelvis are serious in themselves and may result in long-term disability. Even more important, however, is the fact that they are frequently complicated by damage to the soft tissues – urethra, bladder, bowel, blood vessels and nerves – and this can be fatal. Genitourinary complications occur in about 10 per cent of pelvic fractures and in this group the mortality is in excess of 10 per cent.

Clinical assessment

A fracture of the pelvis should be suspected and excluded by x-ray in every patient with serious abdominal or lower limb injuries. The patient may be severely shocked due to blood loss and visceral damage; resuscitation should be started even before the examination is complete. Local bruising or abrasions may be obvious; ecchymoses often extend into the thigh and perineum, and there may

be gross swelling of the labia or scrotum. Bleeding from the urethra or genitalia suggests serious visceral damage. Abdominal tenderness and guarding suggest intraperitoneal bleeding, possibly due to rupture of the spleen or liver.

Pain may be elicited if the pelvic ring is sprung by gentle but firm pressure – first from side to side on the iliac crests, then outwards on the anterior superior iliac spines, and then directly on the symphysis pubis. During a rectal examination the coccyx and sacrum can be felt; more important, the position of the prostate may indicate a urethral injury.

A ruptured bladder should be suspected in patients who do not void or in whom a bladder is not palpable after adequate intravenous fluid replacement.

Neurological examination is essential. There may be damage to the lumbosacral plexus.

X-ray

A good anteroposterior view of the pelvis is mandatory, but ideally five views should be obtained: the standard anteroposterior view, an inlet view, an outlet view and two oblique views. A CT scan is invaluable for the diagnosis of sacroiliac disruption. Three-dimensional CT re-formation of the pelvic image gives the most accurate picture of the injury; this is the method of choice wherever the facilities are available.

If there is evidence of abdominal injury, and the patient has haematuria, an intravenous urogram is performed to exclude renal injury. This will also show whether there is any ureteric or major bladder damage.

When a urethral injury is suspected, a urethrogram should be undertaken using 25–30 ml of water-soluble contrast agent with suitable aseptic technique.

The types of fracture

Pelvic fractures fall into four groups: (1) isolated fractures with an intact pelvic ring;

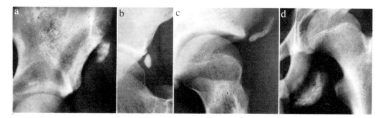

29.14 Avulsion injuries of the pelvis These all result from powerful muscle action. (a) Avulsion of sartorius attachment; this should not be confused with (b) an os acetabuli, which is well defined on all sides. (c) Avulsion of rectus origin. (d) Avulsion of hamstring origin – the clinical condition is much less alarming than the x-ray.

(2) fractures with a broken ring – these may be stable or unstable; (3) fractures of the acetabulum – although these are ring fractures, involvement of the joint raises special problems and therefore they are considered separately; and (4) sacrococcygeal fractures.

Isolated fractures

AVULSION FRACTURES A piece of bone is pulled off by violent muscle contraction; this is usually seen in sportsmen and athletes. The sartorius may pull off the anterior superior iliac spine, the rectus femoris the anterior inferior iliac spine, the adductor longus a piece of the pubis, and the hamstrings part of the ischium. All are essentially muscle injuries, needing only rest for a few days and reassurance.

DIRECT FRACTURES A direct blow to the pelvis, usually after a fall from a height, may fracture the ischium or the iliac blade. Bed rest until pain subsides is usually all that is needed.

STRESS FRACTURES Fractures of the pubic rami are fairly common (and often quite painless) in severely osteoporotic or osteomalacic patients.

Fractures of the pelvic ring

The innominate bones and the sacrum form a ring which is held together by the weak symphyseal joint anteriorly and the strong sacroiliac and iliolumbar ligaments posteriorly. Because of the rigidity of the adult pelvis, a break at one point in the ring must be accompanied by disruption at a second point. (Try breaking a ring-shaped biscuit at one point only!). Exceptions are comminuted fractures due to direct blows (including fractures of the acetabular floor), or ring fractures in children, whose symphysis and sacroiliac joints are springy. Often, however, the second break is not visible, in which case the ring is *stable*. A fracture or joint disruption that is markedly displaced, and all obvious double ring fractures, are *unstable*.

SIGNS OF INSTABILITY

Noticeable pelvic deformity
Excessive mobility of the pelvic brim
Severe soft-tissue damage
X-ray signs of sacroiliac displacement or double-ring fractures

---

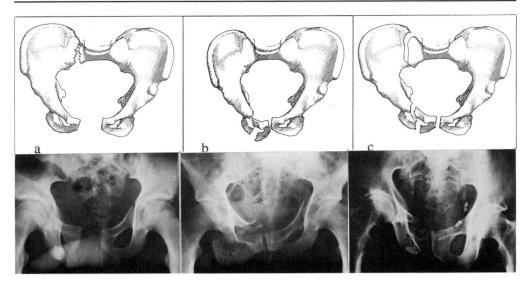

29.15 Pelvic ring fractures   The three important types of injury are shown. (a) Anteroposterior compression with lateral rotation may cause the 'open book' injury. (b) Lateral compression causing the ring to buckle and break; the pubic rami are fractured, sometimes on both sides. (c) Vertical shear, with disruption of the sacroiliac region on one side.

Mechanisms of injury

The basic mechanisms of pelvic ring injury are anteroposterior compression, lateral compression, vertical shear and combinations of these.

ANTEROPOSTERIOR COMPRESSION The pubic rami are fractured or the innominate bones are sprung apart, with disruption of the symphysis – the so-called 'open book' injury; posteriorly the sacroiliac ligaments are partially torn, or there may be a fracture of the posterior part of the ilium, but this is very rarely unstable. The injury is usually caused by a frontal collision between a pedestrian and a car.

LATERAL COMPRESSION   Side-to-side compression of the pelvis causes the ring to buckle and break. This is usually due to a side-on impact in a road accident or a fall from a height. Anteriorly the pubic rami are fractured, and posteriorly there is a severe sacroiliac strain or a fracture of the ilium, either on the same side as the

fractured pubic rami or on the opposite side of the pelvis. If the sacroiliac injury is much displaced, the pelvis will be unstable.

VERTICAL SHEAR   The innominate bone on one side is displaced vertically, fracturing the pubic rami and disrupting the sacroiliac region on the same side. This occurs typically when someone falls from a height onto one leg. These are usually severe, unstable injuries with gross tearing of the soft tissues and retroperitoneal haemorrhage.

COMPLEX INJURIES   In severe pelvic injuries there may be combinations of the above.

Clinical features

With isolated fractures and stable injuries the patient is not severely shocked but has pain on attempting to walk. There is localized tenderness but seldom any damage to pelvic viscera.

With unstable injuries the patient is severely shocked, in great pain and unable to stand; he may also be unable to pass urine. There may be blood at the external meatus. Tenderness is widespread and attempting to move the ilium is very painful. One leg may be partly anaesthetic because of sciatic nerve injury. These are extremely serious injuries, carrying a high risk of associated visceral damage.

Emergency treatment

As with all major injuries, the first priority is to ensure that the airway is clear and ventilation is unimpaired.

Shock and blood loss should be treated immediately and throughout the period of assessment. If the blood pressure cannot be restored, a diagnostic peritoneal aspiration should be carried out to exclude intra-abdominal bleeding. Occasionally an emergency laparotomy is necessary to deal with visceral injuries.

If the patient cannot pass urine he *must not be catheterized*: gentle retrograde urethrography is harmless and may show a urethral tear. Urogenital damage is particularly likely in bilateral pubic rami fractures. If the urethra is ruptured, urinary drainage should be provided by suprapubic cystostomy.

Treatment of the fractures

Undisplaced ring fractures

These injuries can usually be treated by 4 weeks' rest in bed. Throughout this period exercises are encouraged.

Displaced fractures without sacroiliac disruption

Disruption of the symphysis pubis (the 'open book' injury)   If displacement is not marked, it can be reduced simply by nursing the patient on his side or in a canvas sling for 6–8 weeks. For more severe degrees of displacement, or if urogenital surgery is being done, external fixation is better. Threaded pins are driven into the wing of each ilium and these are then clamped to a metal frame; using a winch apparatus in the frame, the two halves of the pelvis can be drawn together. The fixator is retained for 6–8 weeks but the patient can get up and walk around.

Pubic rami fractures   These are usually due to lateral compression, so a sling would be quite inappropriate. If displacement is not severe, bed rest and leg traction for 3–6 weeks will suffice. For severe displacement, external fixation provides more stability.

Displaced fractures with sacroiliac disruption

All vertical shear injuries, and some of the more severe compression injuries, disrupt the sacroiliac joint or produce unstable fractures around the joint. The fracture or dislocation must be stabilized, either by internal fixation with plates and screws (a difficult task) or by combined external fixation and prolonged traction in bed (8–12 weeks). If the symphysis is disrupted, it, too, can be fixed with small plates and screws.

Complications

Urogenital damage   Compression fractures are the usual cause of urogenital tract damage; but with all pelvic ring disruptions, damage must be excluded. All that needs to be provided urgently in a seriously ill patient is adequate urinary drainage, which is accomplished by suprapubic cystostomy. Definitive repair can be delayed while the patient's general condition improves and expert urological advice is sought.

Nerve injury   Displacement of the sacroiliac joint or fracture of the sacrum may injure the lumbosacral plexus. The damage is usually permanent and some weakness will have to be accepted.

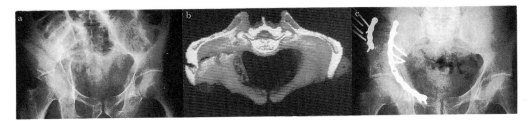

29.16 Pelvic fractures – imaging   (a) The plain x-ray gives useful but limited information. (b) In this case the three-dimensional CT scan was much better and enabled the operative treatment (c) to be planned with precision. (Courtesy of Mr R. N. Brueton and Dr R. L. Guy.)

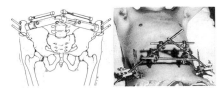

29.17   Pelvic fractures – external fixation
Displaced fractures can often be reduced and held by external fixation.

Persistent sacroiliac pain This is fairly common after unstable pelvic fractures and may occasionally necessitate arthrodesis of the sacroiliac joint.

Fractures of the acetabulum

Fractures of the acetabulum occur when the head of the femur is driven into the pelvis. This is caused either by a blow on the side (as in a fall from a height) or by a blow on the front of the knee, usually in a dashboard injury when the femur also may be fractured.

The types of fracture

There are four main types of acetabular fracture: anterior, posterior, transverse and combinations of these.

Anterior column fracture The fracture runs through the anterior part of the acetabulum separating a segment between the anterior inferior iliac spine and the obturator foramen. It is uncommon, does not involve the weight-bearing area and has a good prognosis.

Posterior column fracture This fracture runs upwards from the obturator foramen into the sciatic notch, separating the posterior ischiopubic column of bone and breaking the weight-bearing part of the acetabulum. It is usually associated with a posterior dislocation of the hip and may injure the sciatic nerve. Treatment is more urgent and usually involves internal fixation to obtain a stable joint.

Transverse fracture This is an uncomminuted fracture running transversely through the acetabulum and separating the iliac portion above from the pubic and ischial portions below. It is usually fairly easy to reduce and to hold reduced.

Complex fractures Some acetabular fractures are complex injuries which damage either the anterior or the posterior segments (or both) as well as the roof of the acetabulum. The joint surface is disrupted; the fractures are difficult to reduce and the end result is likely to be less than perfect.

Clinical features

There has usually been a severe injury – either a traffic accident or a fall from a height. Associated fractures are not uncom-

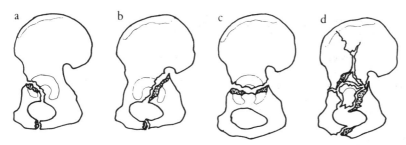

29.18 Acetabular fractures   The four types of injury: (a) fracture of the anterior column; (b) fracture of the posterior column; (c) transverse fracture, which usually lies just above the cotyloid notch; and (d) a composite fracture. The transverse fractures (occasionally) and the composite fractures (almost always) damage the weight-bearing surface and may cause post-traumatic osteoarthritis.

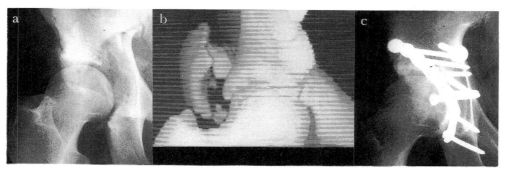

29.19 Acetabular fractures (a) Before and (c) after reduction and fixation. (b) The three-dimensional MRI shows the large posterior fragment which needed accurate repositioning. (Courtesy of Mr R. N. Brueton and Dr R. L. Guy.)

mon and, because they may be more obvious, are liable to divert attention from the more urgent pelvic injuries. Whenever a fractured femur, a severe knee injury or a fractured calcaneum is diagnosed, the pelvis and hips also should be x-rayed.

The patient may be severely shocked, and the complications associated with pelvic fractures should be sought. There may be bruising around the hip and the limb may lie in internal rotation (if the hip is dislocated). No attempt should be made to examine movements at the hip.

X-RAY   Several views of the hip, and sometimes a CT scan as well, may be needed before the fracture can be accurately visualized.

Treatment

Emergency treatment should consist only of counteracting shock and reducing a dislocation. Traction is then applied to the limb (10 kg will suffice) and during the next 3 or 4 days the patient's general condition is brought under control. Definitive treatment of the fracture is delayed until he is fit and operating facilities are optimal; but the delay should not exceed 7 days.

With simple anterior or posterior fractures closed reduction under general anaesthesia is attempted. If this is successful, traction is maintained for a further 6 weeks. If closed reduction fails and adequate surgical expertise is available, operative reduction and internal fixation with plates and screws is advisable.

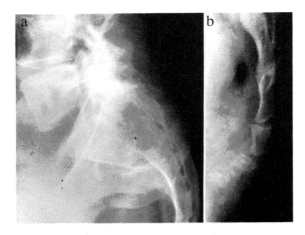

29.20   Sacrococcygeal   fractures   (a)
Fractured sacrum; (b) fractured coccyx.

Complex fractures are difficult to reduce, and in elderly patients operative intervention is not advised unless a persistent posterior dislocation needs to be stabilized. In younger patients, however, the likelihood of osteoarthritis is so great that operative reduction and fixation is justified. It should not be attempted in the absence of ideal operating facilities, ample blood for transfusion and adequate surgical expertise.

If comminution is so severe that the architecture cannot be restored, again operation should not be attempted. Traction is continued and exercises started as soon as possible. If necessary, arthroplasty of the hip can be carried out years later when union is complete and function has stabilized.

Complications

Nerve injury With posterior fractures the sciatic nerve may be injured. The nerve is usually not severed, so the chances of eventual recovery are good.

Avascular necrosis As in all severe injuries of the hip, femoral head necrosis may occur. The changes take months or even years to develop. If this progresses to fragmentation

and collapse of the head, arthroplasty may be indicated.

Osteoarthritis Secondary osteoarthritis of the hip is a common (late) complication, especially if the fracture involves the weight-bearing surface. The fractures must be united before operative treatment is contemplated.

Injuries to the sacrum and coccyx

A blow from behind or a fall onto the 'tail' may fracture the sacrum or coccyx, or sprain the joint between them.

If the fracture is displaced, reduction is worth attempting. The lower fragment may be pushed backwards per rectum. The reduction is stable, which is fortunate. The patient is allowed to resume normal activity, but is advised to use a U-shaped cushion when sitting.

Persistent pain, especially on sitting, is common after coccygeal injuries. If the pain is not relieved by the use of a cushion or by the injection of local anaesthetic into the tender area, excision of the coccyx may be considered.

Posterior dislocation of the hip

Four out of five traumatic hip dislocations are posterior. Usually this occurs in a road accident when someone seated in a truck or car is thrown forward, striking the knee against the dashboard. The femur is thrust upwards and the femoral head is forced out of its socket; often a piece of bone at the back of the acetabulum is sheared off as well (fracture-dislocation).

Special features

In a straightforward case the diagnosis is easy: the leg is short and lies adducted, internally rotated and slightly flexed. However, if one of the long bones is fractured – usually the femur – the hip injury can easily be missed. *The golden rule is to x-ray the pelvis in every case of massive injury*, and, with femoral fractures, to insist on an x-ray that includes the hip. The lower limb should be examined for signs of sciatic nerve injury.

X-RAY In the anteroposterior film the femoral head is seen out of its socket and above the acetabulum. Multiple views (and sometimes even a CT scan) may be needed to exclude a fracture of the acetabular rim or the femoral head.

Treatment

The dislocation must be reduced under general anaesthesia. An assistant steadies the

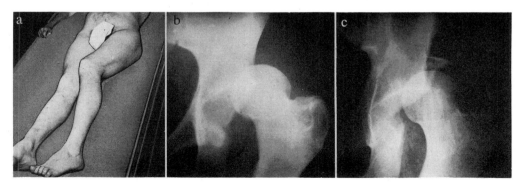

30.1 Posterior dislocation (a, b) Uncomplicated posterior dislocation; reduction is usually straightforward, but it is important to be sure that no loose bony fragments remain in the joint. (c) Associated acetabular fracture which may need open reduction and fixation.

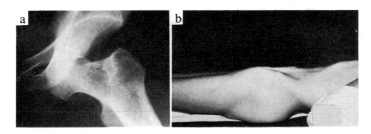

30.2 Anterior dislocation
(a) The femoral head is displaced and the hip is abducted. (b) There is a prominent lump in front of the hip.

pelvis; the surgeon flexes the patient's hip and knee to 90 degrees and pulls the thigh vertically upwards. X-rays are essential to confirm reduction and to exclude a fracture. If it is suspected that bone fragments have been trapped in the joint, CT is needed.

Reduction is stable, but the hip has been severely injured and needs to be rested. The simplest way is to apply traction and maintain it for 3 weeks. Movement and exercises are begun as soon as pain allows. At the end of 3 weeks the patient is allowed to walk with crutches.

Complications

Fractured acetabulum A fragment of the acetabulum may have been sheared off; if it is large or imperfectly reduced, it should be fixed in place by screws. If fragments of bone have entered the joint they should be removed by operation. The acetabulum is thoroughly washed out to get rid of debris.

Fractured femoral head The dislocation may have sheared off a segment of the femoral head. If it does not fall back into place when the dislocation is reduced, it must either be replaced and fixed in position with a screw or removed altogether to allow free movement of the joint.

Nerve injury The sciatic nerve is sometimes damaged but it usually recovers spontaneously. However, if a fracture has to be fixed, the nerve should be explored at the same time to ensure that it is not trapped by the bone fragments.

Avascular necrosis The blood supply of the femoral head is seriously impaired in at least

10 per cent of traumatic hip dislocations. Avascular necrosis shows on x-ray as increased density, but this is not seen for at least 6 weeks, and sometimes very much longer. If the femoral head shows signs of fragmentation, an operation may be needed: in younger patients, realignment osteotomy is often the method of choice; in patients aged over 50, hip replacement should be considered.

Osteoarthritis Secondary osteoarthritis may occur due to any of the following: (1) cartilage damage, (2) retained fragments in the joint, (3) deformity of the acetabulum or femoral head, (4) femoral head necrosis.

Anterior dislocation

This is rare compared with posterior dislocation. The leg lies externally rotated, abducted and slightly flexed. Seen from the side, the anterior bulge of the dislocated head is unmistakable.

X-RAY In the anteroposterior view the dislocation is usually obvious, but occasionally the head is almost directly in front of its normal position; any doubt is resolved by a lateral film.

Treatment The manoeuvres employed are almost identical with those used to reduce a posterior dislocation, except that while the flexed thigh is being pulled upwards, it should be adducted. The subsequent treatment is similar to that for posterior dislocation. Avascular necrosis is the only complication.

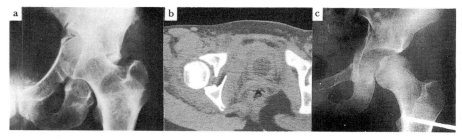

30.3 Central dislocation (a) The plain x-ray gives a good picture of the displacement, but (b) a CT scan shows the pelvic injury much more clearly. (c) Skeletal traction is an effective method of reduction.

Central dislocation

This is not a true dislocation because the femoral head does not really come out of its socket; it is driven through the medial wall of the acetabulum into the pelvis.

X-RAY   Usually the floor of the acetabulum is shattered and comminuted; sometimes the acetabulum is split and a large segment of bone is displaced medially.

Treatment   An attempt should always be made to reduce the dislocation. Even if secondary osteoarthritis is inevitable, a more or less normal anatomy will make reconstructive surgery easier. Strong traction is applied and, if successful, maintained for 4–6 weeks. The hip is then mobilized and the patient is allowed up on crutches.

If secondary osteoarthritis develops, this may need operative treatment; usually an arthroplasty is in order but in a very young patient arthrodesis may be wiser.

Fracture of the femoral neck

This injury occurs mainly among elderly women whose bones are osteoporotic. The patient may fall, but often merely catches her foot and twists the hip; the femoral neck is broken by the rotational force. In most cases the fracture is markedly displaced and completely unstable; in some the fragments are impacted and the patient may even walk about, albeit with some pain.

In Garden's classification, Stage I is an incomplete impacted fracture, Stage II is a complete but undisplaced fracture, Stage III is a complete fracture with moderate displacement and Stage IV is a severely displaced fracture. Left untreated, a comparatively benign-looking Stage I fracture may rapidly disintegrate to Stage IV.

Special features

There is usually a history of a fall, followed by pain in the hip. The patient lies with the limb in lateral rotation, and the leg looks short.

X-RAY   Two questions must be answered: Is there a fracture? And is it displaced? Usually the break is obvious but an impacted fracture can be missed by the unwary. Displacement is judged by the abnormal shape of the bone shadows and the degree of mismatch of the trabecular lines in the femoral head and neck. This assessment is important because impacted or undisplaced fractures have a good prognosis whereas displaced fractures have a high rate of nonunion and avascular necrosis.

Treatment

Operative treatment is almost mandatory. Displaced fractures will not unite without

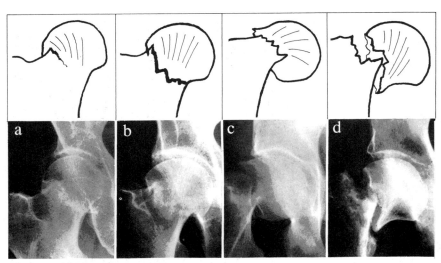

30.4 Garden's classification of femoral neck fractures   (a) Stage I: incomplete (so-called abducted or impacted). (b) Stage II: complete without displacement. (c) Stage III: complete with partial displacement – fragments still connected by posterior retinacular attachment; the femoral trabeculae are malaligned. (d) Stage IV: complete with full displacement – the proximal fragment is free and lies correctly in the acetabulum so that the trabeculae appear normally aligned.

internal fixation, and in any case old people should be got up and active without delay if pulmonary complications and bed sores are to be prevented. Impacted fractures can be left to unite, but there is always a risk that they may become displaced, even while lying in bed, so fixation is safer.

What if operation is considered dangerous? Lying in bed on traction may be even more dangerous, and leaving the fracture untreated too painful; the patient least fit for operation may need it most.

The principles of treatment are accurate reduction, secure fixation and early activity. Under anaesthesia the fracture is manipulated and reduction is checked by x-ray. If it is satisfactory, the fracture is securely fixed with cannulated pins or screws, or with a sliding ('dynamic') compression screw which attaches to the femoral shaft. Impacted fractures can be fixed as they lie.

What if the fracture cannot be accurately reduced? In old people the femoral head should be removed and replaced by a metal prosthesis. In patients under 60 it is worth trying open reduction rather than sacrificing the joint.

From the first postoperative day the patient should sit up in bed or in a chair. She is encouraged to begin walking with crutches as soon as possible.

Fractures in children   If the fracture is undisplaced it can be held in a plaster cast until it unites. If it is displaced it should be reduced and fixed with threaded pins or screws.

Complications

General complications   There is a high incidence of general complications in these elderly and often frail patients. Thromboembolism, pneumonia and bed sores are constant dangers, not to mention the disorders that might have been present before the fracture.

Avascular necrosis   There is a high incidence of avascular necrosis in Garden III and IV fractures. The reason is simple. The femoral head derives its blood supply from three

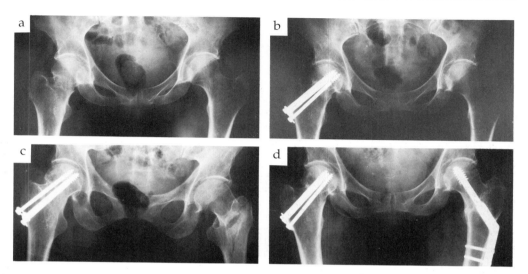

30.5 Fractured femoral neck – treatment   This elderly woman was osteoporotic but otherwise well, until she stumbled and fractured the right femoral neck (a). The fracture was fixed with three long screws (b) and united soundly. Then, a year later, she tripped and sustained an intertrochanteric fracture on the left side (c). This needed more extensive fixation – a large screw fitted to a plate attached to the femoral shaft (d).

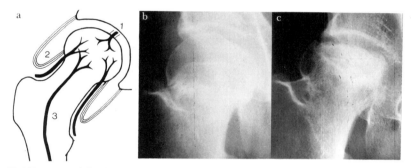

30.6 Fracture of the femoral neck – avascular necrosis   (a) The blood supply to the femoral head comes from (1) a vessel in the ligamentum teres, (2) the retinacular vessels and (3) the nutrient artery. Fracture of the femoral neck interrupts at least one source of supply and may seriously compromise the others. Even (b) an impacted fracture, if it is displaced in marked valgus, can lead to avascular necrosis (c).

sources: the nutrient artery, vessels reflected from the capsule, and vessels in the ligamentum teres. When the femoral neck is fractured and severely displaced, the branches from the nutrient artery are severed, the retinacular vessels from the capsule are torn, and the remaining blood supply via the ligamentum teres may be insufficient to prevent ischaemia of the femoral head. The bone dies and eventually collapses, with distortion of the femoral head and irreversible damage to the joint.

Whether the fracture unites or not, collapse of the femoral head will cause pain and progressive loss of function. The treatment is total joint replacement.

Non-union More than one-third of all femoral neck fractures fail to unite, and the risk is particularly high in those that are severely displaced. There are many causes: poor blood supply, imperfect reduction, inadequate fixation, and the tardy healing that is characteristic of intra-articular fractures. The bone at the fracture site is ground away, the fragments fall apart and the nail or screw cuts out of the bone or is extruded laterally. The patient complains of pain, shortening of the limb and difficulty with walking. The x-ray shows the sorry outcome.

Treatment of non-union depends on the age of the patient. In those under 50 an attempt may be made to secure union by placing a bone graft across the fracture and reinserting a fixation device. In older patients, prosthetic replacement of the femoral head, or total replacement of the joint, must be considered.

Osteoarthritis Subarticular bone necrosis or femoral head collapse may lead, after several years, to secondary osteoarthritis. If the symptoms warrant it, the joint should be replaced.

Intertrochanteric fractures

As with femoral neck fractures, these injuries are common in elderly, osteoporotic women. However, in sharp contrast to the intracapsular neck fractures, the extracapsular intertrochanteric fractures unite very easily and seldom cause avascular necrosis.

Following a fall the patient is in pain and unable to stand. The limb is shortened and lies in external rotation.

X-RAY   The fracture may be comminuted and severely displaced, but in some cases the fracture line can hardly be seen.

Treatment

These fractures are almost always treated by internal fixation – not because they fail to

unite with conservative treatment (they unite quite readily), but (1) to obtain the best possible position, and (2) to get the patient up and walking as soon as possible. The fracture is reduced under x-ray control and then fixed with an angled nail-plate and screws.

Complications

Malunion Fractures that are severely displaced or unstable may unite in some degree of external rotation and varus angulation (even after internal fixation). This is seldom so disabling as to require treatment.

Femoral shaft fractures

A spiral fracture is usually caused by a fall in which the foot is anchored while a twisting force is transmitted to the femur. An angulation force or a direct injury may cause a transverse fracture, which is particularly common in motorcycle accidents. Fracture occurring after middle life should be viewed with suspicion; it may be pathological.

Special features

The patient is usually a young adult. Shock is severe, and with closed fractures fat embolism is common. The leg is rotated externally and may be shortened and deformed. The thigh is swollen and bruised.

X-RAY   The fracture, usually in the middle third of the shaft, may be spiral or transverse, or there may be a separate triangular ('butterfly') fragment. Displacement may occur in any direction. Occasionally there are two transverse fractures, and so a segment of the femur is isolated.

The pelvis should always be x-rayed to avoid missing an associated hip injury or pelvic fracture.*

*Fractured femur – x-ray the pelvis

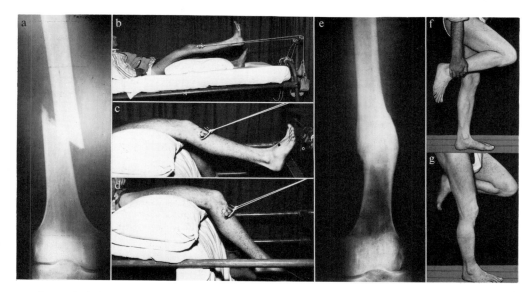

30.7 Femoral shaft fractures (1) Skeletal traction without a splint can be satisfactory. The patient with this rather unstable fracture (a) can lift his leg and exercise his knee (b, c, d). At no time was the leg splinted, but clearly the fracture has consolidated (e), and the knee range (f) is only slightly less than that of the uninjured left leg (g).

Treatment

At the site of the accident, shock should be treated and the fracture splinted before the patient is moved. The injured limb may be tied to the other leg or to any convenient splint. For transport a Thomas' splint is ideal: the leg is pulled straight and threaded through the ring of the splint; the shod foot is tied to the cross-piece so as to maintain traction; and the limb and splint are firmly bandaged together.

CLOSED FRACTURES Definitive treatment depends on the age of the patient, the level of the fracture and the type of fracture. Within each category there is a choice between *closed methods*, which are safe but irksome and prolonged, and *open treatment*, which is quick and convenient but not without risk.

Initially skin traction is applied while the patient is resuscitated. Definitive treatment should be commenced as soon as possible, and certainly within the first week.

For children, continuous skin traction is the method of choice. Infants under 12 kg weight are most easily managed by 'gallows traction' (see Figure 30.8); the feet should be checked frequently for circulatory problems. Older children are better suited to Russell's traction (see Figure 24.4). Union occurs within 2–4 weeks and at that stage a hip spica is applied. Consolidation is normally complete by 4–8 weeks.

For adults, the choice lies between balanced skeletal traction (see page 246) and internal fixation. *Traction* can hold most fractures in reasonable alignment and joint mobility can be ensured by active exercises. The position of the fragments is checked repeatedly by x-ray and the system is adjusted as necessary. Once union is well advanced (around 8 weeks) a *plaster spica* or *functional brace* is applied and retained until the fracture is consolidated (around 16 weeks). Some residual deformity is almost inevitable; but up to 2 cm of shortening, 10 degrees of angulation and 15 degrees of

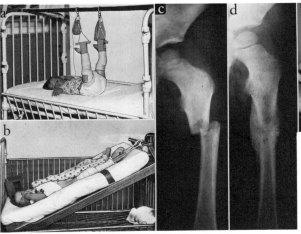

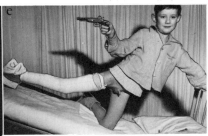

30.8 Femoral shaft fractures (2) (a–d) Traction without a splint is certainly adequate in children, and skin traction is sufficient. (e) Clearly this fracture has united.

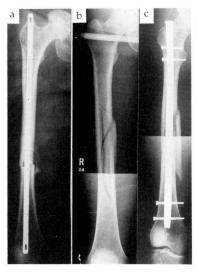

30.9 Femoral shaft fractures (3) (a) Most surgeons use intramedullary nailing. If the fracture is unstable (b), the nail should be anchored by locking screws (c).

anterior bowing can usually be tolerated without significant loss of function.

However, non-operative treatment is unreliable for fractures in the upper half of the femur. For these, *internal fixation* with a long intramedullary nail is preferred. Other indications are pathological fractures,

multiple fractures and fractures associated with vascular injury.

Ideally, nailing should be done 'closed', i.e. by inserting the nail from the proximal end of the bone, under x-ray control, without exposing the fracture. If the fracture is comminuted, or if it is either very high or very low, locking screws can be added proximally and distally to prevent movement of the unstable fragment.

After operation, exercises are begun and within a week or two the patient can be allowed to walk with the aid of crutches and limited weight-bearing. Full weight-bearing is resumed when the x-ray shows that the fracture has united.

OPEN FRACTURES   Open femoral fractures should be carefully assessed for (1) skin loss; (2) wound contamination; (3) muscle ischaemia; and (4) injury to vessels and nerves.

The immediate treatment is similar to that of closed fractures. Antibiotics are started and wound cleansing and debridement are carried out with as little delay as possible. The major decision then is how to stabilize the fracture. With small, clean wounds and little delay from the time of injury, the fracture can be treated as for a closed injury, with the addition of prophylactic antibiotics. With large wounds, contaminated wounds, skin loss or tissue destruction, internal fixation should be avoided; after debridement the wound should be left open and the fracture stabilized by applying an external fixator. Some weeks later, once the wound has healed or has been successfully skin-grafted, a further decision can be made about the need for internal fixation (see also page 253).

Complications

All the complications described in Chapter 25, with the exception of visceral injury and avascular necrosis, are encountered in femoral shaft fractures. The more common ones are listed here with brief comments.

Shock One or two litres of blood can be lost even with a closed fracture, and shock may be severe. Prevention is better than cure; most patients will require a transfusion.

Fat embolism This is so common in young people with closed fractures of the femur that its presence should be assumed in every case. Treatment is supportive, with the emphasis on preventing hypoxia and maintaining blood volume.

Vascular injury The vascular lesion takes priority and the vessel must be repaired or grafted without delay. At the same operation the fracture is fixed by an intramedullary nail.

Thromboembolism Prolonged traction in bed predisposes to thrombosis. Movement and exercises are important in preventing this. Constant vigilance is needed and anticoagulant treatment is started immediately if thigh vein or pelvic thrombosis is diagnosed.

Infection In open injuries, and following internal fixation, there is always a risk of infection. Prophylactic antibiotics, and careful attention to the principles of fracture surgery, should keep the incidence below 2 per cent. Management is discussed on page 15.

Delayed union and non-union It is said that a fractured femur should unite in 100 days plus or minus 20! If union is delayed much beyond this time, the fracture may need bone grafting. Certainly if the x-ray shows

that the bone ends are becoming sclerotic, rigid internal fixation and the addition of cancellous bone grafts are needed.

Malunion Until the x-ray shows solid union the fracture is too insecure to permit weight-bearing; the bone will bend and what previously seemed a satisfactory reduction may end up with lateral or anterior bowing. This is more likely if the fragments were not straight to begin with: in an adult, no more than 15 degrees of angulation should be accepted. If malunion is marked, the mechanical effect on the hip or knee may predispose to secondary osteoarthritis. Shortening is seldom a major problem; if it occurs the shoe can be built up.

Joint stiffness It is surprising how often the knee is affected after a femoral shaft fracture. The joint may be injured at the same time, or it stiffens due to soft-tissue adhesions during treatment; hence the importance of exercise and knee movements.

Supracondylar fractures of the femur

Supracondylar fractures may occur in adults of any age who sustain a sufficiently severe injury, but they often occur with lesser trauma in older, osteoporotic individuals. The fracture is just above the condyles and the pull of the gastrocnemius attachments may tilt the distal fragment backwards.

Special features

The knee is swollen and deformed; movement is too painful to be attempted. The tibial pulses should always be palpated.

X-RAY The fracture is just above the femoral condyles and is transverse or comminuted. The distal fragment is often tilted backwards.

NOTE The entire femur must be x-rayed so as not to miss a proximal fracture or dislocated hip.

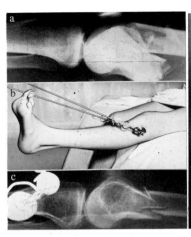

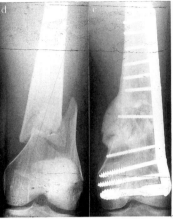

30.10   Supracondylar fractures (a, b, c) These fractures can sometimes be treated successfully by skeletal traction through the upper tibia; if there is much posterior displacement (endangering the popliteal vessels) it may be corrected by vertical traction through a second pin above the knee. (d) If the bone is not too osteoporotic, (e) internal fixation is a good alternative.

Treatment

If the fracture is only slightly displaced, or if it reduces easily with the knee in flexion, it can be treated quite satisfactorily by traction and splintage. At 4–6 weeks, when the fracture is beginning to unite, traction can be replaced by a cast-brace and the patient allowed up and partially weight-bearing with crutches.

If closed reduction fails, open reduction and internal fixation with a dynamic screw and plate may be successful. This does not necessarily lead to earlier mobilization because the bone is often osteoporotic and the patient may be old and frail, but nursing in bed is easier and knee movements can be started sooner.

The equivalent injury in childhood or adolescence is a fracture-separation of the distal femoral epiphysis. Manual reduction is usually fairly easy and a few weeks in plaster suffices.

Condylar fractures

One or both of the femoral condyles may be fractured. The knee is swollen and has the doughy feel of a haemarthrosis.

X-RAY   One condyle may be fractured and shifted upwards; occasionally the condyles are split apart and there may be a supracondylar fracture, too.

Treatment

The haemarthrosis must be aspirated as soon as possible. Because the articular surface is involved, accurate reduction is important. Open reduction and internal fixation are therefore often employed.

Complications

Stiffness of the knee is common. It usually responds to prolonged physiotherapy, although movement may not be fully restored.

Osteoarthritis   As with other intra-articular fractures, secondary osteoarthritis is a late complication.

Tibial plateau fractures

These fractures all involve the articular surface of the tibia. The guiding principle in their management is simple: knee function is more important than a pretty x-ray.

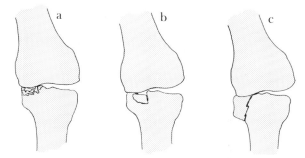

30.11 Tibial plateau fractures   The three common types of fracture: (a) comminuted fracture with many small fragments; (b) depression of part of the articular surface; (c) separation of a large condylar segment.

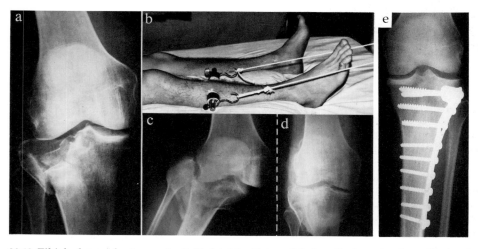

30.12 Tibial plateau fractures   (a–d) Skeletal traction well below the knee is often effective in reducing these fractures, especially when combined with early movements. (e) The alternative is internal fixation, which certainly produces a satisfying x-ray.

Many of these injuries are caused by cars running into pedestrians (hence the term 'bumper fracture') or by falls from a height in which the knee is forced into valgus or varus. In older people, especially those with osteoporosis, the angulation force crushes or splits the bone; in younger people with strong bones, the tibial surface may remain intact and the force ruptures the collateral ligaments.

Usually it is the lateral tibial condyle that suffers – sometimes the medial, and occasionally both. The three commonest types of fracture are: (1) fragmentation of the entire lateral tibial plateau; (2) depression of

a localized part of the plateau, the rest of the surface remaining intact; (3) separation of a single large segment of one condyle.

Special features

The patient is nearly always an adult. The joint is swollen and has the doughy feel of a haemarthrosis. It is tender over the fracture, and also on the opposite side if a ligament is injured.

X-RAY   Multiple views (and, sometimes, tomography) are needed to show the true extent of the fracture. Stress films under general anaesthesia are required if ligament rupture is suspected.

Treatment

Treatment by traction is simple and usually produces a well-functioning knee, but slight residual angulation is not uncommon. On the other hand, obsessional surgery to restore a shattered surface may produce a good x-ray appearance – and a stiff knee. Wisdom lies somewhere in between.

Minimally displaced fractures The haemarthrosis is aspirated and a compression bandage applied. CPM and active exercises are begun but weight-bearing is delayed until the fracture has healed (6–8 weeks).

Comminuted lateral plateau fracture This is the most common injury. After aspiration and compression bandaging, skeletal traction is applied via a threaded pin passed through the tibia. The leg is cradled on pillows and, with 5 kg of traction in place, active exercises are practised assiduously. With movement the intact femoral condyle 'moulds' the comminuted fragments into shape. At 6 weeks (earlier if cast-bracing is used) the pin is removed and the patient allowed up on crutches, but full weight-bearing is deferred for another 6 weeks.

Depressed fracture with part of surface intact The object here is to get the intact part of the tibial articular surface back to its normal level. If it is badly depressed it should be reduced. This can sometimes be done closed by strong lateral compression; if this is successful, tibial traction is applied as for a comminuted fracture. If closed reduction fails, open reduction and fixation is worth while. This is done by pushing the fragmented portion upwards from below, packing the subchondral area with bone grafts and securing the entire condyle with a contoured buttress plate and screws. Postoperatively, active exercises are begun as soon as possible and 2 weeks later the patient is allowed up in a cast-brace which is retained until the fracture has united.

Fracture with a single large condylar fragment The large fragment should be fixed back in position with screws or thin bolts. Active exercises are started soon afterwards but the knee is protected in a cast-brace for 6–8 weeks.

Complications

Compartment syndrome With severe condylar fractures there is a significant risk of developing a compartment syndrome. The leg and foot should be examined repeatedly for signs of ischaemia.

Valgus deformity This is compatible with good function but carries the risk of lateral compartment degeneration in later life.

Joint stiffness Failure to regain full knee bend is an important cause of disability, and is minimized by starting movements early.

Fractured patella

The key to the management of patellar fractures is the state of the extensor mechanism.

Three types of fracture are seen: (1) an undisplaced crack across the patella, which is probably due to a direct blow; (2) a comminuted or 'stellate' fracture, due to a fall or a direct blow on the front of the knee; and (3) a transverse fracture with a gap between the fragments – this is an indirect traction injury due to forced, passive flexion of the knee while the quadriceps muscle is contracted; the entire extensor mechanism is torn across and active knee extension is impossible.

Special features

The knee is painful and swollen; sometimes the gap can be felt. Usually there is blood in the joint. It is helpful to establish whether the patient can actively extend the knee, as this will influence the choice of treatment.

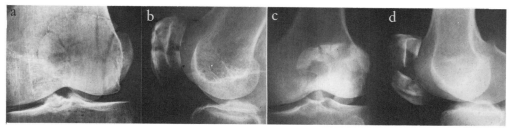

30.13 Fractured patella – stellate   Provided the posterior surface is smooth, a stellate fracture of the patella (a, b) can be treated by activity. With gross displacement (c, d) the possibilities are wiring or excision.

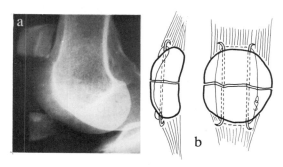

30.14 Fractured patella – transverse   The separated fragments (a) are transfixed by Kirschner wires; malleable wire is then looped around the protruding ends of the K-wires and tightened over the front of the patella (b).

X-RAY   The three types of fracture are usually clearly distinguishable, but it is important not to confuse a crack fracture with a congenital bipartite patella in which a smooth line extends obliquely across the superolateral angle of the bone.

Treatment

Undisplaced or minimally displaced crack   If there is a haemarthrosis it is aspirated. The extensor mechanism is intact and treatment is mainly protective. A plaster cylinder holding the knee straight is worn for 4–6 weeks and during this time quadriceps exercises are practised every day.

Comminuted (stellate) fracture   The extensor expansions are intact and the patient may be able to lift the leg. However, the under-surface of the patella is irregular and there is a serious risk of damage to the patellofemoral joint. For this reason many people advocate patellectomy however

slight the displacement. To others it seems reasonable to preserve the patella if the fragments are not severely displaced; a backslab is applied but removed for daily exercises to mould the fragments into position and to preserve mobility.

Displaced transverse fracture   The lateral expansions are torn and the entire extensor mechanism is disrupted. Operation is essential; the fragments are held apposed by internal fixation (using the tension band principle) and the extensor expansions are repaired. A plaster backslab is worn until active extension of the knee is regained, but flexion and extension exercises are practised each day.

Dislocation of the patella

While the knee is flexed and the quadriceps muscle relaxed, the patella may be forced

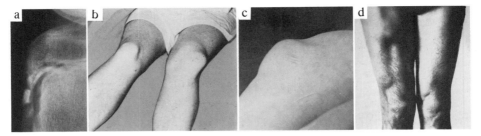

30.15 Other extensor mechanism injuries These tend to occur at progressively higher levels with increasing age. (a) Osgood–Schlatter's disease; (b) patellar dislocation; (c) ruptured quadriceps tendon; (d) ruptured rectus femoris.

laterally by direct violence. It may perch temporarily on the ridge of the lateral femoral condyle and then either slip back into position or be displaced to the outer side, where it lies with its anterior surface facing laterally.

Special features

The knee usually collapses and the patient may fall to the ground. There is obvious (if somewhat misleading) deformity: the displaced patella is not easily noticed but the uncovered medial femoral condyle is unduly prominent and may be mistaken for the displaced patella. The patella can be felt on the outer side of the knee. Neither active nor passive movement is possible.

X-RAY   The patella is seen to be laterally displaced and rotated. In 5 per cent of cases there is an associated osteochondral fracture.

Treatment

The patella is easily pushed back into place, and anaesthesia is not always necessary. If there is much bruising medially the quadriceps expansion is torn, and immediate operative repair may prevent later recurrent dislocation.

With the knee straight, a plaster backslab is applied. It is worn for 3 weeks. When the backslab has been removed, flexion is easily regained.

Recurrent dislocation

After the first episode the patella may dislocate repeatedly, and with less and less difficulty. This is seen particularly in young girls; predisposing factors are generalized joint laxity, marked genu valgum and an unduly high patella. The condition is discussed on page 203.

Knee ligament injuries

The bony parts of the knee joint are inherently unstable and abnormal displacements are prevented mainly by the surrounding ligaments and muscles. These structures may be damaged if the tibia and femur are forcibly angulated or rotated upon each other. Such injuries are common in footballers, skiers and gymnasts, and in the victims of road accidents.

The medial ligaments are most commonly affected, the usual cause being a twisting injury with the knee rotated and thrust into valgus. The tissues rupture layer by layer: first the superficial capsular ligament, then the medial collateral ligament, and then – as the tibia rotates externally – the anterior cruciate ligament. Similar injuries occur (though much less often) on the lateral side when the knee is forced into varus, and to the posterior cruciate ligament when the tibia is thrust backwards in relation to the femur.

Special features

The patient gives a history of a twisting or wrenching injury and may even claim to have heard the tissues snap. The knee is painful and (often) swollen – and, in contrast to the story in meniscal injury, the swelling appears almost immediately. Tenderness is most acute over the torn ligament, and stressing one or other side of the joint may produce excruciating pain.

To distinguish between partial and complete ruptures is critical because their treatment is totally different; *so, if there is doubt, examination under anaesthesia is mandatory.* Each of the ligaments is tested for laxity and compared with that of the uninjured knee (see page 196). The important movements are: (1) sideways tilting, examined with the knee at 30 degrees of flexion, and with the knee straight; (2) anteroposterior glide, tested with the knee flexed 20 degrees and 90 degrees; and (3) rotation of the flexed knee.

X-RAY   Plain films may show that the ligament has avulsed a small piece of bone. Stress films (if necessary, under anaesthesia) demonstrate if the joint hinges open on one side.

ARTHROSCOPY   Arthroscopy may be necessary to diagnose a torn cruciate ligament.

Treatment

Partial tears   The intact fibres splint the torn ones and spontaneous healing will occur. The hazard is adhesions, so active exercises are prescribed from the start, facilitated by aspirating a tense effusion and injecting local anaesthetic into the tender area. Weight-bearing is permitted but the knee is protected from rotation or angulation strain by a posterior splint.

Complete tears   Healing can occur provided the torn ends are closely apposed and the joint held still in plaster. However, for young people and for athletes operative repair is preferred. In either case, the knee has to be immobilized in a full-length cast for 3–4 weeks, after which a hinged brace is used.

Complications

Adhesions   If the knee with a partial ligament tear is not actively exercised, torn fibres stick to intact fibres and to bone. The knee 'gives way' with catches of pain; localized tenderness is present and pain on medial or lateral rotation. The obvious confusion with a torn meniscus can be resolved by the grinding test (page 198), or by manipulation and injection under anaesthesia (which will cure ligament pain) or by arthroscopy.

Instability   As the sequel to an injury the knee may continue to give way. The instability tends to get worse and eventually degenerative arthritis may follow.

Dislocation of the knee

The knee can be dislocated only by considerable violence, as in a road accident. The cruciate ligaments and one or both collateral ligaments are torn.

There is severe bruising, swelling and gross deformity. The circulation in the foot must be examined because the popliteal artery may be torn or obstructed. Distal sensation and movement should be tested to exclude lateral popliteal nerve injury.

X-RAY   In addition to the dislocation there may be fractures of the tibial spine or the tip of the fibula, due to ligament avulsion. If the circulation is threatened an arteriogram should be obtained.

Treatment

Reduction under general anaesthesia is urgent. If closed manipulation fails, open reduction must be performed. A plaster cast is worn for about 12 weeks, during which time quadriceps exercises are encouraged.

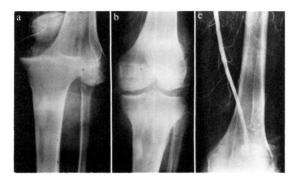

30.16 Knee dislocation and vascular trauma (a) This patient was admitted with a dislocated knee. After reduction the x-ray (b) looked satisfactory, but the arteriogram (c) showed vascular cut-off at the level of the patella.

Fractured tibia and fibula

A twisting force causes a spiral fracture of both bones at different levels; an angulatory force produces transverse or short oblique fractures, usually at the same level. With an indirect injury one of the bone fragments may puncture the skin; a direct injury crushes or splits the skin over the fracture. Motorcycle accidents are the most common cause.

Special features

Because the tibia is subcutaneous, fractures are commonly open. Those in the lower third of the tibia tend to heal slowly.

X-RAY   The x-ray must include the knee and ankle, or fractures at widely different levels may be missed.

Treatment

CLOSED FRACTURES   *Closed treatment* is satisfactory in most cases. If the tibial fracture is undisplaced (or minimally displaced), a full-length cast from upper thigh to metatarsal necks is applied without further ado (displacement of the fibular fracture is unimportant and can be ignored). If the fragments are displaced, they are manipulated under general anaesthesia and with x-ray control; apposition need not be

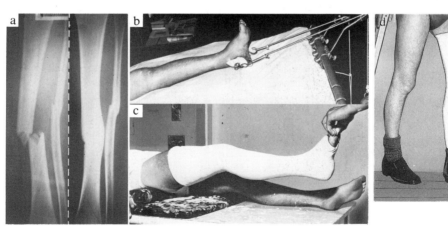

30.17 Fractured tibia and fibula – closed treatment   Most fractures of the tibia and fibula can be treated successfully by closed methods (a). Traction (b) is seldom used except as a temporary measure. A full-length plaster (c, d) will permit early weight-bearing; however, the long cast may be changed to a patellar-tendon-bearing cast after 3–4 weeks.

complete but alignment must be perfect. A full-length plaster is applied, with the knee slightly flexed and the ankle at a right-angle. Minor degrees of angulation can still be corrected by making a transverse cut in the plaster and wedging it into a better position. The limb is elevated and the patient is kept under observation for 48–72 hours; if there is undue swelling the plaster is split. After 2 weeks the position is checked by x-ray and, if it is satisfactory, the patient is allowed to walk with crutches, taking partial weight. The cast is retained (or renewed if it becomes loose) until the fracture unites – which is around 8 weeks in children but seldom under 12 weeks in adults.

Exercise Right from the start, the patient is taught to exercise the muscles of the foot, ankle and knee. When he gets up, an overboot with a rockered sole is fitted, and he is taught to walk correctly. When the plaster is removed, a crepe bandage is applied and the patient is told that he may either elevate and exercise the limb or walk correctly on it, but he must not let it dangle idly.

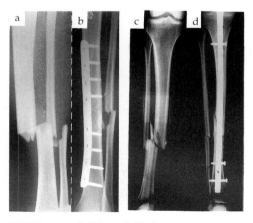

30.18 Fractured tibia and fibula – open treatment
(a, b) Plating of this subcutaneous fracture is easily performed but it requires a long wound and stripping of soft tissues (with the attendant risk of infection). (c, d) 'Closed' intramedullary nailing (if necessary with interlocking screws) is preferable; active movements and weightbearing can be started soon after operation.

Functional bracing With transverse fractures (which are relatively stable) the full-length cast may be changed after 3 or 4 weeks to a functional below-knee cast which is carefully moulded to bear upon the upper tibia and patellar tendon. This liberates the knee and allows full weight-bearing.

Internal fixation Internal fixation is indicated when closed reduction fails or when an unstable (spiral or comminuted) fracture keeps displacing in the plaster. Internal fixation is applied, either by a plate and screws or by a long intramedullary nail. After plating, partial weight-bearing only is permitted until there are signs of fracture healing. After intramedullary nailing, weight-bearing can be started within a week or two.

External fixation Tibial fractures are ideally suited to immobilization by external fixation. This is a great help when the fracture is severely comminuted or when there is marked soft-tissue damage. Partial weight-bearing is permitted; after 6 weeks the fixator is removed and a functional brace is applied and retained until healing is complete.

OPEN FRACTURES *Antibiotics* are started immediately and the wound is *debrided* and cleaned. Grade I and Grade II injuries can usually be closed and are then treated as for closed fractures. *All other grades of injury are left open* and the fracture is *stabilized*. The safest method is external fixation, though this carries a significant risk of pin-track infection and/or fracture displacement. There is now a trend towards the use of intramedullary nails, without prior reaming, for Grade III injuries. The better the stability the lower the risk of infection.

The wound is inspected every few days; as soon as it is clean and granulating it is closed by either direct suture or skin grafting. From then on treatment is as for closed fractures.

Complications

Infection Open fractures are always at risk; even a small perforation should be treated with respect and debridement carried out before the wound is closed. Larger lacerations require wide excision and the wound should be left open until the risk of infection has passed (see page 253).

Vascular injury Fractures of the proximal half of the tibia may damage the popliteal artery (see page 256). This is an emergency of the first order, requiring exploration and repair.

Compartment syndrome Proximal third fractures are inclined to cause bleeding and progressive soft-tissue expansion within the fascial compartments of the leg, thus precipitating muscle ischaemia (see page 257). A tight plaster on a swollen leg may have the same effect. Operative decompression of all the affected compartments is essential.

Delayed union and non-union If union is unduly slow, cast fixation should be reviewed and weight-bearing should be encouraged. If the fracture is still mobile after 4 months, intramedullary fixation and bone grafting are indicated.

Malunion Marked angulation is not only unsightly but may also predispose to osteoarthritis. Anything over 20 degrees should be corrected by osteotomy.

Joint stiffness If a full-length cast is used, stiffness is inevitable. Fortunately it usually responds to intensive physiotherapy; however, if soft-tissue damage is severe, full movement may never be regained.

Algodystrophy Algodystrophy differs from simple stiffness in that the joints are often painful and tender, there may be associated vascular changes and the bones are osteoporotic. Treatment is discussed on page 261.

Fracture of the tibia alone

Except in children, this is uncommon. Its importance lies in the fact that, with displacement, there is an increased tendency to non-union because the intact fibula holds the fragments apart. If this happens, the fibula may need to be divided. Otherwise management is as for fractures of both bones.

Fatigue fracture of the tibia

Repetitive stress may cause a fatigue fracture of the tibia. This is seen in army recruits, runners and ballet dancers, who complain of pain in the front of the leg. There is local tenderness and slight swelling.

X-RAY   For the first 4 weeks there may be nothing abnormal about the x-ray, but a bone scan shows increased activity. After some weeks periosteal new bone may be seen, with a small transverse defect in the cortex. There is a danger that these appearances may be mistaken for those of an osteosarcoma, with tragic consequences. If the diagnosis of stress fracture is kept in mind, such mistakes are unlikely.

Treatment

The patient is told to avoid the stressful activity. Usually after 8–10 weeks the symptoms settle down.

Ankle ligament injuries

The patient stumbles and the foot is twisted and inverted. As a rule, there is only a partial tear (or strain) of the lateral ligament. Sometimes, however, the ligament is completely torn and the joint subluxates; the talus momentarily tilts into inversion, then snaps back into position.

Bruising may be severe (suggesting a complete tear) or may be faint and only appear a day or two after the injury (more likely with a strain). The ankle is always swollen. Tenderness is usually maximal on the lateral aspect of the joint. Passive inversion is painful, but only with a complete tear of the ligament is the movement excessive.

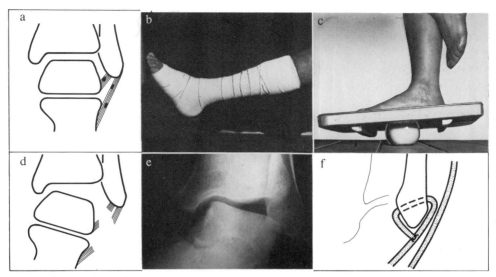

30.19 Ankle sprains The most common is a partial tear of the lateral ligament (a). In treatment a crêpe bandage (b) is more efficient than adhesive strapping. The balancing board (c) is a useful method of strengthening the muscles.
A complete tear of the lateral ligament (d) causes recurrent giving way; a strain film reveals talar tilt (e). The operation shown in (f), which utilizes the peroneus brevis, is simple and effective.

Pain may prevent this from being demonstrated and, if the injury is severe, inversion should be tested again under local or general anaesthesia. There may also be excessive anteroposterior movement at the ankle.

X-RAY The x-ray appearance of the resting ankle is normal whether the joint has been strained or subluxed, for a subluxation reduces itself. X-ray films with both ankles inverted (if necessary, using local or general anaesthesia) will show whether the talus tilts unduly.

Treatment

An ankle strain should be treated by activity. A crepe bandage is applied and active exercises are begun immediately and persevered with until full movement is regained.

A complete tear can be treated by plaster immobilization for 8–10 weeks. However, in 'high-demand' patients (athletes, dancers), operative repair followed by 6 weeks of plaster immobilization may be preferable.

Complications

Adhesions Following an ankle strain, adhesions are liable to form. The patient complains that the ankle 'gives way' and lets him down. If active exercises fail to restore full painless movement, the joint should be manipulated under anaesthesia.

Recurrent subluxation If a complete tear of the lateral ligament was undiagnosed, and consequently unsplinted, the ligament fails to repair and subluxation becomes recurrent. Stress x-rays will show the degree of talar tilt. Often this requires no treatment apart from adjustment of the shoes (raising and extending the outer side of the heel). If disability is marked, operative reconstruction of the ligament may be undertaken.

Fractures around the ankle

Fractures and fracture-dislocations of the ankle are common. One such injury was

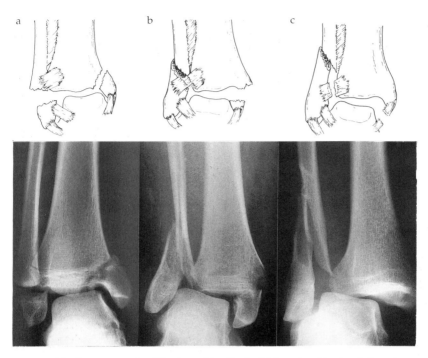

30.20 Ankle fractures – classification   The Danis–Weber classification is based on the level of the fibular fracture. (a) Type A – a fracture below the syndesmosis. (b) Type B – a fracture at the syndesmosis, often associated with disruption of the anterior fibres of the tibiofibular ligament. (c) Type C – the fibular fracture is above the syndesmosis; the tibiofibular ligament must be torn, resulting in an unstable fracture-subluxation.

described by Percivall Pott in 1768, and the group as a whole is now referred to colloquially as Pott's fracture.

Normally the talus is seated firmly in the mortise made up of the distal tibia and the medial and lateral malleoli. If it is twisted and tilted in the mortise, one or both of the malleoli can be pushed off or pulled off by the strong collateral ligaments. If a malleolus is pushed off, it fractures obliquely; if it is pulled off, it fractures transversely. Clearly the movements producing these injuries are either forced inversion or forced eversion, often with the added component of rotation or vertical compression. Simply stated, *eversion and external rotation* will push the lateral malleolus (an oblique fracture) and pull on the medial side (a ruptured ligament or a transverse fracture),

whilst *adduction or inversion* will push the medial malleolus (oblique fracture) and pull the lateral structures (ruptured ligament or transverse fracture).

Another important point is the level of the fibular fracture: if this is below the distal tibiofibular joint, the syndesmosis is intact and after reduction the ankle will be relatively stable. If it is above the tibiofibular joint, the syndesmotic ligaments must have been torn; this is an unstable fracture-subluxation of the ankle requiring open reduction and fixation.

Special features

The patient may have stumbled over an unexpected obstacle or stair, or may have

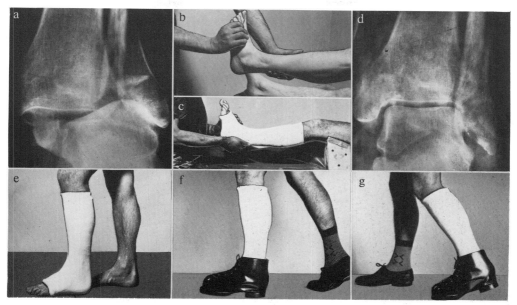

30.21 Ankle fractures – closed treatment An external rotation fracture below the tibiofibular syndesmosis (a) is reduced by traction followed by internal rotation (b); a below-knee plaster is applied, moulded and held till it has set (c). The check x-ray is usually satisfactory (d). The plaster must be plantigrade, i.e. with the sole at right angles to the leg (e); a rockered boot permits an almost normal gait (f, g).

fallen from a height. The ankle is twisted severely under the leg. Swelling and bruising appear rapidly and deformity may be marked. The site of tenderness is important; if both sides are tender, an injury (bony or ligamentous) must be suspected on both sides.

X-RAY From a study of the fracture pattern, the type of injury can be deduced (*see* above), and treatment depends upon its correct identification. Special views may be needed to show whether the tibiofibular joint has sprung apart (diastasis).

Treatment

The principles of treatment are the same for all ankle fractures:

– The shape of the mortise must be restored by accurate reduction of the bones.
– Swelling is rapid and severe; if the fracture is not reduced within a few hours, definitive treatment may have to be deferred for several days while the leg is elevated so that the swelling can subside.
– After reduction – whether closed or open – the leg must be held in plaster for 6–8 weeks or until the fractures unite.

Isolated fracture of one malleolus Often this means that the ligament on the opposite side of the joint has been injured; even if displacement is not marked, the ankle must be immobilized for about 6 weeks. A large medial malleolar fragment should be accurately replaced by open operation and internally fixed with a long oblique screw.

Fractures of both malleoli below the tibiofibular joint The tibiofibular syndesmosis is intact. Closed reduction can be accurate provided the mechanism of injury has been analysed from the x-ray. Treatment in plaster may be adequate, but a large medial malleolar fragment may need open reduction and a single screw.

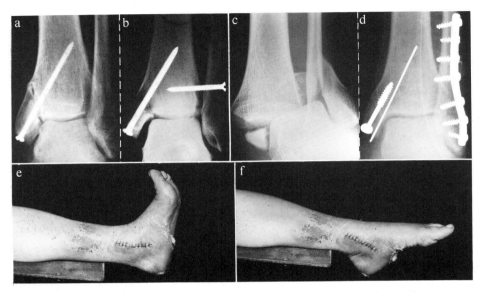

30.22 Ankle fractures – open treatment   (a) A large medial fragment needs a malleolar screw; (b) if diastasis is present, a tibiofibular screw may be added; (c, d) if the fibula is displaced its length must be restored and held by internal fixation; (e) and (f) show this patient exercising his ankle a few days after operation, and before the walking plaster was applied.

Fractures of both malleoli with the fibular fracture above the tibiofibular joint This unstable injury always requires operative treatment. The key is to restore the length of the fibula and fix it with a plate and screws. If the medial malleolar fragment is large, it, too, will need a screw. If the medial malleolus is intact but the talus is tilted, then the medial collateral ligament must be torn and it may have to be repaired. It is essential to ensure that the tibiofibular syndesmosis is completely reduced and held reduced, if necessary by transverse screws between the fibula and the tibia.

Fractures involving the roof of the mortise A single displaced posterior fragment should be accurately repositioned and fixed with a screw. A badly comminuted fracture is beyond salvaging; it should be managed by calcaneal traction and active exercises to maintain ankle movement.

Complications

Joint stiffness After prolonged plaster immobilization the ankle may be stiff. Oedema can be minimized by bandaging the foot and ankle firmly and by encouraging exercises. Occasionally, manipulation under anaesthesia is needed.

Osteoarthritis The ankle is a fairly forgiving joint, but if the articular surfaces are badly damaged or inaccurately restored, secondary osteoarthritis may develop. If pain and stiffness are severe, the joint can be arthrodesed.

Fracture-separation of the distal tibial and fibular epiphyses

Physeal injuries are quite common in children and almost a third of these occur around the ankle.

The foot is fixed to the ground or trapped in a crevice and the leg twists to one or the other side. The tibial (or fibular) physis is wrenched apart, usually resulting in a Salter–Harris type 1 or 2 fracture (see page 255).

Type 3 and 4 fractures are uncommon but dangerous. The epiphysis is split vertically and one piece of the epiphysis may be displaced; if it is not accurately reduced it will inevitably result in abnormal growth and deformity of the ankle.

Special features

Following a sprain the ankle is painful, swollen, bruised and acutely tender.

X-RAY   Undisplaced physeal fractures are easily missed. Even a hint of physeal widening should be regarded with great suspicion and the child x-rayed again after a week.

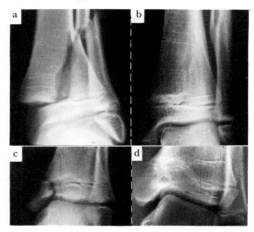

30.23   Ankle   fractures   in   children   (a) Salter–Harris type 2 injury; after reduction (b) growth has proceeded normally. (c) Salter–Harris type 3 injury; (d) the medial side of the physis has not grown – presumably it was bridged by bone.

Treatment

Salter–Harris type 1 and 2 injuries are treated closed. If it is displaced, the fracture is gently reduced under general anaesthesia; the limb is immobilized in a full-length cast for 3 weeks and then in a below-knee walking cast for a further 3 weeks.

Type 3 or 4 fractures, if undisplaced, can be treated in the same manner, but the ankle must be re-x-rayed after 5 days to ensure that the fragments have not slipped. Unless reduction is perfect, the fracture should be reduced open and fixed with thin transverse or oblique cancellous screws (which will have to be removed after about 4 months). Postoperatively the leg is immobilized in a below-knee cast for 6 weeks.

Complications

Malunion   Imperfect reduction may result in deformity – usually valgus. In children under 10 years old, mild deformities may be accommodated by further growth and modelling. In older children the deformity should be corrected by osteotomy.

Asymmetrical growth   Fractures through the epiphysis may result in fusion of the physis. The bony bridge is usually in the medial half of the growth plate; the lateral half goes on growing and the distal tibia gradually veers into varus. CT is helpful in showing where it is. If the bridge is small it can be excised and replaced by a pad of fat in the hope that physeal growth may be restored. If more than half of the physis is involved, or the child is near the end of the growth period,   supramalleolar   osteotomy   is indicated.

Shortening   Damage to the physis may result in shortening. If this promises to be marked, leg length equalization will be necessary.

Talar injuries

Talar injuries are rare and due to considerable violence, usually a car accident or falling from a height. The injuries include

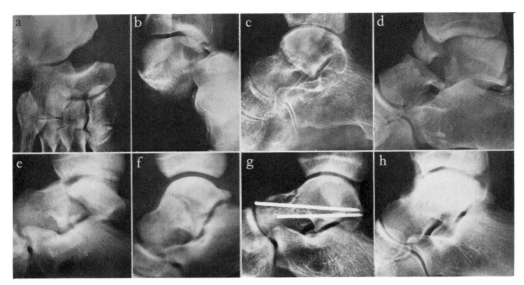

30.24 Talar fractures and dislocations   (a, b) Two views of subtalar dislocation. (c) Talar fracture without displacement, and (d) with considerable displacement. (e, f) Talar fracture before and after reduction by forced plantarflexion. (g) Another method of treatment, by open reduction and internal fixation. (h) Avascular necrosis of the posterior half of the talus following fracture.

fractures (of the head, neck, body or lateral process of the talus), dislocations (midtarsal, subtalar or total dislocation of the talus) and fracture-dislocations (talar fractures combined with dislocation). Tarsal injuries are often missed; good x-rays are needed to define the injury accurately.

Treatment

When displacement is no more than trivial, reduction is not needed. A split plaster is applied and, when the swelling has subsided, is replaced by a complete plaster in the plantigrade position. This is worn for 6–8 weeks.

With displaced fractures and fracture-dislocations, reduction is urgent. Closed manipulation is tried first, but should this fail there must be no hesitation in performing open reduction. The reduced fracture can be stabilized with one or two Kirschner wires. A below-knee plaster is needed for 6–8 weeks.

Complications

Avascular necrosis   Fractures of the neck of the talus often result in avascular necrosis of the body (the posterior fragment). The fracture may fail to unite and the posterior half of the bone eventually collapses. The ankle may need to be arthrodesed.

Fractures of the calcaneum

The patient usually falls from a height, often from a ladder, onto one or both heels. The calcaneum is driven up against the talus and is split or crushed. The same accident may also have damaged the spine, pelvis or hip, which must always be examined in calcaneal injuries.

Extra-articular fractures involve the calcaneal processes or the posterior part of the bone. They are easy to manage and have a good prognosis.

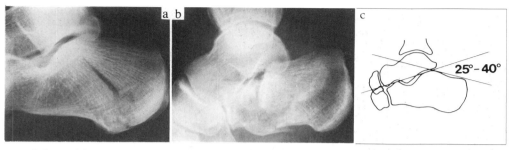

30.25 Calcaneal fractures   (a) Crack fracture with little displacement and no joint involvement. (b) Crush fracture, with flattening of the calcaneum and distortion of the talocalcaneal joint. (c) Böhler's angle is normally 25–40 degrees; compare the appearance in (b).

Intra-articular fractures cleave the bone obliquely and run into the superior articular surface; secondary cracks cause further disruption of the bone. The articular facet is split apart and there may be severe comminution.

Special features

The foot is painful, swollen and bruised; the heel may look broad and squat. The tissues are thick and tender, and the normal concavity below the lateral malleolus is lacking. The subtalar joint cannot be moved but ankle movement is possible.

X-RAY   Crack fractures can be missed unless special views of the calcaneum are obtained. Extra-articular fractures are usually quite obvious. Intra-articular fractures, also, can often be identified in the plain films, and if there is displacement of the fragments the lateral view may show flattening of the tuber-joint angle (Böhler's angle). However, for accurate definition of intra-articular fractures, CT is needed.

   With severe injuries – and especially with bilateral fractures – it is essential to x-ray the spine and pelvis as well.

Treatment

For all except the most minor injuries, the patient is admitted to hospital so that the leg and foot can be elevated and treated with ice-packs until swelling subsides. This also gives time to obtain the necessary x-rays and CT scans.

Undisplaced fractures are treated closed. Exercises are encouraged from the outset. When the swelling subsides, a firm bandage is applied and the patient is allowed up non-weight-bearing on crutches for 4–6 weeks.

Displaced avulsion fractures of the tuberosity should be reduced and fixed with screws; the foot is then immobilized in slight equinus to relieve tension on the tendo Achillis. Weight-bearing can be permitted after 4–6 weeks.

Displaced intra-articular fractures are best treated by open reduction and internal fixation with plates and screws. Bone grafts are used to fill any defects. If there is much bleeding from the bone, the wound should be drained. Postoperatively the foot is lightly splinted and elevated. Exercises are begun as soon as pain subsides and after 2–3 weeks the patient can be allowed up non-weight-bearing on crutches. Partial weight-bearing is permitted only when the fracture has healed (seldom before 8 weeks), and full weight-bearing about 4 weeks after that.

Complications

Broadening of the heel is quite common and may cause problems with shoe fitting.

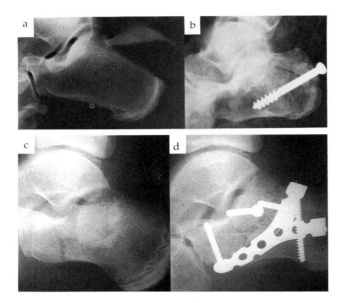

30.26 Calcaneal fractures – open treatment Avulsion fracture (a) treated by screw fixation (b).

(c, d) Displaced intra-articular fracture treated by open reduction and internal fixation.

Talocalcaneal stiffness and osteoarthritis Displaced intra-articular fractures may lead to joint stiffness and, eventually, osteoarthritis. This can usually be managed conservatively, but persistent or severe pain may necessitate subtalar arthrodesis. If the calcaneocuboid joint is also involved, a triple arthrodesis is better.

Mid-tarsal and tarsometatarsal injuries

Falls in which the foot is twisted or forced into equinus may cause a variety of injuries, from a relatively benign ligamentous strain to fracture-dislocation of the tarsal or tarsometatarsal joints. Crushing injuries are worse, because they are accompanied by severe soft-tissue damage; bleeding into the fascial compartments may cause ischaemia of the foot.

Special features

The foot is bruised and swollen. With a strain, pain is elicited by moving the forefoot; with a fracture or dislocation, all attempts at movement will be resisted. The foot should be carefully examined for signs of ischaemia.

X-RAY   Multiple views are necessary to show the extent of the injury.

Treatment

Ligamentous strains The foot may be bandaged until acute pain subsides. Thereafter, movement is encouraged.

Undisplaced fractures The foot is elevated to counteract swelling. After 3 or 4 days a below-knee cast is applied and the patient is allowed up on crutches with limited weight-bearing. The plaster is retained for 4–6 weeks.

Fracture-dislocation These are severe injuries. Under general anaesthesia, the dislocation can usually be reduced by closed manipulation, but holding it is a problem. If there is the least tendency to redisplacement, Kirschner wires or Steinmann pins are run across the joints to fix them in position. The foot is immobilized in a below-knee plaster

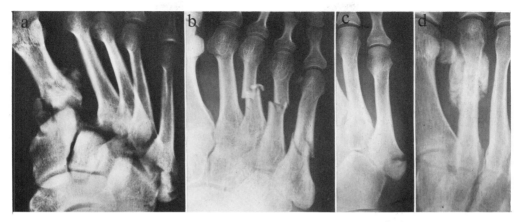

30.27 Metatarsal injuries   (a) Tarsometatarsal dislocation is a serious injury which may endanger the circulation of the foot. (b) Transverse fractures of several metatarsal shafts. (c) Avulsion fracture of the base of the fifth metatarsal. (d) Florid callus in a stress fracture.

for 6–8 weeks. Exercises are then begun and should be practised assiduously; it may be 6–8 months before function is regained.

Metatarsal fractures

Metatarsal fracture may be caused by a direct blow, by a severe twisting injury or by repetitive stress. In the usual case there is a history of injury and the foot is painful and somewhat swollen. X-ray examination will show the fracture.

Treatment A walking plaster may be applied, mainly for comfort, and is retained for 3 weeks. The fracture unites readily.

In the unlikely event of severe displacement, reduction and Kirschner wire fixation may be justified.

Stress injury (march fracture)

In a young adult (often a recruit or a nurse) the foot may become painful after overuse. A tender lump is palpable just distal to the mid-shaft of a metatarsal bone, usually the second. The x-ray appearance may at first be normal but a radioisotope scan will show an area of intense activity in the bone. Later a hairline crack may be visible, and later still a mass of callus or periosteal new bone is seen.

No displacement occurs and neither reduction nor splintage is necessary. The forefoot may be supported with Elastoplast and normal walking is encouraged.

NOTE: Similar lesions occur in osteoporotic patients after operations that shorten the big toe, throwing extra stress on the adjacent metatarsals. Elderly patients should be warned about this possibility.

Fractured toes

A heavy object falling on the toes may fracture phalanges. If the skin is broken it must be covered with a sterile dressing. The fracture is disregarded and the patient encouraged to walk in a suitably mutilated boot.

Fractured sesamoids

One of the sesamoids (usually the medial) may fracture from either a direct injury (landing from a height on the ball of the foot) or sudden traction; chronic, repetitive stress is more often seen in dancers and runners.

The patient complains of pain directly over the sesamoid. There is a tender spot in the same area and sometimes pain can be exacerbated by passively hyperextending the big toe.   X-rays will usually show the fracture (which must be distinguished from a smooth-edged bipartite sesamoid).

Treatment is often unnecessary, though a local injection of lignocaine helps for pain. If discomfort is marked, the foot can be immobilized in a short-leg walking cast for 2–3 weeks. Occasionally, intractable symptoms call for excision of the offending ossicle.

Index